EAT RIGHT
COOK RIGHT
4
YOUR TYPE

EAT RIGHT
COOK RIGHT
4
YOUR TYPE

Dr. Peter J. D'Adamo
with Catherine Whitney

PRENTICE HALL

Library of Congress Cataloging-in-Publication Data

D'Adamo, Peter.
    Eat right & cook right 4 your type : the customized diet and cookbook that will shed pounds, improve your health, and increase longevity / Peter J. D'Adamo, with Catherine Whitney.—Exclusive deluxe ed.
        p.   cm.
    Includes index.
    ISBN 0-13-033977-6
    1. Blood groups. 2. Nutrition. 3. Cookery. 4. Health. I. Title: Eat right and cook right for your type. II. Whitney, Catherine (Catherine A.) III. Title.
    QP98.D333 2001
    613—dc21   00–068478
                                                                                                              CIP

© 2001 by Peter D'Adamo and Catherine Whitney

Printed in the United States of America

10 9 8 7 6 5 4 3 2 1

ISBN 0-13-033977-6

ATTENTION: CORPORATIONS AND SCHOOLS

Prentice Hall books are available at quantity discounts with bulk purchase for educational, business, or sales promotional use. For information, please write to: Prentice Hall Special Sales, 240 Frisch Court, Paramus, New Jersey 07652. Please supply: title of book, ISBN, quantity, how the book will be used, date needed.

PRENTICE HALL
Paramus, NJ 07652
On the World Wide Web at http://www.phdirect.com

Acknowledgments

THERE ARE MANY PEOPLE TO THANK, AS NO SCIENTIFIC PURSUIT is solitary. Along the way, I have been driven, inspired, and supported by all of the people who placed their confidence in me. In particular, I give deep thanks to my wife, Martha Mosko D'Adamo, for her love and friendship; my daughters, Claudia and Emily, for the joy they bring me; my parents, James D'Adamo, Sr., N.D., and Christiana, for teaching me to trust in my intuition; my brother, James D'Adamo, Jr., and his wife, Ann; and my sister, Michele, for believing in me.

I am also more grateful than I can express to:

Joseph Pizzorno, N.D., for teaching me to trust in the science of natural medicine.

Catherine Whitney, my writer, who imparted a style and organization to the raw material characteristic of a true wordsmith.

My literary agent, Janis Vallely, who saw the promise of my work and didn't allow it to languish somewhere in a dusty file cabinet.

Amy Hertz, my editor at Riverhead/Putnam, whose vision turned the blood type science into a meaningful mainstream program.

I am also thankful to:

Dorothy Mosko and Sally Cardy Mosko, for their invaluable assistance in the preparation of the manuscripts.

Paul Krafin, Catherine Whitney's partner, who crafted prose in a poetic yet practical way.

Jane Dystel, Catherine's literary agent, whose advice was always on target.

My good friend and colleague, Gregory Kelly, N.D., who has provided invaluable clinical support and a sharp scientific mind to assure the most current and medically valid information.

Scott Carlson, my assistant, who makes the office run smoothly; Carolyn Knight, R.N., my invaluable nurse and my wonderfully supportive staff: Wendy Carlson, Melissa Danelowski, and Richard Tuzzio.

Cheryl Miller, Martine Lloyd Warner, and Garbielle Lloyd Sindorf, who developed many wonderful recipes that are right for each blood type.

Eric and Olga Butterworth, for their great friendship and support of my work.

Gail Winston, the editor who long ago, out of the clear blue sky, rang me up and asked me if I wanted to write a book about natural medicine.

I am thankful to the dedicated staff at Prentice Hall, for bringing this special deluxe edition into being. In particular, I'd like to acknowledge the efforts of Debora Yost, Gene Brissie and Eve Mossman.

Special thanks to the professionals who have given their support to this work, in particular Michael Finney; Jay Fiano; Michael Schacter, M.D.; Thomas Kruzel, N.D.; William Mitchell, N.D.; Jeffrey Bland, Ph.D.; Jonathan Wright, M.D.; Steve Shapiro; Alan Datner, M.D.; Dr. Klaus Stadler, of Piper Publishing; and Paul Schulick.

I also wish to thank the research interns at Bastyr University, who expertly sifted through the extensive medical literature pertaining to blood type.

Lastly, I thank all of the wonderful patients, who in their quest for health and happiness, chose to honor me with their trust.

Contents

The Work
of Two Lives

I believed that no two people on the face of the earth were alike; no two people have the same fingerprints, lip prints, or voice prints. No two blades of grass or snowflakes are alike. Because I felt that all people were different from one another, I did not think it was logical that they should eat the same foods. It became clear to me that since each person was housed in a special body with different strengths, weaknesses, and nutritional requirements, the only way to maintain health or cure illness was to accommodate to that particular patient's specific needs.

> *James D'Adamo,*
> *my father*

YOUR BLOOD TYPE IS THE KEY THAT UNLOCKS THE DOOR TO THE mysteries of health, disease, longevity, physical vitality, and emotional strength. Your blood type determines your susceptibility to illness, which foods you should eat, and how you should exercise. It is a factor in your energy levels, in the efficiency with which you "burn" calories, in your emotional response to stress, and perhaps even in your personality.

The connection between blood type and diet may sound radical, but it is not. We have long known that there was a missing link in our comprehension of the process that leads either to the path of wellness or to the dismal trail of disease. There had to be a reason why there were so many paradoxes in dietary studies and disease survival. There also had to be an explanation for why some people were able to lose weight on particular diets, while others were not; why some people retained vitality late in life, while others deteriorated mentally and physically. Blood type analysis has given us a way to explain these paradoxes. And the more we explore the connection, the more valid it becomes.

Blood types are as fundamental as creation itself. In the masterly logic of nature, blood types follow an unbroken trail from the earliest moment of human creation to the present day. They are the signature of our ancient ancestors on the indestructible parchment of history.

Now we have begun to discover how to use the blood type as a cellular fingerprint that unravels many of the major mysteries surrounding our quest for good health. This work is an extension of the recent groundbreaking findings concerning human DNA. Our understanding of blood type takes the science of genetics one step further by stating unequivocally that every human being is utterly unique. There is no right or wrong lifestyle or diet; there are only right or wrong choices to be made based on our individual genetic codes.

How I Found the Missing Blood Type Link

My work in the field of blood type analysis is the fulfillment of a lifetime pursuit—not only my own but also my father's. I am a second-generation naturopathic physician. Dr. James D'Adamo, my father, graduated from naturopathic college (a four-year postgraduate program) in 1957 and later studied in Europe at several of the great spas. He noticed that although many patients did well on strict vegetarian and low-fat diets, which are the hallmarks of "spa cuisine," a certain number of patients did not appear to improve, and some did poorly or even worsened. A sensitive man with keen powers of deduction and insight, my father reasoned that there should be some sort of blueprint that he could use to determine differences in the dietary needs of his patients. He rationalized that since blood was the fundamental source of nourishment to the body, perhaps some aspect of the blood could help identify these differences. My father set about testing this theory by blood-typing his patients and observing individualized reactions when they were prescribed different diets.

Through the years and with countless patients, a pattern began to emerge. He noticed that patients who were Type A seemed to do poorly on high-protein diets that included generous portions of meat, but did very well on vegetable proteins such as soy and tofu. Dairy products tended to produce copious amounts of mucous discharge in the sinuses and respiratory passages of Type As. When told to increase their levels of physical activity and exercise, Type As usually felt fatigued and unwell; when they performed lighter forms of exercise, such as yoga, they felt alert and energized.

On the other hand, Type O patients thrived on high-protein diets, and they felt invigorated by intense physical activities, such as jogging and aerobics. The more my father tested the different blood types, the greater his conviction became that each of them followed a distinct path to wellness.

Inspired by the saying "One man's food is another man's poison," my father condensed his observations and dietary recommendations into a book he titled *One Man's Food*. When the book was published in 1980, I was in my third year of naturopathic studies at Seattle's John Bastyr College. During this time revolutionary gains were being achieved in naturopathic education. The goal of Bastyr College was nothing less than to produce the complete alternative physician, the intellectual and scientific equal of a medical internist, but with specialized naturopathic training. For the first time naturopathic techniques, procedures, and substances could be scientifically evaluated with the benefits of modern technology. I waited for an opportunity to research my father's blood type theory. I wanted to assure myself that it carried valid scientific weight. My chance came in 1982, my senior year, when, for a clinical rounds requirement, I began scanning the medical literature to see if I could find any correlation between the ABO blood types and a predilection for certain diseases, and whether any of this supported my father's diet theory. Since my father's book was based on his subjective impressions of the blood types rather than on an objective method of evaluation, I wasn't certain that I would be able to find any scientific basis for his theories. But I was amazed at what I learned.

My first breakthrough came with the discovery that two major diseases of the stomach were associated with blood type. The first was the peptic ulcer, a condition often related to higher-than-average stomach-acid levels. This condition was reported to be more common in people with Type O blood than in people with other blood types. I was immediately intrigued, since my father had observed that Type O patients did well on animal products and protein diets—foods that require more stomach acid for proper digestion.

The second correlation was an association between Type A and stomach cancer. Stomach cancer was often linked to low levels of stomach-acid production, as was pernicious anemia, another disorder found more often in Type A individuals. Pernicious anemia is related to a lack of vitamin B_{12}, which requires sufficient stomach acid for its absorption.

As I studied these facts I realized that on the one hand, Type O blood predisposed people to an illness associated with too much stomach acid, while on the other hand, Type A blood predisposed people to two illnesses associated with too little stomach acid.

That was the link I'd been looking for. There absolutely was a scientific basis for my father's observations. And so began my ongoing love affair with the science and anthropology of the blood types. In time, I found that my father's initial work on the correlation between blood type, diet, and health was far more significant than even he had imagined.

Four Simple Keys to Unlock Life's Mysteries

I grew up in a family that was mostly Blood Type A, and because of my father's work we ate a basically vegetarian diet consisting of foods such as tofu, steamed vegetables, and salads. As a child I was often embarrassed and felt somewhat deprived, because none of my friends ate weird foods like tofu. To the contrary, they were happily engaged in another kind of "diet revolution" sweeping the 1950s;

their diets consisted of hamburgers, hot dogs, greasy French fries, candy bars, ice cream, and lots of soda.

Today, I still eat the way I did as a child, and I love it. Every day I eat the foods that my Type A body craves, and it's immensely satisfying.

In *Eat Right & Cook Right 4 Your Type* I will teach you about the fundamental relationship between your blood type and the dietary and lifestyle choices that will help you live at your very best. The essence of the blood type connection rests in these facts:

- Your blood type—O, A, B, or AB—is a powerful genetic fingerprint that identifies you as surely as your DNA.
- When you use the individualized characteristics of your blood type as a guidepost for eating and living, you will be healthier, you will naturally reach your ideal weight, and you will slow the process of aging.
- Your blood type is a more reliable measure of your identity than race, culture, or geography. It is a genetic blueprint for who you are, a guide to how you can live most healthfully.
- The key to the significance of blood type can be found in the story of human evolution: Type O is the oldest; Type A evolved with agrarian society; Type B emerged as humans migrated north into colder, harsher territories; and Type AB was a thoroughly modern adaptation, a result of the intermingling of disparate groups. This evolutionary story relates directly to the dietary needs of each blood type today.

What is this remarkable factor, the blood type?

Blood type is one of several medically recognized variations, much like hair and eye color. Many of these variations, such as fingerprint patterns and the more recent DNA analysis, are used extensively by forensic scientists and criminalists, as well as those who research the causes and cures of disease. Blood type is every bit as significant as other variations; in many ways, it's a more useful measure. Blood type analysis is a logical system. The information is simple to learn and easy to follow. I've taught the system to numerous doctors, who tell me they are getting good results with patients who follow its guidelines. Now I will teach it to you. By learning the principles of blood type analysis, you can tailor the optimal diet for yourself and your family members. You can pinpoint the foods that make you sick, contribute to weight gain, and lead to chronic disease.

Early on, I realized that blood type analysis offered a powerful means of interpreting individual variations in health and disease. Given the amount of available research data, it is surprising that the effects of blood type on our health have not received the measure of attention that they deserve. But now I am prepared to make that information available—not just to my fellow scientists and colleagues in the medical community, but to you.

At first glance, the science of blood type may seem daunting, but I assure you it is as simple and basic as life itself. I will tell you about the ancient trail of the evolution of blood types (as riveting as the story of human history), and demystify the science of blood types to provide a clear and simple plan that you will be able to follow.

I realize that this is probably a completely new idea for you. Few people ever even think about the implications of their blood type, even though it is a powerful genetic force. You may be reluctant to wade into such unfamiliar territory, even if the scientific arguments seem convincing. I ask you to do only three things: Talk to your physician before you begin, find out your blood type if you don't already know it, and try your Blood Type Diet for at least two weeks. Most of my patients experience some results within that time period—increased energy, weight loss, a lessening of digestive complaints, and improvement of chronic problems such as asthma, headaches, and heartburn. Give your Blood Type Diet a chance to bring you the benefits I've seen it bring to the more than four thousand people I've put on the diet. See for yourself that blood not only provides your body's most vital nourishment, but now proves itself a vehicle for your future well-being.

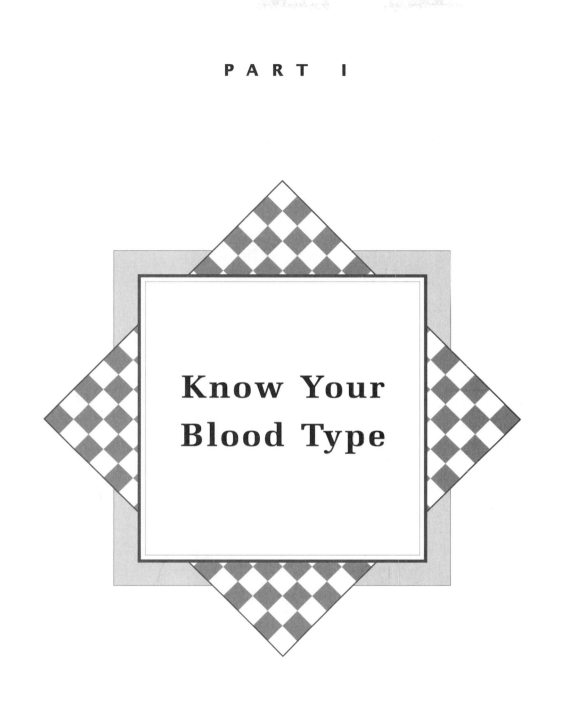

Know Your Blood Type

A Celebration of Individuality

The Four Distinct Types

*B*LOOD IS LIFE ITSELF. IT IS THE PRIMAL FORCE THAT fuels the power and mystery of birth, the horrors of disease, war, and violent death. Entire civilizations have been built on blood ties. Tribes, clans, and monarchies depend on them. We cannot exist without blood—literally or figuratively.

Blood is magical. Blood is mystical. Blood is alchemical. It appears throughout human history as a profound religious and cultural symbol. Ancient peoples mixed it together and drank it to denote unity and fealty. From the earliest times, hunters performed rituals to appease the spirits of the animals they killed by offering up the animal blood and smearing it on their faces and bodies. The blood of the lamb was placed as a mark on the hovels of the enslaved Jews of Egypt so that the Angel of Death would pass over them. Moses is said to have turned the waters of Egypt to blood in his quest to free his people. The symbolic blood of Jesus Christ has been, for nearly two thousand years, central to the most sacred rite of Christianity.

Blood evokes such rich and sacred imagery because it is in reality so extraordinary. Not only does it supply the complex delivery and defense systems that are necessary for our very existence, it also provides a keystone for humanity—a looking glass through which we can trace the faint tracks of our journey.

In the last forty years we have been able to use biological markers such as blood type to map the movements and groupings of our ancestors. By learning how these early people adapted to the challenges posed by constantly changing climates, germs, and diets, we are learning about ourselves. Change in climate and available food produced new blood types. Blood type is the unbroken cord that binds us to one another.

Ultimately, the differences in blood types reflect upon the human ability to acclimate to different environmental challenges. For the most part, these challenges affected the digestive and immune systems: A piece of bad meat could kill you; a cut or scrape could evolve into a deadly infection. Yet the human race survived. And the story of that survival is inextricably tied to our digestive and immune systems. It is in these two areas that most of the distinctions between blood types are found.

The Human Story

The story of humankind is the story of survival. More specifically, it is the story of where humans lived and what they could eat there. It is about food—about finding food and moving to find food. We don't know for certain when the human evolution began. Neanderthals, the first humanoids we can recognize, may have developed 500,000 years ago. Maybe more.

We do know that human prehistory began in Africa, where we evolved from humanlike creatures. Early life was short, nasty, and brutish. People died a thousand different ways—opportunistic infections, parasites, animal attacks, broken bones, childbirth—and they died young.

Early humans must have had a harrowing time providing for themselves in this savage environment. Their teeth were short and blunt—ill suited for attack. Unlike most of their competitors on the food chain, they had no special abilities with regard to speed, strength, or agility. Initially, the chief quality humans possessed was an innate cunning, which later grew to reasoned thought.

> ### Do You Know Your Blood Type?
>
> There are several ways to find out your blood type.
>
> 1. Donate blood. Also note that blood banks will often perform a blood type test for a fee, even if you don't wish to give blood.
> 2. Ask your doctor—but don't be surprised if he or she doesn't know. When blood is drawn for routine cholesterol screening or other factors, blood typing is not normally done unless it has been requested.
> 3. Refer to the back of this book to order an easy, accurate at-home blood type testing kit.

Neanderthals probably ate a rather crude diet of wild plants, grubs, and the scavenged leftovers from the kills of predatory animals. They were more prey than predator, especially when it came to infections and parasitic afflictions. (Many of the parasites, worms, flukes, and infectious microorganisms found in Africa do not stimulate the immune system to produce a specific antibody to them, probably because the early Type O people already had protection in the form of the antibodies they carried from birth.)

As the human race moved around and was forced to adapt its diet to changing conditions, the new diet provoked adaptations in the digestive tract and immune system necessary for it to first survive and later thrive in each new habitat. These changes are reflected in the development of the blood types, which appear to have arrived at critical junctures of human development:

1. The ascent of humans to the top of the food chain (evolution of Type O to its fullest expression).
2. The change from hunter-gatherer to a more domesticated agrarian lifestyle (appearance of Type A).
3. The merging and migration of the races from the African homeland to Europe, Asia, and the Americas (development of Type B).
4. The modern intermingling of disparate groups (the arrival of Type AB).

Each blood type contains the genetic message of our ancestors' diets and behaviors, and though we're a long way away from early history, many of their traits still affect us. Knowing these predispositions helps us to understand the logic of the blood type diets.

O Is for Old

The appearance of our Cro-Magnon ancestors in around 40,000 B.C. propelled the human species to the top of the food chain, making them the most dangerous predators on Earth. They began to hunt in organized packs; in a short time, they were able to make weapons and use tools. These major advances gave them strength and superiority beyond their natural physical abilities.

Skillful and formidable hunters, the Cro-Magnons soon had little to fear from any of their animal rivals. With no natural predators other than themselves, the population exploded. Protein—meat— was their fuel, and it was at this point that the digestive attributes of Blood Type O reached their fullest expression.

Humans thrived on meat, and it took a remarkably short time for them to kill off the big game within their hunting range. There were more and more people to feed, so competition for meat became intense. Hunters began fighting and killing others who were impinging on what they claimed were their exclusive hunting grounds. As always, human beings found their greatest enemy to be themselves. Good hunting areas became scarce. The migration of the human race began.

By 30,000 B.C., bands of hunters were traveling farther and farther in search of meat. When a shift in the trade winds desiccated what had been fertile hunting land in the African Sahara, and when previously frozen northern areas grew warmer, they began to move out of Africa into Europe and Asia.

This movement seeded the planet with its base population, which was Blood Type O, the predominant blood type even today.

By 20,000 B.C. Cro-Magnons had moved fully into Europe and Asia, decimating the vast herds of large game to such an extent that other foods had to be found. Searching each new area for anything edible, it is likely that the carnivorous humans quickly became omnivorous, with a mixed diet of berries, grubs, nuts, roots, and small animals. Populations also thrived along the coastlines and the teeming lakes and rivers of the Earth where fish and other food were abundant. By 10,000 B.C., humans occupied every main landmass on the planet, except for Antarctica.

The movement of the early humans to less temperate climates created lighter skins, less massive bone structures, and straighter hair. Nature, over time, reacclimated them to the regions of the Earth they inhabited. People moved northward, so light skin developed, which was better protected against frostbite than dark skin. Lighter skin was also better able to metabolize vitamin D in a land of shorter days and longer nights.

The Cro-Magnons eventually burned themselves out; their success was anathema. Overpopulation soon exhausted the available hunting grounds. What had once seemed like an unending supply of large game animals diminished sharply. This led to increased competition for the remaining meat. Competition led to war, and war to further migration.

A Is for Agrarian

Type A blood initially appeared somewhere in Asia or the Middle East between 25,000 and 15,000 B.C. in response to new environmental conditions. It emerged at the peak of the Neolithic period, or New Stone Age, which followed the Old Stone Age, or Paleolithic period, of the Cro-Magnon hunters. Agriculture and animal domestication were the hallmarks of its culture.

The cultivation of grains and livestock changed everything. Able to forgo their hand-to-mouth existence and sustain themselves for the first time, people established stable communities and permanent living structures. This radically different lifestyle, a major change in diet and environment, resulted in an entirely new mutation in the digestive tracts and the immune systems of the Neolithic peoples— a mutation that allowed them to better tolerate and absorb cultivated grains and other agricultural products. Type A was born.

Settling into permanent farming communities presented new developmental challenges. The skills necessary for hunting together now gave way to a different kind of cooperative society. For the first time, a specific skill at doing one thing depended on the skills of others doing something else. For example, the miller depended on the farmer to bring in his crops; the farmer depended on the miller to grind his grain. One no longer thought of food as only an immediate source of nourishment or as a sometime thing. Fields needed to be sown and cultivated in anticipation of future reward. Planning and networking with others became the order of the day. Psychologically, these are traits at which Type As excel—perhaps another environmental adaptation.

The gene for Type A began to thrive in the early agrarian societies. The genetic mutation that produced Type A from Type O occurred rapidly—so rapidly that the rate of mutation was comparable to four times that of *Drosophila*, the common fruit fly and current record holder!

What could have been the reason for this extraordinary rate of human mutation from Type O to Type A? It was survival. Survival of the fittest in a crowded society. Because Type A emerged as more resistant to infections common to densely populated areas, urban, industrialized societies quickly became Type A. Even today, survivors of plague, cholera, and smallpox show a predominance of Type A over Type O.

Eventually, the gene for Type A blood spread beyond Asia and the Middle East into western Europe, carried by the Indo-Europeans, who penetrated deeply into the pre-Neolithic populations. The Indo-European hordes originally appeared in south-central Russia, and between 3,500 and 2,000 B.C. pushed southward into the top of southwestern Asia, creating the populations and peoples of Iran and Afghanistan. Ever burgeoning, they moved further westward into Europe. The Indo-European invasion was really the original Diet Revolution. It introduced new foods and lifestyle habits into the simpler immune systems and digestive tracts of the early hunter-gatherers, and those changes were so profound that they produced the environmental stress necessary to spread the Type A gene. In time, the digestive system of the hunter-gatherers lost its ability to digest its carnivorous pre-agricultural diet.

Today, Type A blood is still found in its highest concentration among western Europeans. The frequency of Type A diminishes as we head eastward from western Europe, following the receding trails of the ancient migratory patterns. Type A peoples are highly concentrated across the Mediterranean, Adriatic, and Aegean seas, particularly in Corsica, Sardinia, Spain, Turkey, and the Balkans. The Japanese also have some of the highest concentrations of Type As in eastern Asia, along with a moderately high number of blood Type Bs.

Blood Type A had mutated from Type O in response to the myriad infections provoked by an increased populace and major dietary changes. But Blood Type B was different.

B Is for Balance

Blood Type B developed sometime between 15,000 and 10,000 B.C., in the area of the Himalayan highlands—now part of present-day Pakistan and India.

Pushed from the hot, lush savannahs of eastern Africa to the cold, unyielding highlands of the Himalayas, Blood Type B may have initially mutated in response to climatic changes. It first appeared in India or the Ural region of Asia among a mix of Caucasian and Mongolian tribes. This new blood type was soon characteristic of the great tribes of steppe dwellers, who by this time dominated the Eurasian plains.

As the Mongolians swept through Asia, the gene for Type B blood was firmly entrenched. The Mongolians spread northward, pursuing a culture dependent upon herding and domesticating animals—as their diet of meat and cultured dairy products reflected.

Two distinct Type Bs sprang up as the pastoral nomads pushed into Asia: an agrarian, comparatively sedentary group in the south and the east; and a nomadic, warlike society conquering the north and the west. The nomads were expert horsemen who penetrated far into eastern Europe, and the gene for Type B blood is still in strong evidence in many of the eastern European populations. In the meantime, an entire agriculturally based culture had spread throughout China and southeast Asia. Because of the nature of the land they chose to till, and climates unique to their areas, these peoples created and employed sophisticated irrigation and cultivation techniques that displayed an awesome blend of creativity, intelligence, and engineering.

The schism between the warlike tribes to the north and the peaceful farmers to the south was deep, and its remnants exist to this day in southern Asian cuisine, which uses little if any dairy foods. To the Asian mind, dairy products are the food of the barbarian, which is unfortunate because the diet they have adopted does not suit Type Bs so well.

Of all the ABO types, Type B shows the most clearly defined geographic distribution. Stretching as a great belt across the Eurasian plains and down to the Indian subcontinent, Type B is found in increased numbers from Japan, Mongolia, China, and India up to the Ural Mountains. From there westward, the percentages fall until a low is reached at the western tip of Europe.

The small numbers of Type B in Old and Western Europeans represents western migration by Asian nomadic peoples. This is best seen in the easternmost western Europeans, the Germans and Austrians, who have an unexpectedly high incidence of Type B blood compared with their western neighbors. The highest occurrence of Type B in Germans occurs in the area around the upper and middle Elbe River, which had been nominally held as the dividing line between civilization and barbarism in ancient times.

Modern subcontinental Indians, a Caucasian people, have some of the highest frequencies of Type B blood in the world. The northern Chinese and Koreans have very high rates of Type B blood and very low rates of Type A.

The blood type characteristics of the various Jewish populations have long been of interest to anthropologists. As a general rule, regardless of their nationality or race, there is a trend toward higher-than-average rates of Type B blood. The Ashkenazim and the Sephardim, the two major Jewish sects, share strong levels of Type B blood, and appear to have very few differences. The pre-Diaspora Babylonian Jews differ considerably from the primarily Type O Arabic population of Iraq (the location of the biblical Babylon) in that they are primarily Type B, with some frequency of Type A.

AB Is for Modern

Type AB blood is rare. Emerging from the intermingling of Type A Caucasians with Type B Mongolians, it is found in less than 5 percent of the population, and it is the newest of the blood types.

Until ten or twelve centuries ago, there was no Type AB blood. Then barbarian hordes sliced through the soft underbelly of many collapsing civilizations, overrunning the length and breadth of the Roman Empire. As a result of the intermingling of these Eastern invaders with the last trembling vestiges of European civilization, Type AB blood came to be. No evidence for the occurrence of this blood type extends beyond nine hundred to a thousand years ago, when a large western migration of eastern peoples took place. Blood Type AB is rarely found in European graves prior to A.D. 900. Studies on exhumations of prehistoric graves in Hungary show a distinct lack of this blood group into the Longobard age (fourth to seventh century A.D.). This would seem to indicate that up until that point in time, European populations of Type A and Type B did not come into common contact, or if so, did not mingle or intermarry.

Because Type ABs inherit the tolerance of both Type A and Type B, their immune systems have an enhanced ability to manufacture more specific antibodies to microbial infections. This unique quality of possessing neither anti-A nor anti-B antibodies minimizes their chances of being prone to allergies and other autoimmune diseases such as arthritis, inflammation, and lupus. There is, however, a greater predisposition to certain cancers because Type AB responds to anything A-like or B-like as "self," so it manufactures no opposing antibodies.

Type AB presents a multifaceted, and sometimes perplexing, blood type identity. It is the first blood type to adopt an amalgamation of immune characteristics, some of which make them stronger, and some of which are in conflict. Perhaps Type AB presents the perfect metaphor for modern life: complex and unsettled.

The Blending Grounds

Blood type, geography, and race are woven together to form our human identity. We may have cultural differences, but when you look at blood type, you see how superficial they are. Your blood type is older than your race and more fundamental than your ethnicity. The blood types were not a hit-or-miss act of random genetic activity. Each new blood type was an evolutionary response to a series of cataclysmic chain reactions, spread over eons of environmental upheaval and change.

Although the early racial changes seem to have occurred in a world that was composed almost exclusively of Type O blood, the racial diversifications—coupled with dietary, environmental, and geographical adaptations—were part of the evolutionary engine that ultimately produced the other blood types.

Some anthropologists believe that classifying humans into races invites oversimplification. Blood type is a far more important determinant of individuality and similarity than is race. For example, an African and Caucasian of Type A blood could exchange blood or organs and have many of the same aptitudes, digestive functions, and immunological structures—characteristics they would not share with a member of their own race who was Blood Type B.

Racial distinctions based on skin colors, ethnic practices, geographical homelands, or cultural roots are not a valid way to distinguish peoples. Members of the human race have a lot more in common with one another than we may have ever suspected. We are all potentially brothers and sisters. In blood.

Your Genetic Fingerprint

Why Blood Type Matters

*B*LOOD IS A FORCE OF NATURE, THE ÉLAN VITAL THAT has sustained us since time immemorial. A single drop of blood, too small to see with the naked eye, contains the entire genetic code of a human being. The DNA blueprint is intact and replicated within us endlessly—through our blood.

Our blood also contains eons of genetic memory—bits and pieces of specific programming, passed on from our ancestors in codes we are still attempting to comprehend. One such code rests within our blood type. Perhaps it is the most important code we can decipher in our attempt to unravel the mysteries of blood and its vital role in our existence.

To the naked eye, blood is a homogeneous red liquid. But under the microscope, blood shows itself to be composed of many different elements. The abundant red blood cells contain a special type of iron that our bodies use to carry oxygen and create the blood's characteristic rust color. White blood cells, far less numerous than red, cruise our bloodstreams like ever-vigilant troops, protecting us against infection.

This complex, living fluid also contains proteins that deliver nutrients to the tissues, platelets that help it clot, and plasma that contains the guardians of our immune system.

The Importance of Blood Type

You may be unaware of your own blood type unless you've donated blood or needed a transfusion. Most people think of blood type as an inert factor, something that comes into play only when there is a hospital emergency. But now that you have heard the dramatic story of the evolution of blood type, you are beginning to understand that blood type has always been the driving force behind human survival, changing and adapting to new conditions, environments, and food supplies.

Why is our blood type so powerful? What is the essential role it plays in our survival—not just thousands of years in the past, but today?

Your blood type is the key to your body's entire immune system. It controls the influence of viruses, bacteria, infections, chemicals, stress, and the entire assortment of invaders and conditions that might compromise your immune system.

The word *immune* comes from the Latin *immunis*, which denoted a city in the Roman Empire that was not required to pay taxes. (If only your blood type could give you that kind of immunity!) The immune system works to define "self" and destroy "non-self." This is a critical function, for without it your immune system could attack your own tissues by mistake or allow a dangerous organism access to vital areas of your body. In spite of all its complexity, the immune system boils down to two basic functions: recognizing "us" and killing "them." In this respect your body is like a large invitation-only party. If the prospective guest supplies the correct invitation, the security guards allow him to enter and enjoy himself. If an invitation is lacking or forged, the guest is forcibly removed.

Enter the Blood Type

Nature has endowed our immune system with very sophisticated methods to determine if a substance in the body is foreign or not. One method involves chemical markers called *antigens*, which are found on the cells of our bodies. Every life-form, from the simplest virus to humans themselves, has unique antigens that form a part of

IF YOU ARE	YOU HAVE THIS ANTIGEN(S) ON YOUR CELLS
Blood Type A	A
Blood Type B	B
Blood Type AB	A and B
Blood Type O	no antigens

its chemical fingerprint. One of the most powerful antigens in the human body is the one that determines your blood type. The different blood type antigens are so sensitive that when they are operating effectively, they are the immune system's greatest security system. When your immune system sizes up a suspicious character (i.e., a foreign antigen from bacteria), one of the first things it looks for is your blood type antigen to tell it whether the intruder is friend or foe.

Each blood type possesses a different antigen with its own special chemical structure. Your blood type is named for the blood type antigen you possess on your red blood cells.

Visualize the chemical structure of blood types as antennae of sorts, projecting outward from the surface of our cells into deep space. These antennae are made from long chains of a repeating sugar called fucose, which by itself forms the simplest of the blood types, Blood Type O. The early discoverers of blood type called it "O" as a way to make us think of "zero" or "no real antigen." This antenna also serves as the base for the other blood types, A, B, and AB.

- Blood Type A is formed when the O antigen, or fucose, plus another sugar called N-acetyl-galactosamine, is added. So fucose plus N-acetyl-galactosamine equals Blood Type A.
- Blood Type B is also based on the O antigen, or fucose, but has a different sugar, named D-galactosamine, added on. So fucose plus D-galactosamine equals Blood Type B.
- Blood Type AB is based on the O antigen, fucose, plus the two sugars, N-acetyl-galactosamine and D-galactosamine. So fucose plus N-acetyl-galactosamine plus D-galactosamine equals Blood Type AB.

The Four Blood Types and Their Antigens

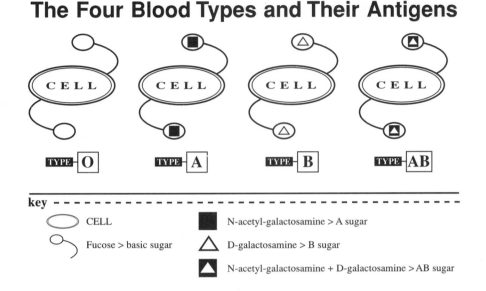

key

⬯ CELL

⟋◯ Fucose > basic sugar

■ N-acetyl-galactosamine > A sugar

△ D-galactosamine > B sugar

◣ N-acetyl-galactosamine + D-galactosamine > AB sugar

The four blood types and their antigens. Type O is the stalk, fucose; Type A is fucose plus the sugar N-acetyl-galactosamine; Type B is fucose plus the sugar D-galactosamine; Type AB is fucose plus the A-sugar and the B-sugar.

At this point you may be wondering about other blood type identifiers, such as positive and negative, or secretor/non-secretor. Usually, when people tell their blood types they say, "I'm A positive." Or "I'm O negative." These variations, or subgroups, within blood types play relatively insignificant roles. More than 90 percent of all the factors associated with your blood type are related to your primary type—O, A, B, or AB. (See the back of this book for details on the meaning of the subgroups.) We will concentrate on your blood type itself.

Antigens Create Antibodies (Immune System "Smart Bombs")

When your blood type antigen senses that a foreign antigen has entered the system, the first thing it does is create antibodies to that antigen. These antibodies, specialized chemicals manufactured by the cells of the immune system, are designed to attach to and tag the foreign antigen for destruction.

Antibodies are the cellular equivalent of the military's "smart bomb." The cells of our immune system manufacture countless varieties of antibodies, and each is specifically designed to identify and attach to one particular foreign antigen. A continual battle wages between the immune system and intruders that try to change or mutate their antigens into some new form the body will not recognize. The immune system responds to this challenge with an ever-increasing inventory of antibodies.

When an antibody encounters the antigen of a microbial interloper, a reaction called agglutination (literally, gluing) occurs. The antibody attaches to the viral antigen and makes it very sticky. When cells, viruses, parasites, and bacteria are agglutinated, they stick together and clump up, which makes the job of their disposal all the easier. As microbes must rely on their slippery powers of evasion, this is a very powerful defense mechanism. It is rather like handcuffing criminals together; they become far less dangerous than when they are allowed to move around freely. Sweeping the system of odd cells, viruses, parasites, and bacteria, the antibodies herd the undesirables together for easy identification and disposal.

The system of blood type antigens and antibodies has other ramifications besides detecting microbial and other invaders. Nearly one hundred years ago, Dr. Karl Landsteiner, a brilliant Austrian physician and scientist, also found that blood types produced antibodies to other blood types. His revolutionary discovery explained why some people could exchange blood, while others could not. Until Dr. Landsteiner's time, blood transfusions were a hit-or-miss affair. Sometimes they "took," and sometimes they didn't, and nobody knew why. Thanks to Dr. Landsteiner, we now know which blood types are recognized as friend by other blood types, and which are recognized as foe.

Dr. Landsteiner learned that:

- Blood Type A carried anti-B antibodies. Type B would be rejected by Type A.
- Blood Type B carried anti-A antibodies. Type A would be rejected by Type B.

IF YOU ARE	YOU CARRY ANTIBODIES AGAINST
Blood Type A	Blood Type B
Blood Type B	Blood Type A
Blood Type AB	No antibodies
Blood Type O	Blood Types A and B

Thus, Type A and Type B could not exchange blood.

■ Blood Type AB carried no antibodies. The universal receiver, it would accept any other blood type! But because it carried both A and B antigens, it would be rejected by all other blood types.

Thus, Type AB could receive blood from everyone, but could give blood to no one. Except another Type AB, of course.

■ Blood Type O carried anti-A and anti-B antibodies. Type A, Type B, and Type AB would be rejected.

Thus, Type O could not receive blood from anyone but another Type O. But free of A-like and B-like antigens, Type O could give blood to everyone else. Type O is the universal donor!

The "anti-other-blood-type" antibodies are the strongest antibodies in our immune system, and their ability to clump—agglutinate— the blood cells of an opposing blood type is so powerful that it can be immediately observed on a glass slide with the unaided eye. Most of our other antibodies require some sort of stimulation (such as a vaccination or an infection) for their production. The blood type antibodies are different: They are produced automatically, often appearing at birth and reaching almost adult levels by four months of age.

But there was much more to the agglutination story. It was also found that many foods agglutinate the cells of certain blood types (in a way similar to rejection) but not others, meaning that a food that may be harmful to the cells of one blood type may be beneficial to the cells of another. Not surprisingly, many of the antigens in these foods had A-like or B-like characteristics. This discovery provided the scientific link between blood type and diet. Remarkably, however, its revolutionary implications would lie dormant, gathering dust for most of this century—until a handful of scientists, doctors, and nutritionists began to explore the connection.

Lectins: The Diet Connection

A chemical reaction occurs between your blood and the foods you eat. This reaction is part of your genetic inheritance. It is amazing but true that today your immune and digestive systems still maintain a favoritism for foods that your blood type ancestors ate.

We know this because of a factor called lectins. Lectins, abundant and diverse proteins found in foods, have agglutinating properties that affect your blood. Lectins are a powerful way for organisms in nature to attach themselves to other organisms in nature. Lots of germs, and even our own immune systems, use this super glue to their benefit. For example, cells in our liver's bile ducts have lectins on their surfaces to help them snatch up bacteria and parasites. Bacteria and other microbes have lectins on their surfaces as well, which work rather like suction cups, so that they can attach to the slippery mucosal linings of the body. Often the lectins used by viruses or bacteria can be blood type specific, making them a stickier pest for people of that blood type.

So, too, with the lectins in food. Simply put, when you eat a food containing protein lectins that are incompatible with your blood type antigen, the lectins target an organ or bodily system (kidneys, liver, brain, stomach, etc.) and begin to agglutinate blood cells in that area.

Here's an example of how a lectin agglutinates in the body. Let's say a Type A person eats a plate of lima beans. The lima beans are digested in the stomach through the process of acid hydrolysis. However, the lectin protein is resistant to acid hydrolysis. It doesn't get digested, but stays intact. It may interact directly with the lining of the stomach or intestinal tract, or it may get absorbed into your bloodstream along with the digested lima bean nutrients. Different lectins target different organs and body systems.

Once the intact lectin protein settles someplace in your body, it literally has a magnetic effect on the cells in that region. It clumps the cells together and they are targeted for destruction, as if they, too, were foreign invaders. This clumping can cause irritable bowel syndrome in the intestines or cirrhosis in the liver, or block the flow of blood through the kidneys—to name just a few of the effects.

Lectins: A Dangerous Glue

You may remember the bizarre assassination of Gyorgi Markov in 1978 on a London street. Markov was killed by an unknown Soviet KGB agent while waiting for a bus. Initially, the autopsy could not pinpoint how it was done. After a thorough search, a tiny gold bead was found embedded in Markov's leg. The bead was found to be permeated with a chemical called ricin, which is a toxic lectin extracted from castor beans. Ricin is so potent an agglutinin that even an infinitesimally small amount can cause death by swiftly converting the body's red blood cells into large clots that block the arteries. Ricin kills instantaneously.

Fortunately, most lectins found in the diet are not quite so life threatening, although they can cause a variety of other problems, especially if they are specific to a particular blood type. For the most part our immune systems protect us from lectins. Ninety-five percent of the lectins we absorb from our typical diets are sloughed off by the body. But at least 5 percent of the lectins we eat are filtered into the bloodstream, where they react with and destroy red and white blood cells. The actions of lectins in the digestive tract can be even more powerful. There they often create a violent inflammation of the sensitive mucous of the intestines, and this agglutinative action may mimic food allergies. Even a minute quantity of a lectin is capable of agglutinating a huge number of cells if the particular blood type is reactive.

This is not to say that you should suddenly become fearful of every food you eat. After all, lectins are widely abundant in legumes, seafood, grains, and vegetables. It's hard to bypass them. The key is to avoid the lectins that agglutinate your particular cells—determined by blood type. For example, gluten, the most common lectin found in wheat and other grains, binds to the lining of the small intestine, causing substantial inflammation and painful irritation in some blood types—especially Type O.

Lectins vary widely, according to their source. For example, the lectin found in wheat has a different shape from the lectin found in soy, and attaches to a different combination of sugars; each of these foods is dangerous for some blood types, but beneficial for others.

Nervous tissue as a rule is very sensitive to the agglutinating effect of food lectins. This may explain why some researchers feel that allergy-avoidance diets may be of benefit in treating certain types of nervous disorders, such as hyperactivity. Russian researchers have noted that the brains of schizophrenics are more sensitive to the attachment of certain common food lectins.

Injections of lentil lectin into the knee joint cavities of non-sensitized rabbits resulted in the development of arthritis that was indistinguishable from rheumatoid arthritis. Many people with arthritis feel that avoiding the nightshade vegetables such as tomatoes, eggplant, and white potatoes seems to help their arthritis. That's not surprising, as most nightshades are very high in lectins.

Food lectins can also interact with the surface receptors of the body's white cells, programming them to multiply rapidly. These lectins are called mitogens because they cause the white cells to enter mitosis, the process of reproduction. They do not clump blood by gluing cells together; they merely attach themselves to things, like fleas on a dog. Occasionally an emergency room physician will be faced with a very ill but otherwise apparently normal child who has an extraordinarily high white blood cell count. Although pediatric leukemia is usually the first thing to come to mind, the astute physician will ask the parent, "Was your child playing in the yard?" If the answer is yes, "Was he eating any weeds or putting plants in his mouth?" Often it will turn out that the child was eating the leaves or shoots of the pokeweed plant, which contains a lectin with the potent ability to stimulate white cell production.

Blood Type-Specific Food Lectins

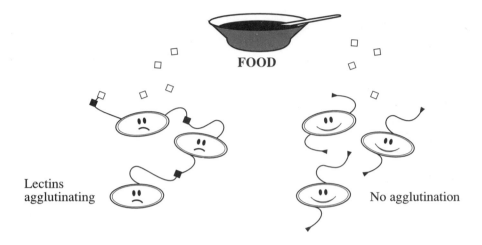

FOOD

Lectins agglutinating

No agglutination

Since each blood type antigen possesses a unique shape, many lectins interact with one specific blood type because they fit the shape of that particular blood type. In the example above, food lectins from a steaming plate of lima beans interact and agglutinate Type A cells (on the left) because they fit the shape of the A antigen. The antigen for Type B blood (on the right), a different sugar molecule with a different shape, is not affected. Conversely, a food lectin (such as buckwheat) that can specifically attach to and agglutinate cells of Blood Type B would not fit Type A blood.

How to Detect Your Harmful Lectins

I often have the experience of hearing patients insist that they are following the Blood Type Diet to the letter and staying away from all the lectins targeted for their blood type—but I know differently. When I challenge their assurance, usually they will drop all signs of protest and say in amazement, "How do you know?"

I know because the effects of lectins on different blood types are not just a theory. They're based on science. I've tested virtually all common foods for blood type reactions, using both clinical and laboratory methods. I can purchase isolated lectins from foods such as

The Indican Test

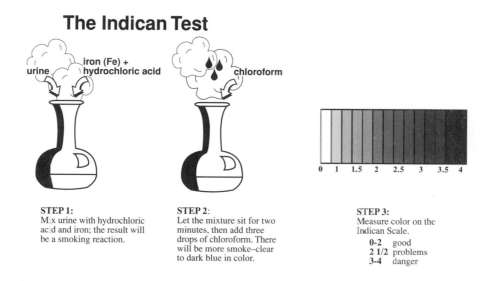

STEP 1:
Mix urine with hydrochloric acid and iron; the result will be a smoking reaction.

STEP 2:
Let the mixture sit for two minutes, then add three drops of chloroform. There will be more smoke–clear to dark blue in color.

STEP 3:
Measure color on the Indican Scale.
0-2 good
2 1/2 problems
3-4 danger

peanuts, lentils, meat, or wheat from chemical laboratories, and the results are visible under the microscope: I can see them agglutinating cells in the affected blood type.

There is also a more direct scientific barometer that can be used to measure the presence of lectins in your system. The barometer is a simple urine test called the Indican Scale. The Indican Scale measures a factor called bowel putrefaction. When the liver and intestines don't properly metabolize proteins, they produce toxic by-products called indols. The level of these toxic by-products is shown on the Indican Scale.

If you avoid foods containing toxic lectin proteins or foods that are difficult for your particular blood type to digest, your Indican Scale will be low.

If, on the other hand, you regularly consume foods that are high in lectins or difficult to digest, your Indican Scale will be high—meaning that you have a high carcinogenity of substances in your body.

My patients with high Indican Scale results often protest that they usually follow the diet, easing up only occasionally. They can't believe that their Indican Scale numbers are so high.

Here's the reason: The Indican Scale shows that a carcinogen entering your system is magnified to ninety times the effect of someone for whom it is not toxic. For example, if a Type A eats a processed or cured food, such as bologna, the nitrites are magnified ninety times in the negative affect they have because Type As are particularly susceptible to stomach cancer and the toxic effects of nitrites.

The average person comes into my office with a 2H on the scale—more than enough toxicity to indicate a problem. The good news is, after only two weeks of faithfully following the Blood Type Diet, that person's Indican Scale number will drop to 1 or even 0.

This may be the first time you've ever heard of the Indican Scale, but it has been widely used in conventional medicine for the last fifty years, and all commercial laboratories perform it. Ironically, only a year ago, several major laboratory groups discontinued its use because not enough people were requesting it. I am certain that as people begin to better understand the blood type–lectin association, the Indican Scale will be revived. Meanwhile, ask your medical doctor or naturopath to perform the test.

Make the Right Choices

Your Guide to Maximum Health

*Y*OUR BLOOD TYPE PLAN LETS YOU ZERO IN ON THE health and nutrition information that corresponds to your exact biological profile. Armed with this new information, you can now make choices about your diet, exercise regimen, and general health that are based on the dynamic natural forces within your own body. The next four sections supply highly specific diet, supplement, and exercise plans for each of the blood types. These sections are followed, in Part III, by a thorough breakdown of every common health condition and disease, with your particular blood type susceptibilities and remedies. If you follow your Blood Type Plan carefully, you can:

- Avoid many common viruses and infections.
- Lose weight, as your body rids itself of toxins and fats.
- Fight back against life-threatening diseases such as cancer, cardiovascular disease, diabetes, and liver failure.
- Avoid many of the factors that cause rapid cell deterioration, thus slowing down the aging process.

The Blood Type Plan is not a panacea. But it is a way to restore the natural protective functions of your immune system, reset your metabolic clock, and clear your blood of dangerous agglutinating lectins. It is literally the best thing you can do to halt the rapid cell deterioration that produces symptoms of aging. And if you have medical problems, this plan can make a critical difference. Depending on the severity of the condition and on the level of compliance with the plan, every person will realize some benefits. That has been my experience, and the experience of my colleagues who use this system with thousands of patients. It makes perfect scientific sense.

In this chapter I will introduce the elements you will find in your Blood Type Plan. They include:

- The Blood Type Diet
- Meal Planning
- The Weight-Loss Factor
- The Supplement Advisory
- The Stress/Exercise Profile
- The Personality Question

The Blood Type Diet

Your blood type diet is the restoration of your natural genetic rhythm. The groundwork for the Blood Type Diets was prepared for us many thousands of years ago. Perhaps if we had continued to follow the inherent, instinctual messages of our biological natures, our current condition would be very different. However, human diversity and the sweeping forces of technology intervened.

As we know, most, if not all, early humans were Type O hunters and gatherers who fed on animals, insects, berries, roots, and leaves. The range of dietary choices was extended when humans learned how to raise animals for their own use and how to cultivate crops. But it was not necessarily a smooth and orderly process because not every society adapted well to this change. In many of the early Type O societies, such as the Missouri Valley Indians, the change from a meat-eating diet to an agrarian diet was accompanied by changes in skull formation and the appearance for the first time of dental cavities. Their systems were simply not suited to the newly introduced foods.

Even so, for a long period of time, the traditional agrarian diet provided ample nutrients to avoid malnutrition and support large pop-

Blood Type and the USDA Food Pyramid

For certain blood types, the Food Pyramid recommendations make a fair amount of sense. Fundamentally, however, the pyramid is based on the reductionistic model we discussed earlier, meaning that it doesn't take into consideration dietary variations. For example, Type Os should not follow the basic pyramid recommendation of six to eleven servings of grain-based foods each day. And only Type B will benefit by eating the recommended amount of dairy foods. The Food Pyramid is probably closest to the needs of Type A. However, even foods within categories—which are not distinguished from one another in this model—can have a huge affect. For example, while Type Bs thrive on regular portions of meat, chicken can cause havoc in their digestive and immune systems.

My best advice is that you shouldn't try to fit a square peg into a round hole. Create your own Food Pyramid based on the foods that are listed on your blood type charts. All types should eat the recommended three to five servings of fruits and vegetables daily, but there is a wide divergence of choices in the level above, with two to three servings of dairy products recommended as well as two to three servings of meat, poultry, fish, beans, eggs, and nuts. For some blood types, such recommendations can be a very poor choice, indeed! The top of the pyramid, in which fats, oils, and sweets are located, recommends using these items sparingly, ignoring the fact that for many people 40 percent or more of their diets are from this section. The Food Pyramid was created to help Americans understand what a healthy diet entails. As with many other things, we've grown more sophisticated in our assessments of such recommendations. They seem well-meaning but inadequate. The pyramid really was created to provide minimal nutritional standards that would avoid malnutrition. As with many guidelines, the data are far too broad to really shed light on individual needs.

ulations. This changed as advances in agricultural and food-processing techniques began to alter foodstuffs even further and remove them more and more from their natural state. For example, the refining of rice with new milling techniques in twentieth-century Asia caused a scourge of beriberi, a thiamine-deficiency disease, which resulted in millions of deaths.

A more current example is the change from breast feeding to bottle feeding in developing Third World countries. This change to highly refined, processed infant formula has been responsible for a great deal of malnutrition, diarrhea, and a lowering of the natural immune factors passed on through mother's milk.

Today, it is well accepted that nutrition—or the foods we eat—has a direct impact on the state of our health and general well-being. But confusing, and often conflicting, information about nutrition has created a virtual minefield for health-conscious consumers.

How are we to choose which recommendations to follow, and which diet is the right diet? The truth is, we can no more choose the right diet than we can choose our hair color or gender. It was already chosen for us many thousands of years ago.

I believe that much of the confusion is the result of a cavalier "one diet fits all" premise. Although we have seen with our own eyes that certain people respond very well to particular diets while others do not, we have never made a commitment—in science or nutrition—to study the specialized characteristics of populations or individuals that might explain the variety of responses to any given diet. We've been so busy looking at the characteristics of food that we have failed to examine the characteristics of people.

Your blood type diet works because you are able to follow a clear, logical, scientifically researched and certified dietary blueprint based on your cellular profile.

Each of the blood type diets includes sixteen food groups:

- Meats and poultry
- Seafood
- Dairy and eggs
- Oils and fats
- Nuts and seeds
- Beans and legumes
- Cereals
- Breads and muffins
- Grains and pasta

- Vegetables
- Fruit
- Juices and fluids
- Spices
- Condiments
- Herbal teas
- Miscellaneous beverages

Each of these groups divides foods into three categories: HIGHLY BENEFICIAL, NEUTRAL, and AVOID. Think of the categories this way:

- Highly Beneficial is a food that acts like a Medicine.
- Neutral is a food that acts like a Food.
- Avoid is a food that acts like a Poison.

There are a wide variety of foods in each diet, so don't worry about limitations. When possible, show preference for the highly beneficial foods over the neutral foods, but feel free to enjoy the neutral foods that suit you; they won't harm you from the standpoint of lectins, and they contain nutrients that are necessary for a balanced diet.

At the top of each food category, you will see a chart that looks something like this:

BLOOD TYPE O		WEEKLY ▪ IF YOUR ANCESTRY IS		
Food	Portion	African	Caucasian	Asian
All seafood	4–6 oz.	1–4x	3–5x	4–6x

The portion suggestions according to ancestry are not meant as firm rules. My purpose here is to present a way to fine-tune your diet even more, according to what we know about the particulars of your ancestry. Although people of different races and cultures may share a blood type, they don't always have the same frequency of the gene. For example, a Type A person may be AA, meaning both parents were As, or AO, meaning one parent was O. Overall, people of Caucasian ancestry tend to have more AA genes; people of African ancestry tend to have more OO genes; and people of Asian ancestry tend to have more BB or AA genes. That is one reason why many people of African descent are lactose intolerant, even if they are Type B (a blood type that benefits from dairy foods).

There are also geographic and cultural variations. For example, people of Asian ancestry are not traditionally exposed to dairy products, so Type Bs of Asian descent may need to incorporate them more slowly into their diets as they adjust their systems to them.

These refinements also take into account typical differences in the size and weight of various peoples. Use the refinements if you think they're helpful; ignore them if you find that they're not. In any case, try to formulate your own plan for portion sizes.

At the back of each Blood Type Diet are three sample menus and several recipes to give you an idea of how you might incorporate the diet into your life.

The Weight-Loss Factor

Being overweight was anathema to our ancient ancestors, whose bodies were machines that consumed and expended the fuel they needed. Today, obesity has become one of the biggest health problems in most industrialized societies. For this reason, losing weight has become an obsession, and naturally many of my patients are interested in the weight-loss aspects of the Blood Type Diet. I always tell them that this diet was not specifically designed for weight loss; it was designed for optimum performance. Having said that, I add that weight loss is one of the natural side effects of the body's restoration. Because the Blood Type Diet is tailored to the cellular composition of your body (as opposed to being a generic, one-size-fits-all recommendation), specific foods will cause weight gain or weight loss for you, even though they may have a different effect on a person of another blood type.

My patients often ask me about current diet plans that are in vogue. The latest are the high-protein diets, which have made a recent comeback. By severely limiting carbohydrates, high-protein diets force the burning of fats for energy and the production of ketones, which indicate a high rate of metabolic activity. It doesn't surprise me that the patients who tell me they have lost weight on high-protein diets are usually Type Os and Type Bs. You don't see many Type As who do well on these diets; their systems are biologically unsuited to metabolize meat as efficiently as Type Os and Type Bs. Nor do Type ABs lose weight on high-protein diets, since these diets lack the balance of A-like foods that Type ABs require.

On the other hand, the principles of a macrobiotic diet, which encourage the consumption of natural foods such as vegetables, rice, whole grains, fruits, and soy, might be best suited for Type As, providing they eat the recommended grains and legumes.

The bottom line: Anytime you see a new diet plan that claims to work the same way for everyone, be skeptical. Listen to your blood type. Appreciate your individuality.

Let me tell you about the weight-loss potential of each of the blood type diets. Actually, the greatest problem most of my patients encounter is that they lose too much weight very quickly and I have to make adjustments in their diets to slow down the rate of weight loss. Too much weight loss may seem to be the least of your problems if you've always struggled with your weight. But remember, your ultimate goal is optimum health and performance, and that means achieving a balance between your weight and your height and shape. Excessive weight loss indicates a malnourished state that will weaken your immune system— exactly what you are trying to avoid. So use these guidelines wisely.

The dynamics of weight loss are related to the changes your body makes when you follow your genetically tailored diet. There are two factors.

First, as your body makes the dramatic shift of eliminating foods that are poorly digested or toxic, the first thing it does is try to flush out the toxins that are already there. Those toxins are deposited mainly in the fat tissue, so the process of eliminating toxins also means eliminating fat.

The second factor is the effects that specific foods have on the bodily systems that control weight. Depending on your blood type, the lectin activity of certain foods may do the following:

- Inflame the digestive tract lining.
- Interfere with the digestive process, causing bloating.
- Slow down the rate of food metabolism, so you don't efficiently burn calories for energy.
- Compromise the production of insulin.
- Upset the hormonal balance, causing water retention (edema), thyroid disorders, and other problems.

Each blood type has its own reactions to certain foods; these are outlined in your Blood Type Diet. In the first few weeks you'll need to experiment with the guidelines. I've found that many people approach their diet religiously in the beginning. They eat only the HIGHLY BENEFICIAL foods, and don't consume even NEUTRAL foods. The result is inevitably a rather unhealthy weight loss. They look gaunt and unwell because they're not getting the full range of nutrients needed for a healthy diet. A better approach is to eliminate all the foods on your AVOID list and reduce or eliminate those NEUTRAL foods that are prone to cause weight gain for your blood type. That will leave you with a balanced diet and a healthier method of weight loss.

The Role of Supplements

Your Blood Type Plan also includes recommendations about vitamin, mineral, and herbal supplements that can enhance the effects of your diet. This is another area in which there is great confusion and misinformation. Popping vitamins, minerals, exotic preparations, and herbal tinctures is a popular thing to do these days. It's hard not to be seduced by the vast array of remedies overflowing the shelves of your local health food store. Promising energy, weight loss, pain relief, sexual potency, strength, longevity, and mental power—along with cures for headaches, colds, nerves, stomach pain, arthritis, chronic fatigue, heart disease, cancer, and every other ailment in the book—these tempting panaceas seem to be the answer we've all been looking for.

But as with food, nutritional supplements don't always work the same way for everyone. Every vitamin, mineral, and herbal supplement plays a specific role in your body. The miracle remedy your Type B friend raves about may be inert or even harmful for your Type A system.

It can be dangerous to self-prescribe vitamin and mineral supplements—many of which act like drugs in your body. For example, even though they are all readily available, vitamin A, vitamin D, vitamin K, and vitamin B_3 (niacin) should be administered only under the care of a physician.

However, there are many natural substances in plants, called phytochemicals, that are more effective and less damaging than vitamins and minerals. Your Blood Type Plan recommends individualized phytochemical regimens for each blood type.

You may be unfamiliar with the term *phytochemicals*. Modern science has discovered that many of these phytochemicals, once called "weeds" or "herbs," are sources of high concentrations of biologically active compounds. These compounds are widely available in other plants, but in far smaller amounts. Many phytochemicals—which I prefer to think of as food concentrates—are antioxidants, and several of them are many times more powerful than vitamins. Interestingly, these phytochemical antioxidants exhibit a remarkable degree of tissue preference, which vitamins do not enjoy. For example, the milk thistle plant *(Silybum marianum)* and the spice turmeric *(Curcuma longa)* both have an antioxidant capability hundreds of times stronger than vitamin E, and they deposit with a great degree of preference for liver tissue. These plants are very beneficial for disorders characterized by inflammation of the liver, such as hepatitis and cirrhosis.

Your specialized program of vitamins, minerals, and phytochemicals will round out the dietary aspect of your program.

The Stress/Exercise Connection

It is not only the foods you eat that determine your well-being. It is also the way your body uses those nutrients for good or ill. That's where stress comes in. The concept of stress is very prominent in modern society. We often hear people remark, "I'm so stressed," or, "My problem is too much stress." Indeed, it is true that unbridled stress reactions are associated with many illnesses. Few people realize, though, that it is not the stress itself but our reaction to the stress in our environment that depletes our immune systems and leads to illness. This reaction is as old as human history. It is caused by a natural chemical response to the perception of danger. The best way to describe the stress reaction is to get a mental picture of how the body responds to stress.

Imagine this. You are man before the dawn of civilization. You lie bundled in the dark night, pressed together with your kind, sleeping. Suddenly, a huge wild animal appears in your midst. You feel its hot, rank breath on your flesh. You see it snatch your companion with its powerful claws and tear him apart with its fierce teeth. Do you grab a weapon and try to fight? Or do you turn and run for your life?

The body's response to stress has been developed and refined over thousands of years. It is a reflex, an animal instinct, our survival mechanism for dealing with life-or-death situations. When danger of any kind is sensed, we mobilize our fight-or-flight response, and we either confront what is alarming us or flee from it—mentally or physically.

Now imagine another scenario. You are in bed asleep. All is peaceful and silent. Suddenly, there is a thunderous explosion nearby. Your walls, roof, and windows shudder. You are awake now, aren't you? And how do you feel? Probably very frightened and most definitely in some kind of heart-pounding high gear.

Alarmed, your pituitary and adrenal glands flood your bloodstream with their excitant hormones. Your pulse quickens. Your lungs suck in more oxygen to fuel your muscles. Your blood sugar soars to supply a burst of energy. Digestion slows. You break into a sweat. All of these biological responses happen in an instant, triggered by stress. They prepare you—in the same way they prepared our ancient ancestors—for fight or flight.

The moment ends. The danger passes. Your body begins to change again. In the secondary, or resistance, stage of stress, your body starts to calm down and compose itself after all of the furor caused by the release of so many chemicals. The resistance stage is usually reached when whatever caused the alarm is identified and dealt with. And then, if whatever caused the initial stress is resolved, all of the reactions disappear, and everything is once again copacetic with the body's complex response system.

If whatever caused the initial stress continues, however, the body's ability to adapt to the stress becomes exhausted. It shuts down.

Unlike our ancestors, who faced intermittent acute stresses, such as the threat of predators or starvation, we live in a highly pressured, fast-paced world that imposes chronic, prolonged stress. Even though our stress response may be less acute than that of our ancestors, the fact that it is happening continuously may make the consequences even worse. Experts generally agree that the stresses of contemporary society and the resultant diseases—of the body, the mind, and the spirit—are very much a product of our industrialized culture and unnatural style of living.

The artificial pressures and stresses of a modern technological society exhaust our built-in survival mechanisms and overwhelm us. We have become socially and culturally conditioned to suppress and thwart our most natural responses. More stress hormones are being released into our blood than we can possibly use.

What is the outcome? Stress-related disorders cause 50 to 80 percent of all illnesses in modern life. We know how powerfully the mind influences the body and the body influences the mind. The entire range of these interactions is still being explored. Problems known to be exacerbated by stress and the mind-body connection are ulcers, high blood pressure, heart disease, migraine headaches, arthritis and other inflammatory diseases, asthma and other respiratory diseases, insomnia and other sleep disorders, anorexia nervosa and other eating disorders, and a variety of skin problems ranging from hives to herpes, from eczema to psoriasis. Stress is disastrous to the immune system, leaving the body open to myriad opportunistic health problems.

However, certain stresses, such as physical or creative activity, produce pleasant emotional states that the body perceives as an enjoyably heightened mental or physical experience.

Although each of us reacts to stress in a unique way, no one is immune to its effects, especially if they are prolonged and unwanted. Many of our internal reactions to stress are ancient tunes being called up and played by our bodies—the environmental stresses that shaped the evolution of the various blood types. The cataclysmic changes in locale, climate, and diet imprinted these stress patterns into the genetic memory of each blood type, and even today determine its internal response to stress.

My father has devoted the past thirty-five years to studying the stress patterns and natural energy levels of the different blood types and devising blood type–specific exercise programs that draw from the biological profiles of each. In the process, he has observed thousands of people, adults and children alike, and his empirical observations have taken on a valid shape. His findings are remarkably consistent with everything else we know about what makes each blood type function well.

The most revolutionary aspect of my father's work is the discovery that different blood types need different forms of physical activity, or exercise, to cope with their responses to stress.

Your Blood Type Plan includes a description of your own blood type stress patterns, along with the recommended course of exercise that will turn stress into a positive force. This element provides a crucial complement to your diet.

The Personality Question

With so many physiological connections to blood type, it is not surprising that people might speculate about less tangible characteristics that might be attributed to blood type—such as personality, attitudes, and behavior.

I have experienced this personally on many occasions. People often remark about the fact that I have followed in my father's footsteps to become a naturopath. "You're a chip off the old block," some will say. Or, "I guess you inherited your father's passion for healing." And sometimes, "It looks like the D'Adamos have medical genes."

Even when the observation is made partially in jest, I sense that most people truly believe that I have inherited something besides my physiological characteristics from my father—that it isn't just an accident that I am drawn to the same work that he is drawn to.

The idea that certain inherited traits, mannerisms, emotional qualities, and life preferences are buried in our genetic makeup is well accepted, although we aren't sure how to gauge this inheritance scientifically. We don't know (yet!) of any genes for personality.

Some might argue that the way we behave has more to do with nurture than with nature. But perhaps it is both.

Recently, Beverly, a longtime patient, brought her adult daughter in to see me. Beverly had told me earlier that she was young and unmarried when her daughter was born, and she gave her up for adoption. For thirty years, Beverly never knew what had become of her daughter—until the day a familiar-looking young woman appeared on her doorstep, having found her birth mother through a search organization. It turned out that Beverly's daughter was raised on the West Coast, in a very different environment from Beverly's. Yet I was astounded to watch the two of them together. They were mother and daughter in every way. They possessed exactly the same mannerisms and accents (even though Beverly was a New Yorker and her daughter was a Californian), and they seemed to share a similar sense of humor. Amazingly, Beverly's daughter had chosen the same profession as her mother. Both were human resource managers for their companies. If ever there was evidence of a genetic connection to personality, it was sitting in my office.

Of course, I realize this evidence is anecdotal, not scientific. Most of the research into this aspect of blood types is just that. Still, the connection intrigues us because it makes some sense that there might be a causal relationship between what occurs at the cellular level of our beings and our mental, physical, and emotional tendencies as expressed by our blood type.

Evolutionary changes altered the immune systems and digestive tracts of humans, resulting in the development of the blood types. But the mental and emotional response systems were also altered by evolutionary changes, and, with this alteration, very different psychological patterns and behaviors emerged.

Each blood type waged a difficult, and very distinct, battle for its existence some far time ago. The driven loner Type O would have failed miserably in the orderly, cooperative environment of Type A— a big reason for the blood type adaptation in the first place. Would it be such a surprise to find many of these primitive characteristics hidden in some deep remove of our psyches?

Highly Regarded in Japan

The belief that personality is determined by one's blood type is held in high regard in Japan. Termed *ketsu-eki-gata*, Japanese blood type analysis is serious business. Corporate managers use it to hire workers, market researchers use it to predict buying habits, and most people use it to choose friends, romantic partners, and lifetime mates. Vending machines that offer on-the-spot blood type analysis are widespread in train stations, department stores, restaurants, and other public places. There is even a highly respected organization, the ABO Society, dedicated to helping individuals and organizations make the right decisions, consistent with blood type.

The leading proponent of the blood type–personality connection is a man named Toshitaka Nomi, whose father first pioneered the theory. In 1980, Nomi and Alexander Besher wrote a book called *You Are Your Blood Type*, which has sold more than 6 million copies in Japan. It contains personality profiles and suggestions for the various blood types—right down to what you should do for a living, whom you should marry, and the dire consequences that might befall you if you should ignore this advice.

It makes for fun reading—not unlike astrology, numerology, or other methods of finding your place in the uncertain scheme of things. I think, however, that most of the advice in the book should be taken with a grain of salt. For instance, I don't believe that a soul mate or a romantic partner should be chosen by blood type. I am Type A and I am deeply in love with my wife, Martha, who is Type O. I would hate to think that we might have been kept forever apart because of some psychic incompatibility in our blood types. We do just fine, even though mealtimes can be a little chaotic.

Furthermore, as with all attempts to label people, this one has ominous undertones. Once you say, "Type A is this," or "Type B is that," the unavoidable next step is to say, "Type B is superior," or "Only a Type O can be president." Caste systems develop. A variation of this happens every day in Japan—for example, when a company advertises that it is looking for Type Bs to fill middle management positions.

So what is the value of this speculation, and why am I including it here? It's very simple. Although I think the Japanese *ketsu-eki-gata* is extreme, I can't deny that there is probably an essential truth to the theories about a relationship between our cells and our personalities.

Modern scientists and doctors have clearly acknowledged the existence of a biological mind–body connection, and we've already demonstrated the relationship between your blood type and your response to stress earlier in this chapter. The idea that your blood type may relate to your personality is not really so strange. Indeed, if you look at each of the blood types, you can see a distinct personality emerging—the inheritance of our ancestral strengths. Perhaps this is just another way for you to play to those strengths.

The characterizations and suggestions I will make about your "blood type personality" are based on the pooled impressions made from empirical observations of thousands of people over many years. Perhaps this data will provide a fuller picture of the vital force of blood type. Just don't let it become a source of limitation—rather, let it be a source of fulfillment.

By playing to your blood type's strengths, you may be able to achieve greater efficiency and accuracy in your work, and greater emotional happiness and security in your life.

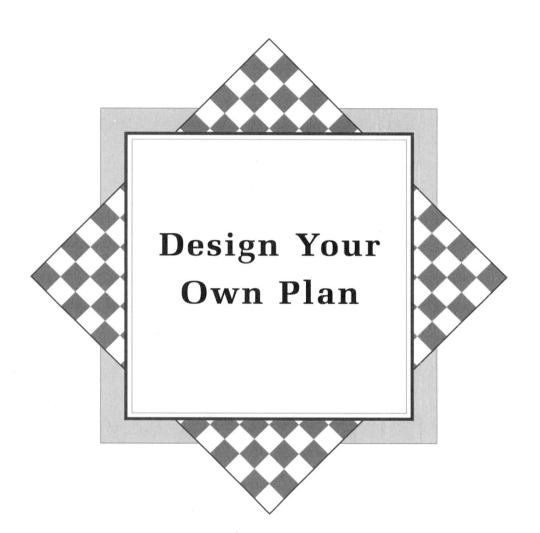

Design Your Own Plan

The Type O Program

Reach for Meat

TYPE O: *The Hunter*

- Meat eater
- Hardy digestive tract
- Overactive immune system
- Intolerant to dietary and environmental adaptations
- Responds best to stress with intense physical activity
- Requires an efficient metabolism to stay lean and energetic

---

The Type O Diet

Type Os thrive on intense physical exercise and animal protein. The digestive tracts of all Type Os retain the memory of ancient times. The high-protein hunter-gatherer diet and the enormous physical demands placed on the systems of early Type Os probably kept most primitive humans in a mild state of ketosis—a condition in which the body's metabolism is altered. The combination of ketosis, calorie deprivation, and constant physical activity was the key to the survival of the human race.

Dietary recommendations today generally discourage the consumption of too much animal protein because saturated fats have been proven to be a risk factor for heart disease and cancer. Of course, most of the meat consumed today is shot through with fat and tainted by the use of hormones and antibiotics.

Fortunately, organic and free-range meats are becoming more widely available. The success of the Type O Diet depends on your use of lean, chemical-free meats, poultry, and fish.

Type Os don't find dairy products and grains quite so user friendly as do most of the other blood types because their digestive systems still have not adapted to them fully.

The Weight-Loss Factor

You will lose weight initially on the Type O Diet by restricting your consumption of grains, breads, legumes, and beans. The leading factor in weight gain for Type Os is the gluten found in wheat germ and whole wheat products. It acts on your metabolism to create the exact opposite of the state of ketosis. Instead of keeping you lean and in a high-energy state, the gluten lectins inhibit your insulin metabolism, interfering with the efficient use of calories for energy. Eating gluten is like putting the wrong kind of octane in your car. Instead of fueling the engine, it clogs the works. (To a lesser extent, corn has the same effect, although it's not nearly as influential as wheat in precipitating Type O weight gain.) I have seen overweight Type Os, who had been unsuccessful with other diets, quickly lose weight solely by eliminating wheat from their diets.

Other factors contribute to weight gain in Type Os. Certain beans and legumes, especially lentils and kidney beans, contain lectins that deposit in your muscle tissues, making them more alkaline and less "charged" for physical activity. Type Os are leaner when their muscle tissues are in a state of slight metabolic acidity. In this state, you use calories more rapidly. (Before you jump to broad conclusions about other blood types, remember that each blood type has a unique set of factors. Metabolic acidity is not good for everyone.)

A third factor in Type O weight gain is related to thyroid regulation. Type Os have a tendency to have low levels of thyroid hormone. This condition, called hypothyroidism, occurs because Type Os often exhibit insufficient levels of iodine—a chemical element whose sole purpose is thyroid hormone production. The symptoms of hypothyroidism include weight gain, fluid retention, muscle loss, and fatigue.

In addition to moderating food portions and choosing leaner meats for maximum weight-control benefits, Type Os need to highlight certain foods for their beneficial effects and avoid others for their hindering effects. Here's a quick guide:

Foods That Encourage Weight Gain

WHEAT GLUTEN	*interferes with insulin efficiency*
	slows metabolic rate
CORN	*interferes with insulin efficiency*
	slows metabolic rate
KIDNEY BEANS	*impair calorie utilization*
NAVY BEANS	*impair calorie utilization*
LENTILS	*inhibit proper nutrient metabolism*

CABBAGE	*inhibits thyroid hormone*
BRUSSELS SPROUTS	*inhibit thyroid hormone*
CAULIFLOWER	*inhibits thyroid hormone*
MUSTARD GREENS	*inhibit thyroid production*

Foods That Encourage Weight Loss

KELP	*contains iodine*
	increases thyroid hormone production
SEAFOOD	*contains iodine*
	increases thyroid hormone production
*IODIZED SALT	*contains iodine*
	increases thyroid hormone production
LIVER	*B-vitamin source*
	aids efficient metabolism
RED MEAT	*aids efficient metabolism*
KALE, SPINACH, BROCCOLI	*aid efficient metabolism*

It is preferable that you obtain your iodine from sources such as seafood and kelp, as sodium can contribute to high blood pressure and water retention.

Incorporate these guidelines into the total picture of the Type O Diet, which follows.

Meats and Poultry

BLOOD TYPE O	WEEKLY ▪ IF YOUR ANCESTRY IS		
Food	*Portion**	*African*	*Caucasian*	*Asian*
Lean red meats	4–6 oz. (men) 2–5 oz. (women and children)	5–7x	4–6x	3–5x
Poultry	4–6 oz. (men) 2–5 oz. (women and children)	1–2x	2–3x	3–4x

The portion recommendations are merely guidelines that can help refine your diet according to ancestral propensities.

Eat lean beef, lamb, turkey, chicken, or the recommended fish as often as you wish. The more stressful your job or demanding your exercise program, the higher the grade of protein you should eat. But beware of portion sizes. Our ancestors didn't feast on sixteen-ounce steaks; meat was too precious and scarce for that. Try to consume no more than six ounces at any one meal.

Type Os can efficiently digest and metabolize meats because they tend to have high stomach acid content. This was an essential component in the survival of early Type Os. However, you must be careful to balance your meat proteins with the appropriate vegetables and fruits to avoid over-acidification, which can cause ulcers and irritation of the stomach lining.

One note: If you are a Type O of African descent, emphasize lean red meats and game over fattier, more domestic choices such as lamb or chicken. The gene for Type O developed in Africa, and your ancestors were the original Type Os. You'll benefit by refining your protein consumption in favor of the varieties of meat that were available to your African ancestors.

Highly Beneficial

Beef	Heart/Sweetbreads	Mutton
Beef, Ground	Lamb	Veal
Buffalo	Liver	Venison

Neutral

Chicken	Grouse	Rabbit
Cornish hens	Guinea hen	Squab
Duck	Ostrich	Squirrel
Goat	Partridge	Turkey
~~Goose~~	Pheasant	

Avoid

Bacon	Ham	Quail
Goose	Pork	

Seafood

BLOOD TYPE O		WEEKLY ■ IF YOUR ANCESTRY IS		
Food	*Portion*	*African*	*Caucasian*	*Asian*
All seafood	4–6 oz.	1–4x	3–5x	4–6x

Seafood, the second most concentrated animal protein, is best suited for Type Os of Asian and Eurasian descent, since seafood was a staple of your coastal ancestors' diet.

Richly oiled cold-water fish, such as cod, herring, and mackerel, are excellent for Type Os. Certain blood clotting factors evolved as humans adapted to environmental changes, and were not inherent to the blood of early Type Os. For this reason, Type Os often have "thin" blood, which resists clotting. Even though fish oils tend to have a blood-thinning effect, they are very good for your type. I suspect that this is because the way your blood type genes influence your blood "thickness" (through clotting factors) is different from the way fish oils influence blood viscosity (through the adhesion of platelets). Fish oils can also be very effective in the treatment of inflammatory bowel disease, such as colitis or Crohn's disease, to which Type Os are susceptible. Many seafoods are also excellent sources of iodine, which regulates the thyroid function. Type Os typically have unstable thyroid functions, which cause metabolic problems and weight gain.

Make seafood a major component of your Type O diet.

Highly Beneficial

Bluefish	Rainbow	Striped bass
Cod	trout	Sturgeon
Hake	Red snapper	Swordfish
Halibut	Salmon	Tilefish
Herring	Sardine	White perch
Mackerel	Shad	Whitefish
Pike	Snapper	Yellow perch
	Sole	Yellowtail

Neutral

Abalone
Anchovy
Beluga
Bluegill bass
Carp
Clam
Crab
Crayfish
Eel
Flounder
Frog
Gray sole

Grouper
Haddock
Lobster
Mahimahi
Monkfish
Mussels
Ocean perch
Oysters
Pickerel
Porgy
Sailfish
Scallop

Sea bass
Sea trout
Shark
Shrimp
Silver perch
Smelt
Snail
Squid (calamari)
Tuna
Turtle
Weakfish

Avoid

Barracuda
Catfish
Caviar
Conch

Herring (pickled)
Lox (smoked salmon)
Octopus

Dairy and Eggs

BLOOD TYPE O		WEEKLY ▪ IF YOUR ANCESTRY IS		
Food	*Portion*	*African*	*Caucasian*	*Asian*
Eggs	1 egg	0	3–4x	5x
Cheeses	2 ounces	0	0–3x	0–3x
Yogurt	4–6 ounces	0	0–3x	0–3x
Milk	4–6 ounces	0	0–1x	0–2x

Type Os should severely restrict your use of dairy products. Your system is ill designed for their proper metabolism, and there are no highly beneficial foods in this group.

If you are a Type O of African ancestry, you should eliminate dairy foods and eggs altogether. They tend to be even more difficult for you to digest; indeed, many African-Americans are lactose intolerant.

Food allergies are not digestive problems. They are immune system reactions to certain foods. Your immune system literally creates an antibody that fights the intrusion of the food into your system. Food intolerances, on the other hand, are digestive reactions that can occur for many reasons, including cultural conditioning, psychological associations, poor-quality food, additives, or just some undefinable quirk in your own system. It makes sense that African-Americans might be lactose intolerant, since their hunter-gatherer African ancestors had no lactose in their diets.

Other Type Os may eat four or five eggs a week and small amounts of dairy, but it is generally a poor protein source for your blood type. Be sure, however, to take a daily calcium supplement, especially if you are a woman, since dairy foods are the best natural source of absorbable calcium.

Neutral

Butter	Ghee (clarified)	Mozzarella cheese
Farmer cheese	butter)	Rice milk
Feta cheese	Goat cheese	

Avoid

American cheese	Emmenthal cheese	Parmesan cheese
Blue cheese	Goat milk	Provolone cheese
Brie	Gouda cheese	Neufchatel cheese
Buttermilk	Gruyère cheese	Ricotta cheese
Camembert	Ice cream	Skim or 2% milk
Casein	Jarlsburg cheese	String cheese
Cheddar cheese	Kefir	Swiss cheese
Colby cheese	Monterey jack	Whey
Cottage cheese	cheese	Whole milk
Cream cheese	Munster cheese	Yogurt, all varieties
Edam cheese		

Oils and Fats

BLOOD TYPE O		WEEKLY • IF YOUR ANCESTRY IS		
Food	*Portion*	*African*	*Caucasian*	*Asian*
Oils	Tablespoon	1–5x	4–8x	3–7x

Type Os respond well to oils. They can be an important source of nutrition and an aid to elimination. You will increase their value in your system if you limit your use to the monounsaturated variety, such as olive oil and flaxseed oil. These oils have positive effects on the heart and arteries, and may even help reduce blood cholesterol.

Highly Beneficial

Linseed (Flaxseed) oil
Olive oil

Neutral

Almond oil	Canola oil	Walnut oil
Black currant seed oil	Cod liver oil	
	Sesame oil	

Avoid

Castor oil	Evening primrose oil	Soy oil
Coconut oil		Sunflower oil
Corn oil	Peanut oil	Wheat germ oil
Cottonseed oil	Safflower oil	

Nuts and Seeds

BLOOD TYPE O		WEEKLY • IF YOUR ANCESTRY IS		
Food	*Portion*	*African*	*Caucasian*	*Asian*
Nuts and seeds	6–8 nuts	2–5x	3–4x	2–3x
Nut butters	Tablespoon	3–4x	3–7x	2–4x

Type Os can find a good source of supplemental vegetable protein from some varieties of nuts and seeds. However, these foods should in no way take the place of high-protein meats. You certainly don't need them in your diet, and should be very selective in their use, as they are high in fat. Certainly you should avoid them if you're trying to lose weight.

Since nuts can sometimes cause digestive problems, be sure to chew them thoroughly, or use nut butters, which are easier to digest, especially if you have the colon problems that are more frequently experienced by Type Os.

Highly Beneficial

Flax seed	Walnuts
Pumpkin Seeds	

Neutral

Almonds	Macadamia	Sesame butter
Almond butter	Pecans	(tahini)
Filbert	Pignola (pine)	Sesame seed
Hickory	Safflower seed	~~Sunflower seed~~

Avoid

Brazil	Peanuts	Poppy seed
Cashew	Peanut butter	Sunflower butter
Chestnut	Pistachios	Sunflower seed
Litchi		

Beans and Legumes

BLOOD TYPE O	WEEKLY ▪ IF YOUR ANCESTRY IS			
Food	*Portion*	*African*	*Caucasian*	*Asian*
All recommended beans and legumes	1 cup, dry	1–2x	1–2x	2–6x

Type Os don't utilize beans particularly well, although those of Asian ancestry do a bit better because they are culturally acclimated to them. In general, beans inhibit the metabolism of other more important nutrients, such as those found in meat. They also tend to make muscle tissue slightly less acidic, and Type Os usually perform better when muscle tissues are somewhat more acidic. This is not to be confused with the acid/alkaline reaction that occurs in your stomach. In that case, the few highly beneficial beans are exceptions. They actually promote the strengthening of the digestive tract and promote healing of ulcerations—a Type O problem because of the high levels of stomach acid. Even so, eat beans in moderation, as an occasional side dish.

Highly Beneficial

Beans, adzuki	Peas, black-eyed

Neutral

Beans, black	Beans, lima	Peas, green
Beans, broad	Beans, mung	Peas, pods
Beans, cannellini	Beans, northern	Soy, bean
Beans, fava	Beans, red	Soy, cheese
Beans, garbanzo	Beans, snap	Soy, milk
Beans, green	Beans, string	Soy, tempeh
Beans, jicama	Beans, white	Soy, tofu

Avoid

Beans, copper	Beans, pinto	Lentils, green
Beans, kidney	Beans, tamarind	Lentils, red
Beans, navy	Lentils, domestic	

Cereals

BLOOD TYPE O		WEEKLY ■ IF YOUR ANCESTRY IS		
Food	Portion	African	Caucasian	Asian
All recommended cereals	1 cup, dry	2–3x	2–3x	2–4x

Type Os do not tolerate whole wheat products at all, and you should eliminate them completely from your diet. They contain lectins that react with both your blood and your digestive tract and interfere with the proper absorption of beneficial foods. Wheat products are a primary culprit in Type O weight gain. The glutens in wheat germ interfere with Type O metabolic processes. Inefficient or sluggish metabolism causes food to convert to energy more slowly, and so store itself as fat. Although oat products are on the avoid list for Type Os, you may experiment with them if you're suffering from digestive problems, or are trying to lose weight.

Neutral

Amaranth	Kamut	Rice, puffed
Buckwheat	Millet, puffed	Spelt
Cream of rice	Rice bran	

Avoid

Barley	Farina	Seven-grain
Cornflakes	Grape nuts	Shredded wheat
Cornmeal	Oat bran	Wheat bran
Cream of wheat	Oatmeal	Wheat germ
Familia		

Breads and Muffins

BLOOD TYPE O	WEEKLY ■ IF YOUR ANCESTRY IS			
Food	Portion	African	Caucasian	Asian
Breads, crackers	1 slice	0–4x	0–2x	0–4x
Muffins	1 muffin	0–2x	0–1x	0–1x

Breads and muffins can be a source of trouble for Type Os, since most of them contain some wheat. It may be difficult at first to eliminate your morning muffin or daily sandwich; these have become staples of the American diet. Even wheat-free breads can be troublesome for Type Os if you eat them often enough; your genetic makeup is not assimilated to the consumption of grains.

Two exceptions are Essene and Ezekiel bread, which are usually found in the freezer section of your local health food store. These sprouted seed breads are assimilable to Type Os because the gluten lectins (principally found in the seed coats) are destroyed by the sprouting process. Unlike commercially produced sprouted breads, Ezekiel and Essene breads are live foods with many beneficial enzymes intact.

Highly Beneficial

Essene bread
Ezekiel bread

Neutral

Brown rice bread	Millet	Rye vita
Fin crisp	Rice cakes	Soy flour bread
Gluten-free bread	100% Rye bread	Spelt bread
Ideal flat bread	Rye crisps	Wasa bread

Avoid

Bagels, wheat	Matzos, wheat	Wheat bran
Corn muffins	Multi-grain bread	muffins
Durum wheat	Oat bran muffins	Whole wheat
English muffins	Pumpernickel	bread
High-protein	Sprouted wheat	
bread	bread	

Grains and Pasta

BLOOD TYPE O		WEEKLY ▪ IF YOUR ANCESTRY IS		
Food	*Portion*	*African*	*Caucasian*	*Asian*
Grains	1 cup, dry	0–3x	0–3x	0–3x
Pastas	1 cup, dry	0–3x	0–3x	0–3x

There are no grains or pastas that could be classified highly beneficial for Type Os.

Most pasta is made with semolina wheat, so you'll need to select very carefully if you want an occasional pasta dish. Pastas made from buckwheat, Jerusalem artichoke, or rice flour are better tolerated by Type Os. But these foods are not essential to your diet and should be limited in favor of more effective animal and fish foods. Again, you may occasionally use oat flour if you have no digestive problems, or you don't need to lose weight.

Neutral

Barley flour	Quinoa	Rice, wild
Buckwheat	Rice, basmati	Rice flour
Kasha	Rice, brown	Rye flour
Pasta, artichoke	Rice, white	Spelt flour

Avoid

Bulgur wheat flour	Graham flour	Sprouted wheat flour
Couscous flour	Oat flour	White flour
Durum wheat flour	Soba noodles	Whole wheat flour
Gluten flour	Pasta, semolina	
	Pasta, spinach	

Vegetables

BLOOD TYPE O	DAILY ▪ ALL ANCESTRAL TYPES	
Food	*Portion*	
Raw	1 cup, prepared	3–5x
Cooked or steamed	1 cup, prepared	3–5x

There are a tremendous number of vegetables available to Type Os, and they form a critical component of your diet. You cannot, however, simply eat all vegetables indiscriminately. Several classes of vegetables cause big problems for Type Os. For example, certain vegetables from the Brassica family—cabbage, Brussels sprouts, cauliflower, and mustard greens—can inhibit the thyroid function, which is already somewhat weak in Type Os.

Leafy green vegetables rich in vitamin K, like kale, collard greens, romaine lettuce, broccoli, and spinach, are very good for Type Os. This vitamin has one purpose only—to help blood clot. Type Os, as we have discussed, lack several clotting factors, and need vitamin K to assist in the process.

Alfalfa sprouts contain components that, by irritating the digestive tract, can aggravate Type O hypersensitivity problems. The molds in domestic and shiitake mushrooms, as well as fermented olives, tend to trigger allergic reactions in Type Os. All of these foods are foreign to the Type O system, which has not been designed to handle them.

The nightshade vegetables, such as eggplant and potatoes, cause arthritic conditions in Type Os because their lectins deposit in the tissue surrounding your joints.

Corn lectins affect the production of insulin, often leading to diabetes and obesity. All Type Os should avoid corn—especially if you have a weight problem or a family history of diabetes.

Tomatoes are a special case. Heavily laced with powerful lectins, called panhemaglutinans (meaning they agglutinate all blood types), tomatoes are trouble for Type A and Type B digestive tracts. However, Type Os can eat tomatoes. They become neutral in your system.

Highly Beneficial

Artichoke, domestic	Collard greens	Kohlrabi
Artichoke, Jerusalem	Dandelion	Lettuce, romaine
Beet leaves	Escarole	Okra
Broccoli	Garlic	Onions, red
Chicory	Horseradish	Onions, Spanish
Onions, yellow	Kale	Seaweed (kelp)
Parsley	Peppers, red	Spinach
Parsnips	Potatoes, sweet	Swiss chard
	Pumpkin	Turnips

Neutral

Arugula
Asparagus
Bamboo shoots
Beets
Bok choy
Brussel sprout
Cabbage, Chinese
Cabbage, red
Cabbage, white
Caraway
Carrots
Celery
Chervil
Daikon radish
Dill
Endive
Fennel

Fiddlehead ferns
Ginger
Lettuce, Bibb
Lettuce, Boston
Lettuce, iceberg
Lettuce, mesclun
Mushroom,
   abalone
Mushroom, enoki
Mushroom,
   Portobello
Mushroom, tree
   oyster
Olives, green
Peppers, green
Peppers, jalapeno
Peppers, yellow

Radicchio
Radishes
Rappini
Rutabaga
Sauerkraut
Scallion
Shallots
Sprouts, mung
Sprouts, radish
Squash, all types
Tempeh
Tofu
Tomato
Water chestnut
Watercress
Yams, all types
Zucchini

Avoid

Avocado
Cauliflower
Corn, white
Corn, yellow
Cucumber
Eggplant
Leek

Mushroom,
   domestic
Mushroom, shiitake
Mustard greens
Olives, black
Olives, Greek
Olives, Spanish

Pickle
Potatoes, red
Potatoes, white
Sprouts, alfalfa
Sprouts, Brussels
Taro
Yucca

Fruit

BLOOD TYPE O	DAILY ▪ ALL ANCESTRY TYPES	
Food	*Portion*	
All recommended fruits	1 fruit or 3–5 oz.	3–4x

Many wonderful fruits are available on the Type O Diet. Fruits are not only an important source of fiber, vitamins, and minerals, but they can be an excellent alternative to breads and pasta for Type Os. If you eat a piece of fruit rather than a slice of bread, your system will be better served—and at the same time you'll be supporting your weight-loss goals.

It may surprise you to find some of your favorite fruits on the Avoid list, and some odd choices on the Highly Beneficial list. The reason that plums, prunes, and figs are so beneficial to your blood type is that most dark red, blue, and purple fruits tend to cause an alkaline rather than an acidic reaction in your digestive tract. The Type O digestive tract has high acidity and needs the balance of the alkaline to reduce ulcers and irritations of the stomach lining. However, just because a fruit is alkaline doesn't mean it's good for you. Melons are also alkaline, but they contain high mold counts, to which Type Os have a proven sensitivity. Most melons should be eaten in moderation, and cantaloupe and honeydew, which have the highest mold counts of all, should be avoided completely.

Oranges, tangerines, and strawberries should be avoided because of their high acid content. Grapefruit also has a high acid content, but you may eat it in moderation because it exhibits alkaline properties after digestion. Most other berries are okay, but stay away from blackberries, which contain a lectin that aggravates Type O digestion. Type Os also have an extreme sensitivity to coconut and coconut-containing products. Stay away from these, and always check food labels to be sure you're not consuming coconut oil. This oil is high in saturated fat and provides little nutritional benefit.

Highly Beneficial

Banana	Figs, fresh	Plums, green
Blueberries	Guava	Plums, red
Cherries	Mango	Prunes
Figs, dried	Plums, dark	

Neutral

Apples	Boysenberries	Cranberries
Apricots	Cherries	Currants, black

Currants, red
Dates, red
Elderberries
Gooseberries
Grapefruit
Grapes, black
Grapes, Concord
Grapes, green
Grapes, red
Kumquat
Lemons
Limes

Loganberries
Melon, canang
Melon, casaba
Melon, Crenshaw
Melon, Christmas
Melon, musk
Melon, Spanish
Melon,
   watermelon
Nectarines
Papayas

Peaches
Pears
Persimmons
Pineapples
Pomegranates
Prickly pear
Raisins
Raspberries
Starfruit
   (carambola)
Strawberries

Avoid

Asian pear
Avocado
Blackberries
Coconuts

Kiwi
Melon, cantaloupe
Melon, honeydew
Oranges

Plantains
Rhubarb
Tangerines

Juices and Fluids

BLOOD TYPE O	DAILY ▪ ALL ANCESTRAL TYPES	
Food	*Portion*	
All recommended juices	8 oz.	2–3x
Water	8 oz.	4–7x

Vegetable juices are preferable to fruit juices for Type Os because of their alkalinity. If you drink fruit juice, choose a low-sucrose variety. Avoid high-sugar juices such as apple juice or apple cider.

Pineapple juice can be particularly helpful in avoiding water retention and bloating, both factors which contribute to weight gain. Black cherry is also a beneficial, high-alkaline juice.

Highly Beneficial

Black Cherry
Guava
Mango

Pineapple
Prune

Neutral

Apricot	Grape	Vegetable juice
Carrot	Grapefruit	(corresponding
Celery	Papaya	with highlighted
Cranberry	Tomato	vegetables)
~~Cucumber~~		Water (with lemon)

Avoid

Apple
Apple cider

Cabbage
Orange

Spices

Your choice of spices can actually improve your digestive and immune systems. For example, kelp-based seasonings are very good for Type Os because they are rich sources of iodine, key to regulating the thyroid gland. Iodized salt is another good source of iodine, but use it sparingly.

The kelp bladder wrack tends to counter the hyperacidity of the Type O digestive tract, reducing the potential for ulcers. The abundant fucose in the kelp protects the intestinal lining of the Type O stomach, preventing ulcer-causing bacteria from adhering. Keep in mind also that kelp is highly effective as a metabolic regulator for Type Os, and is an important aid to weight loss.

Parsley is soothing to your digestive tract, as are certain warming spices, like curry and cayenne pepper. Note, however, that black and white pepper and vinegar are irritants to the Type O stomach.

Sugar products such as honey and sugar will not harm you. Nor will chocolate. But these should all be strictly limited to occasional use as condiments. Avoid corn syrup as a sweetener.

Highly Beneficial

Carob

Curry

Dulse

Kelp (bladder
  wrack)

Parsley

Pepper,
  cayenne

Turmeric

Neutral

Agar

Allspice

Almond extract

Anise

Arrowroot

Barley malt

Basil

Bay leaf

Bergamot

Brown rice syrup

Cardamom

Chervil

Chives

Chocolate

Cinnamon

Clove

Coriander

Cream of tartar

Cumin

Dill

Garlic

Gelatin, plain

Honey

Horseradish

Maple syrup

Marjoram

Mint

Miso

Molasses

Mustard (dry)

Paprika

Pepper,
  peppercorn

Pepper, red
  pepper flakes

Peppermint

Pimiento

Rice syrup

Rosemary

Saffron

Sage

Salt

Savory

Soy sauce

Spearmint

Sucanat

Sugar, white

Sugar, brown

Tamari

Tamarind

Tapioca

Tarragon

Thyme

Vanilla

Wintergreen

Avoid

Capers

Cornstarch

Corn syrup

Nutmeg

Pepper, black
  ground

Pepper, white

Vinegar, apple
  cider

Vinegar, balsamic

Vinegar, red wine

Vinegar, white

Condiments

There are no highly beneficial condiments for Type Os. If you must have mustard or salad dressing on your foods, use them in moderation, and stick to the low-fat, low-sugar varieties.

Although Type Os can have tomatoes occasionally, avoid ketchup that also contains ingredients like vinegar.

All pickled foods are indigestible for Type Os. They severely irritate the Type O stomach lining. My recommendation is that you try to wean yourself from condiments, or replace them with healthier seasonings such as olive oil, lemon juice, and garlic.

Neutral

Apple butter	Mayonnaise	Worcestershire sauce
Jam (from acceptable fruits)	Mustard	
Jelly (from acceptable fruits)	Salad dressing (low-fat, from acceptable ingredients)	

Avoid

Ketchup	Pickles, kosher	Pickles, sour
Pickles, dill	Pickles, sweet	Relish

Herbal Teas

The recommendations regarding herbal teas are based on our general understanding of what makes Type Os sick. Think of herbal teas as a way to shore up your strength against your natural weaknesses. For Type Os, the primary emphasis is on soothing the digestive and immune systems.

Herbs like peppermint, parsley, rose hip, and sarsaparilla all have that effect. On the other hand, herbs like alfalfa, aloe, burdock, and corn silk stimulate the immune system and cause blood thinning, a problem for Type Os.

Highly Beneficial

Chickweed	Hops	Peppermint
Dandelion	Linden	Rose hips
Fenugreek	Mulberry	Sarsaparilla
Fenugreek	Parsley	Slippery elm

Neutral

Catnip	Horehound	Thyme
Chamomile	Licorice root	Valerian
Dong quai	Mullein	Vervain
Elder	Raspberry leaf	White birch
Ginseng	Sage	White oak bark
Green tea	Skullcap	Yarrow
Hawthorn	Spearmint	

Avoid

Alfalfa	Echinacea	Saint John's wort
Aloe	Gentian	Senna
Burdock	Goldenseal	Shepherd's purse
Coltsfoot	Red clover	Strawberry leaf
Corn silk	Rhubarb	Yellow dock

Miscellaneous Beverages

There are very few acceptable beverages for Type Os. You're pretty much limited to the innocuous effects of seltzer and tea. Beer is okay in moderation, but it's not a good choice if you want to lose weight. Modest quantities of wine are allowed, but it shouldn't be a daily ritual. Green tea is allowed as an acceptable substitute for other caffeinated products, but it contains no special curative properties for Type Os. The problem that coffee poses for Type Os is in the increased levels of stomach acid it produces. Type Os have plenty of stomach acid all their own; they really don't need help. If you are a coffee drinker, perhaps you can begin to gradually cut down on the amount you consume each day. Your ultimate goal should be to eliminate drinking coffee altogether. The common withdrawal symptoms such as headache, fatigue, and irritability, won't occur if you wean yourself gradually. Green tea is a good caffeinated alternative.

Highly Beneficial

Seltzer water

Neutral

Beer	Wine, red
Tea, green	Wine, white

Avoid

Coffee, regular	Soda, cola	Tea, black decaf
Coffee, decaf	Soda, diet	Tea, black regular
Liquor, distilled	Soda, other	

Type O
Supplement Advisory

The role of supplements—be they vitamins, minerals, or herbs—is to add the nutrients that are lacking in your diet and to provide extra protection where you need it. The supplement focus for Type Os is:

- Supercharging the metabolism
- Increasing blood-clotting activity
- Preventing inflammation
- Stabilizing the thyroid

The following recommendations emphasize the supplements that help meet these goals, and also warn against the supplements that can be counterproductive or dangerous for Type Os.

Certain common vitamins and minerals are so abundant in Type O foods that they are normally not needed in supplement form. These include vitamin C and iron—although it won't hurt you to take a 500-mg vitamin C supplement every day. Vitamin D supplements are not needed. Many foods are vitamin D fortified, and your best source of all is the natural light of the sun.

All of these recommendations are based on your adherence to the Type O Diet.

Beneficial

VITAMIN B

My father found that Type Os did well on a high-potency vitamin B complex. There's good reason. Type Os tend to have sluggish metabolisms—a holdover from your ancestors' efforts to conserve energy during periods when food was not readily available. Since modern Type Os experience very different conditions, they don't need this conserving effect, but it remains in your blood type memory. A vitamin B complex can have the effect of supercharging your metabolic processes.

Type Os on the correct diet almost never require special vitamin B_{12} or folic acid supplementation. I have, however, successfully treated depression, hyperactivity, and attention deficit disorder (ADD) in many Type Os by using high doses of folic acid and vitamin B_{12} in conjunction with the Type O Diet and exercise program. Those vitamins are responsible for the development of DNA.

If you wish to experiment with a high-potency vitamin B complex, make sure it is free of fillers and binders. Improper binding and compressing can make the pill difficult to absorb in your system. Also avoid using a formula that contains yeast or wheat germ.

Finally, eat plenty of vitamin B–rich foods.

Best B-Rich Foods for Type Os:

meat	nuts
liver, kidney,	dark green,
muscle meats	leafy vegetables
*eggs	fruit
fish	

*in moderation

VITAMIN K

Type Os have lower levels of several blood-clotting factors, which lead to bleeding disorders. Be sure you have plenty of vitamin K in your diet. Since it is generally not recommended as a supplement, pay attention to the foods you eat and choose those that are high in this essential Type O nutrient.

Best K-Rich Foods for Type Os

liver
egg yolks
green leafy vegetables—kale, spinach, and Swiss chard

CALCIUM

Type Os should continually supplement their diet with calcium, since the Type O Diet does not include dairy products which are the best source of this mineral. With the Type O tendency to develop inflammatory joint problems and arthritis, the need for consistent calcium supplementation becomes clear.

Calcium supplementation in high doses (600–1,100 mg elemental calcium) is probably desirable for all Type Os, but it is especially beneficial for Type O children during their growth periods (two to five and nine to sixteen), and for post-menopausal women.

Although the non-dairy sources of calcium are not as beneficial, Type Os should employ them as mainstays of their diets.

Best Calcium-Rich Foods for Type Os

sardines (unboned)
canned salmon (unboned)
broccoli
collard greens

IODINE

Type Os tend to have unstable thyroid metabolisms, due to a lack of iodine. This causes many side effects, including weight gain, fluid retention, and fatigue. Iodine is the key element necessary for the production of thyroid hormone. Although iodine supplements are not recommended, adequate amounts of iodine can be found in the Type O Diet.

Best Iodine-Rich Foods for Type Os

seafood (especially saltwater fish)
kelp (seaweed)
*iodized salt

*in moderation

MANGANESE [with caution]
It is difficult for Type Os to get manganese in their diet because manganese is found primarily in whole grains and legumes. For the most part this isn't a problem, and manganese supplementation is rarely recommended. However, a surprising amount of chronic joint pain (especially in the lower back and knees) in Type O patients has been helped with a short period of manganese supplementation. Never do this on your own! Manganese toxicity can result from inappropriate administration, and it should be used only under a physician's supervision.

Herbs/Phytochemicals: Recommended for Type Os

LICORICE *(Glycyrrhiza glabra).* The high stomach acid typical of Type Os can lead to stomach irritations and ulcers. A licorice preparation called DGL (de-glycyrrhizinated licorice) can reduce your discomfort and aid healing. DGL is widely available in health food stores as a pleasant-tasting powder or in the form of lozenges. Unlike most ulcer medicines, DGL actually heals the stomach lining, in addition to protecting it from stomach acids. Avoid crude licorice preparations, as they contain a component of the plant that can cause elevated blood pressure. This component has been removed in DGL.

BLADDER WRACK *(Fucus vesiculosus).* Bladder wrack (from kelp) is an excellent nutrient for Type Os. This herb, actually a seaweed, has some interesting components, including iodine and large amounts of the sugar fucose. As you may recall, fucose is the basic building sugar of the O antigen. The fucose found in bladder wrack helps protect the intestinal lining of Type Os—especially from the ulcer-causing bacteria, *H. pylori*, which attaches itself to the fucose lining the stomach of Type Os. The fucose in bladder wrack acts on *H. pylori* much as dust would on a piece of adhesive tape: clogging the suction cups on the bacteria, preventing it from attaching to the stomach.

I have also found that bladder wrack is very effective as an aid to weight control for Type Os—especially those who suffer thyroid dysfunctions. The fucose in bladder wrack seems to help normalize the sluggish metabolic rate and produce weight loss. (Note, however, that although bladder wrack has a time-honored reputation as an aid to weight loss for Type Os, it does not work that way for the other blood types.)

PANCREATIC ENZYMES. If you are a Type O who is not used to a high-protein diet, I suggest you take a pancreatic enzyme with large meals for a while, or at least until your system begins to adjust to the more concentrated proteins. Pancreatic enzyme supplements are available at many health food stores, usually in the 4x strength.

Avoid

VITAMIN A

Since your blood type is prone to slower clotting, I would not recommend that Type Os take vitamin A supplements derived from fish oils without first checking with a doctor. These supplements can enhance blood thinning. Instead, take advantage of the rich sources of vitamin A or beta-carotene in your diet.

A-Rich Foods Acceptable for Type Os

yellow, orange, and recommended dark, leafy green
  vegetables

VITAMIN E

Likewise, I would not recommend vitamin E supplements for Type Os because they might also complicate Type O tendencies toward slower blood clotting. Instead, derive vitamin E from foods in your diet.

E-Rich Foods Acceptable for Type Os

vegetable oils
liver
nuts
recommended leafy green vegetables

Type O
Stress/Exercise Profile

The ability to reverse the negative effects of stress lives in your blood type. Stress is not in itself the problem; it's how you respond to stress. Each blood type has a distinct, genetically programmed instinct for overcoming stress.

If you are Type O, you have the immediate and physical response of your hunter ancestors: Stress goes directly to your muscles. Your blood type carries a patterned alarm response that permits explosions of intense physical energy.

When you encounter stress, your body takes over. As your adrenal glands pump their chemicals into your bloodstream, you become tremendously charged up. Given a physical release at this time, any bad stress you are experiencing may be converted into a positive experience.

Healthy Type Os are meant to release the built-up hormonal forces through vigorous and intense physical exercise. Their systems are literally suited for it.

Exercise is especially critical to the health of Type Os, because the impact of stress is direct and physical.

Not only does a regular intense exercise program elevate your spirits, it also enables the Type O to maintain weight control, emotional balance, and a strong self-image. Type Os respond well to heavy exercise—in nearly every way.

Type Os who want to lose weight must participate in highly physical exercise. That is because this type of exercise makes the muscle tissue more acidic and produces a higher rate of fat-burning activity. Acidic muscle tissue is the result of ketosis, which, as we have discussed, was the key to the success of our Type O ancestors. I'd dare to say that there wasn't one overweight Cro-Magnon on the planet!

Type Os who do not express their physical natures with appropriate activity in response to stress are eventually overwhelmed during the exhaustion stage of the stress response. This exhaustion stage is characterized by a variety of psychological manifestations caused by a slower rate of metabolism, such as depression, fatigue, or insomnia. If there is no change, you will leave yourself vulnerable to a number of inflammatory and autoimmune disorders, such as arthritis and asthma, as well as to consistent weight gain and eventual obesity.

The following exercises are recommended for Type Os. Pay special attention to the length of the sessions. To achieve a consistent metabolic effect, you have to get your heart rate up.

You can mix any of these exercises, but be sure you do one or several of them at least four times a week for the best results.

EXERCISE	DURATION	FREQUENCY
Aerobics	40–60 min.	3–4x week
Swimming	30–45 min.	3–4x week
Jogging	30 min.	3–4x week
Weight training	30 min.	3x week
Treadmill	30 min.	3x week
Stair climbing	20–30 min.	3–4x week
Martial arts	60 min.	2–3x week
Contact sports	60 min.	2–3x week
Calisthenics	30–45 min.	3x week
Cycling	30 min.	3x week
Brisk walking	30–40 min.	5x week
Dancing	40–60 min.	3x week
In-line or roller skating	30 min.	3–4x week

Type O
Exercise Guidelines

The three components of a high-intensity exercise program are the warm-up period, the aerobic exercise period, and the cool-down period. A warm-up is very important to prevent injuries, because it brings blood to the muscles, readying them for exercise, whether it is walking, running, biking, swimming, or playing a sport. A warm-up should include stretching and flexibility moves, to prevent tears in the muscles and tendons.

The exercise can be divided into two basic types: isometric exercises, in which stress is created in stationary muscles; and isotonic exercises, such as calisthenics, running, or swimming, which produce muscle tension through a range of movement. Isometric exercises can be used to tone up specific muscles, which can be further strengthened by active isotonic exercise. Isometrics may be performed by pushing or pulling an immovable object or by contracting or tightening opposing muscles.

To achieve maximum cardiovascular benefits from aerobic exercise, you must elevate your heartbeat to approximately 70 percent of your maximum heart rate. Once that elevated rate is achieved during exercise, continue exercising to maintain that rate for thirty minutes. This regimen should be repeated at least three times each week.

To calculate your maximum heart rate:

1. Subtract your age from 220.
2. Multiply the difference by 70 percent (.70). If you are over sixty years of age, or in poor physical condition, multiply the remainder by 60 percent (.60).
3. Multiply the remainder by 50 percent (.50). For example, a healthy fifty-year-old woman would subtract 50 from 220, for a maximum heart rate of 170. Multiplying 170 by .70 would give her 119 beats per minute, which is the top level she should strive for. Multiplying 170 by .50 would give her 85 beats per minute, the lowest number in her range.

Active, healthy individuals under forty and persons under sixty with a low cardiovascular risk can choose their own exercise program from among the recommendations listed.

Remember, your goal is to counter stress with action. Remarkably, for Type Os, the best antidote to fatigue and depression is physical work. Think of your metabolism as a fire. You start a fire first by using little pieces of wood called kindling, and then gradually adding larger and larger pieces of wood until you have an inferno. If you are too tired to imagine doing aerobics for forty-five minutes or an hour, start doing something! As you feel better, add more. At the end, your stress levels will be reduced, your mood will be better, and you'll have renewed energy.

A Final Note:
The Personality Question

Every person with Type O blood carries a genetic memory of strength, endurance, self-reliance, daring, intuition, and an innate optimism. The original Type Os were the epitome of focus, drive, and a strong sense of self-preservation. They believed in themselves. It's a good thing, too, or we might not be here.

If you are a Type O, you may be able to appreciate this inheritance because the things that make you healthy, inspire you, and energize you are very similar to what influenced your ancestors. You're hardy and strong, fueled by a high-protein diet. You respond best to heavy physical exercise—in fact, you become depressed, despondent, and overweight when you are deprived of it.

Perhaps you have also inherited the drive to succeed and the leadership qualities of Type Os—strong, certain and powerful—blushing with good health and optimism.

Former president Ronald Reagan is a Type O who fits the mold quite well. His administration was characterized by a surety, evenness, and an unflagging optimism about the future. You never felt that Reagan suffered much in the way of self-doubt. He forged ahead, for good or ill. He was also a risk taker, as is the way of Type Os. People used to call him the "Teflon president" because he was never felled by the risks he took.

Of course, Reagan didn't exhibit (at least publicly) the sharp, uncompromising, almost brutish style of some leaders. For example, it's not terribly surprising that some famous mafiosos have been

Type Os. Al Capone was a Type O. Now, there's an example of leadership taken to the extreme.

And speaking of risk takers, the penultimate gambler, Jimmy the Greek, was Type O. So is former Soviet president Mikhail Gorbachev—one of the greatest risk takers of modern times.

Great Britain's Queen Elizabeth II is a Type O, as is her son Charles, the Prince of Wales. I find it interesting that the House of Windsor has a history of people with bleeding disorders. Perhaps there's a Type O connection.

The Type A Program

Vegetarians Rule

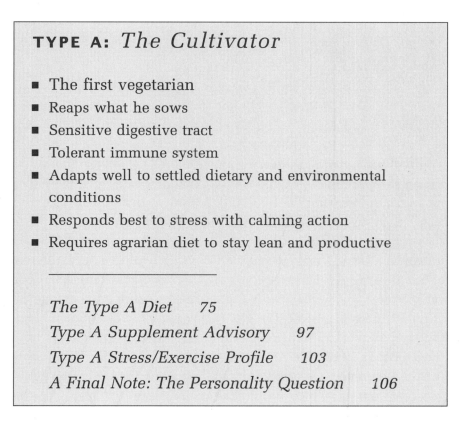

TYPE A: *The Cultivator*

- The first vegetarian
- Reaps what he sows
- Sensitive digestive tract
- Tolerant immune system
- Adapts well to settled dietary and environmental conditions
- Responds best to stress with calming action
- Requires agrarian diet to stay lean and productive

The Type A Diet

Type As flourish on vegetarian diets—the inheritance of their more settled and less warlike farmer ancestors. If you are an average American with Type A blood, you might find it too big an adjustment to move away from the typical meat-and-potato fare to soy proteins, grains, and vegetables. Likewise, you may find it difficult to eliminate overly processed and refined foods, since our civilized diets are increasingly composed of convenient toxins in brightly wrapped packages. But it is particularly important for sensitive Type As to get their foods in as natural a state as possible: fresh, pure, and organic.

I can't emphasize enough how critical this dietary adjustment can be to the sensitive immune system of Type A. Type As are biologically predisposed to heart disease, cancer, and diabetes. In other words, these are your risk factors. But they need not be your destiny. If you follow this diet, you can supercharge your immune system and potentially short-circuit the development of life-threatening diseases. A positive aspect of your genetic ancestry is your ability to utilize the best nature has to offer. It will be your challenge to relearn what your blood already knows.

The Weight-Loss Factor

You will naturally be thinner on the Type A Diet. If you are accustomed to eating meat, you'll lose weight rather rapidly in the beginning as you eliminate the toxic foods from your diet.

In many ways, Type A is the exact opposite of Type O when it comes to metabolism. While animal foods speed up the Type O metabolic rate and make it more efficient, they have a very different effect on Type As. Perhaps you have already noted that when you eat red meat, you feel sluggish and less energized than when you eat vegetable proteins. Some Type As experience fluid retention as their digestive systems slowly process the unwieldy foods. Type Os burn their meat as fuel; Type As ultimately store meat as fat. The reason for the difference is stomach acid. While Type Os have high stomach-acid content, which promotes easy digestion of meat, Type As have low stomach-acid content—an adaptation of their ancestors who survived on an agrarian diet.

Dairy foods are also poorly digested by Type As, and they provoke insulin reactions—another factor in metabolic slowdowns. In addition, dairy foods are very high in saturated fats, the kind that compromise the heart and lead to obesity and diabetes.

Wheat is a mixed factor in the Type A Diet. While Type As may eat wheat, they have to be careful not to eat too much of it or their muscle tissue will become overly acidic. Unlike Type Os, who thrive on slightly acidic tissue, Type As can't utilize the energy so quickly, and calorie metabolism is inhibited. This particular food reaction is a good example of how different foods react in different ways depending on your blood type. Wheat is alkaline in Type Os and acidic in Type As.

In addition to eating a wide variety of healthy, low-fat foods and balancing vegetables and grains, Type As need to highlight certain foods for their beneficial or hindering effects. Here's a quick guide:

Foods That Encourage Weight Gain

MEAT	*poorly digested*
	stored as fat
	increases digestive toxins
DAIRY FOODS	*inhibit nutrient metabolism*
	increase mucous secretions
KIDNEY BEANS	*interfere with digestive enzymes*
	slow metabolic rate
LIMA BEANS	*interfere with digestive enzymes*
	slow metabolic rate
WHEAT (IN OVERABUNDANCE)	*inhibits insulin efficiency*
	impairs calorie utilization

Foods That Encourage Weight Loss

VEGETABLE OILS	*aid efficient digestion*
	prevent fluid retention
SOY FOODS	*aid efficient digestion*
	metabolize quickly
	optimize immune function
VEGETABLES	*aid efficient metabolism*
	increase intestinal mobility
PINEAPPLE	*increases calorie utilization*
	increases intestinal mobility

Incorporate these guidelines into the total picture of the Type A Diet, which follows.

Meats and Poultry

BLOOD TYPE A		WEEKLY ▪ IF YOUR ANCESTRY IS		
Food	Portion*	African	Caucasian	Asian
Lean red meats	4–6 oz. (men) 2–5 oz. (women and children)	0–1x	0x	0–1x
Poultry	4–6 oz. (men) 2–5 oz. (women and children)	0–3x	0–3x	1–4x

The portion recommendations are merely guidelines that can help refine your diet according to ancestral propensities.

To receive the greatest benefits, Type As should eliminate all meats from their diet. Let's be realistic, however. The Western diet is still resolutely protein-driven. The trend in fast-food restaurants seems to be bigger, with more fat and calories than ever before. But, no matter the current trend, I urge you to look at the Type A Diet guidelines with an open mind. This is a way you can begin reducing Type A risk factors for heart disease and cancer in your diet.

Having said that, let me acknowledge that it will probably take time for you to convert to a totally vegetarian diet. Begin by substituting fish for meat several times a week. When you do eat meat, choose the leanest cuts you can find; poultry is preferable to red meat. Prepare meat by broiling or baking.

Stay completely away from processed meat products such as ham, frankfurters, and cold cuts. They contain nitrites, which promote stomach cancer in people with low levels of stomach acid—a Type A trait.

Neutral

Chicken	Guinea hen	Turkey
Cornish hens	Ostrich	
Grouse	Squab	

Avoid

Bacon	Lamb	Quail
Beef	Liver	Rabbit
Buffalo	Mutton	Squirrel
Duck	Partridge	Turtle
Goose	Pheasant	Veal
Ham	Pork	Venison
Heart		

Seafood

BLOOD TYPE A		WEEKLY ■ IF YOUR ANCESTRY IS		
Food	*Portion*	*African*	*Caucasian*	*Asian*
All recommended seafood	4–6 oz.	0–3x	1–4x	1–4x

Type As can eat seafood in modest quantities three or four times a week, but should avoid white fish such as sole and flounder. They contain a lectin that can irritate the Type A digestive tract.

If you are a Type A woman with a family history of breast cancer, consider introducing snails into your diet. The edible snail *Helix pomatia* contains a powerful lectin that specifically agglutinates and is drawn to mutated Type A cells for two of the most common forms of breast cancer, as you will see in Chapter 10. This is a positive kind of agglutination; this lectin gets rid of sick cells.

Seafood should be baked, broiled, or poached to achieve its full nutritional value.

Highly Beneficial

Carp	Red snapper	Silver perch
Cod	Rainbow trout	Snail
Mackerel	Salmon	Whitefish
Monkfish	Sardine	Whiting
Pickerel	Sea trout	Yellow perch

Neutral

Abalone	Sailfish	Swordfish
Brook trout	Sea bass	Tilapia
Mahimahi	Shark	Tuna
Ocean perch	Smelt	Weakfish
Pike	Snapper	White perch
Porgy	Sturgeon	Yellowtail

Avoid

Anchovy	Flounder	Mussels
Barracuda	Frog	Octopus
Beluga	Gray sole	Oysters
Bluefish	Grouper	Scallop
Bluegill bass	Haddock	Shad
Catfish	Hake	Shrimp
Caviar	Halibut	Sole
Clam	Herring (fresh)	Squid (calamari)
Conch	Herring (pickled)	Striped bass
Crab	Lobster	Tilefish
Crayfish	Lox (smoked	
Eel	salmon)	

Eggs and Dairy

BLOOD TYPE A		WEEKLY ∙ IF YOUR ANCESTRY IS		
Food	Portion	African	Caucasian	Asian
Eggs	1 egg	1–3x	1–3x	1–3x
Cheeses	2 oz.	1–3x	2–4x	0
Yogurt	4–6 oz.	0	1–3x	0–3x
Milk	4–6 oz.	0	0–4x	0

Type As can tolerate small amounts of fermented dairy products, but should avoid anything made with whole milk, and also limit egg consumption to occasional organically grown eggs. This will take some planning, as the Western diet is egg, butter, and cream oriented—cakes, pies, cookies, and ice cream being the big favorites.

Your Type A choices should be yogurt, kefir, nonfat sour cream, and cultured dairy products. Raw goat's milk is a good substitute for whole milk.

Most dairy products are not digestible for Type As—for the simple reason that Type A blood creates antibodies to the primary sugar in whole milk—D-galactosamine. D-galactosamine is the essential sugar that, along with fucose, forms the Type B antigen. Since the Type A immune system is designed to reject anything B-like, the antibodies it creates to ward off B antigens will also reject whole-milk products.

If you are a Type A allergy sufferer or are experiencing respiratory problems, be aware that dairy products greatly increase the amount of mucus you secrete. Type As normally produce more mucus than the other blood types, probably because they need the extra protection it provides their somewhat too friendly immune systems. However, too much mucus can be harmful, since various bacteria tend to live off it. An overabundance of mucus inevitably leads to allergic responses, infections, and respiratory problems. This is another good reason to limit your intake of dairy foods.

Neutral

Egg, chicken	Ghee	Mozzarella cheese
Egg, duck	Goat cheese	Ricotta cheese
Egg, goose	Goat milk	Sour cream
Farmer cheese	Kefir	Yogurt
Feta cheese		

Avoid

American cheese	Camembert cheese	Cream cheese
Blue cheese	Casein cheese	Edam cheese
Brie	Cheddar cheese	Emmenthal cheese
Butter	Colby cheese	Gouda cheese
Buttermilk	Cottage cheese	Gruyère cheese

Ice cream	Neufchatel	String cheese
Jarlsberg cheese	Parmesan cheese	Swiss cheese
Monterey jack cheese	Provolone cheese	Whey
	Sherbet	Whole milk
Munster cheese	Skim or 2% milk	

Oils and Fats

BLOOD TYPE A		WEEKLY ■ IF YOUR ANCESTRY IS		
Food	*Portion*	*African*	*Caucasian*	*Asian*
Oils	1 tablespoon	3–8x	2–6x	2–6x

Type As need very little fat to function well, but a tablespoon of olive oil on salads or steamed vegetables every day will aid in digestion and elimination. As a monounsaturated fat, olive oil also has a positive effect on your heart and may actually reduce cholesterol.

The lectins in oils like corn and safflower oil cause problems in the Type A digestive tract—quite the opposite effect of the beneficial oils.

Of course, there are only two oils that are highly beneficial, and frankly, olive oil is far tastier and better suited for cooking than linseed oil.

Highly Beneficial

| Black currant seed oil | Linseed (Flaxseed) oil | Olive oil |
| | | Walnut oil |

Neutral

Almond Oil	Evening primrose oil	Soy oil
Canola oil	Safflower oil	Sunflower oil
Cod liver oil	Sesame oil	Wheat germ oil

Avoid

Castor oil	Cottonseed oil
Coconut oil	Peanut oil
Corn oil	

Nuts and Seeds

BLOOD TYPE A		WEEKLY ▪ IF YOUR ANCESTRY IS		
Food	*Portion*	*African*	*Caucasian*	*Asian*
Nuts and seeds	Small handful	4–6x	2–5x	4–6x
Nut butters	Tablespoon	3–5x	1–4x	2–4x

Many nuts and seeds, such as pumpkin and sunflower seeds, almonds, and walnuts can provide positive supplementation for the Type A Diet. Since Type As eat very little animal protein, nuts and seeds supply an important protein component. Peanuts are the most beneficial. Eat them often because they contain a cancer-fighting lectin. Also eat the peanut skins (not the shells). Pumpkin seeds are also highly beneficial.

If you are Type A and have gallbladder problems, limit yourself to small amounts of nut butters instead of whole nuts.

Highly Beneficial

Peanuts   Walnuts
Peanut Butter
Pumpkin Seeds

Neutral

Almond butter   Nuts, litchi   Sesame seeds
Nuts, almonds   Nuts, macadamia   Sesame butter
Nuts, chestnuts   Nuts, pecan   (tahini)
Nuts, filberts   Nuts, pignola (pine) Sunflower butter
Nuts, hickory   Poppy seeds   Sunflower seeds

Avoid

Brazil nuts
Cashews
Pistachios

Beans and Legumes

BLOOD TYPE A		WEEKLY ▪ IF YOUR ANCESTRY IS		
Food	*Portion*	*African*	*Caucasian*	*Asian*
All recommended beans and legumes	1 cup, dry	4–7x	3–6x	2–5x

Type As thrive on the vegetable proteins found in beans and legumes. Many beans and legumes provide a nutritious source of protein. Be aware, however, that not all beans and legumes are good for you. Some, like the kidney, lima, navy, and garbanzo, contain a lectin that can cause a decrease in insulin production, which is often a factor in both obesity and diabetes.

Tofu is the staple of the Type A Diet. Tofu is a nutritionally complete food that is both filling and inexpensive. Many people in Western societies have an automatic aversion to tofu. I think the real problem with tofu is the way it is usually displayed in the markets, in big plastic tubs of cold water. It doesn't look very appetizing. I've found that tofu displayed this way isn't as good as tofu that is refrigerated. Also, try to purchase tofu in health food stores, where it is likely to be fresher than in supermarkets. Tofu is tasteless; it takes on the flavors of vegetables and spices used in cooking. The best way to prepare it is in a stir-fry with vegetables and flavoring such as garlic, ginger, and soy sauce.

Highly Beneficial

Beans, Adzuki	Beans, soy	Peas, black-eyed
Beans, black	Lentils,	Soy cheese
Beans, fava	domestic	Soy milk
Beans, green	Lentils, green	Tempeh
Beans, pinto	Lentils, red	Tofu

Neutral

Beans, broad	Beans, snap	Peas, pods
Beans, cannellini	Beans, string	Peas, snow
Beans, jicama	Beans, white	
Beans, mung	Peas, green	

Avoid

Beans, copper	Beans, navy
Beans, garbanzo	Beans, red
Beans, kidney	Beans, tamarind
Beans, lima	

Cereals

BLOOD TYPE A		WEEKLY • IF YOUR ANCESTRY IS		
Food	*Portion*	*African*	*Caucasian*	*Asian*
Whole grains	1 cup, dry	6–10x	5–9x	4–8x
Pastas	1 cup, dry	3–5x	4–6x	3–5x

Type As generally do well on cereals and grains, and you can eat these foods one or more times a day. Select the more concentrated whole grains instead of instant and processed cereals. Introduce millet, soy wheat, cornmeal, and whole oats into your diet.

Type As with a pronounced mucus condition caused by asthma or frequent infections should limit wheat consumption, as wheat causes mucus production. You'll have to experiment for yourself to determine how much wheat you can eat.

Wheat-eating Type As must be sure to balance their intake of acid-forming wheat with alkaline foods (see fruits). We're not talking about stomach acid here, but the acid/alkaline balance in your muscle tissues. Type As do best when their tissues are slightly alkaline—in direct contrast with Type Os. While the inner kernel of wheat grain is alkaline in Type Os, it becomes acidic in Type As.

Highly Beneficial

Amaranth
Buckwheat

Neutral

Barley	Kamut	Rice, puffed
Cornflakes	Millet, puffed	Rice bran
Cornmeal	Oat bran	Spelt
Cream of rice	Oatmeal	

Avoid

Cream of wheat	Granola	Shredded wheat
Familia	Grape nuts	Wheat bran
Farina	Seven grain	Wheat germ

Breads and Muffins

BLOOD TYPE A	DAILY ▪ IF YOUR ANCESTRY IS			
Food	*Portion*	*African*	*Caucasian*	*Asian*
Breads, crackers	1 slice	2–4x	3–5x	2–4x
Muffins	1 muffin	1x	1–2x	1x

The Type A guidelines for breads and muffins are similar to those for cereals and grains. They are generally favorable foods, but if you produce excessive mucus or are overweight, these conditions make whole wheat inadvisable. Soy and rice flour are good substitutes for you. However, be aware that sprouted wheat breads sold commercially often contain small amounts of sprouted wheat and are basically whole wheat breads. Read the ingredient labels. Although Essene and Ezekiel breads (found in health food stores) are sprouted wheat breads, the gluten lectin is destroyed in the sprouting process.

Highly Beneficial

Essene bread	Rice cakes	Sprouted
Ezekiel bread	Soy flour bread	wheat bread

Neutral

Brown rice bread	Ideal flat bread	Rye crisps
Corn muffins	Millet	Rye vita
Fin crisp	Oat bran muffins	Spelt bread
Gluten-free bread	Rye bread, 100%	Wasa bread

Avoid

Durum wheat	Matzoh	Wheat bran
English muffins	Multi-grain	muffins
High-protein	bread	Whole wheat
bread	Pumpernickel	bread

Grains and Pasta

BLOOD TYPE A		WEEKLY ▪ IF YOUR ANCESTRY IS		
Food	*Portion*	*African*	*Caucasian*	*Asian*
Grains	1 cup, dry	2–3x	2–4x	2–4x
Pastas	1 cup, dry	2–3x	2–4x	2–4x

Type As have a wonderful cornucopia of choices in grains and pastas. These foods are excellent sources of vegetable protein. They can provide many of the nutrients that the Type A is no longer receiving from animal proteins. Stay away from processed products, such as frozen meals, prepared noodles with sauces, or packaged rice-and-vegetable combinations; instead, gain the full nutritional benefits from whole-grain products. Bake your own cakes, prepare your own pasta, or steam your own rice, using the purest ingredients.

Highly Beneficial

Buckwheat
Flour, oat
Flour, rice
Flour, rye

Noodles, soba
Pasta,
   artichoke

Neutral

Couscous
Flour, barley
Flour, bulgur
   wheat
Flour, durum
   wheat

Flour, gluten
Flour, graham
Flour, spelt
Flour, sprouted
   wheat
Noodles, spelt

Quinoa
Rice, basmati
Rice, brown
Rice, white
Rice, wild

Avoid

Flour, white
Flour, whole wheat

Pasta, semolina
Pasta, spinach

Vegetables

BLOOD TYPE A		DAILY ∙ IF YOUR ANCESTRY IS		
Food	*Portion*	*African*	*Caucasian*	*Asian*
Vegetables, raw	1 cup, cooked	3–6x	2–5x	2–5x
Vegetables, cooked	1 cup, cooked	1–4x	3–6x	3–6x
Soy products	6–8 ounces	4–6x week	4–6x week	5–7x week

Vegetables are vital to the Type A Diet, providing minerals, enzymes, and antioxidants. Eat your vegetables in as natural a state as possible (raw or steamed) to preserve their full benefits.

Most vegetables are available to Type As, but there are a few caveats: Peppers aggravate the delicate Type A stomach, as do the molds in fermented olives. Type As are also very sensitive to the lectins in domestic potatoes, sweet potatoes, yams, and cabbage. Avoid tomatoes, as their lectins have a strongly deleterious effect on the Type A digestive tract. Tomatoes are a rare food—what is called a panhemaglutinan. That means its lectins agglutinate in every blood type. However, Type O doesn't produce antibodies to tomatoes, and can eat them, as can Type AB. They're very bad for Type As and Type Bs, though.

Broccoli is highly recommended for its antioxidant benefits. Antioxidants strengthen the immune system and prevent abnormal cell division. Other vegetables that are excellent for Type As are carrots, collard greens, kale, pumpkin, and spinach.

Use plenty of garlic. It's a natural antibiotic and immune-system booster, and it's good for your blood. Every blood type benefits from the use of garlic, but perhaps Type As benefit most of all, because their immune systems are vulnerable to a number of diseases that garlic ameliorates. Yellow onions are very good immune boosters, too. They contain an antioxidant called quercetin.

Highly Beneficial

Alfalfa sprouts	Escarole	Okra
Aloe	Fennel	Onions, red
Artichoke,	Garlic	Onions, Spanish
domestic	Horseradish	Onions, yellow
Artichoke,	Kale	Parsley
Jerusalem	Kohlrabi	Parsnips
Beet greens	Leek	Pumpkin
Broccoli	Lettuce,	Rappini
Carrots	romaine	Spinach
Chicory	Mushroom,	Sprouts, alfalfa
Collard	maitake	Swiss chard
greens	Mushroom,	Turnip
Dandelion	silver dollar	

Neutral

Arugula
Asparagus
Avocado
Bamboo shoots
Beets
Bok choy
Caraway
Cauliflower
Celery
Chervil
Coriander
Corn, white
Corn, yellow
Cucumber
Daikon radish

Endive
Fiddlehead ferns
Lettuce, Bibb
Lettuce, Boston
Lettuce, iceberg
Lettuce, mesclun
Mushroom,
    abalone
Mushroom,
    enoki
Mushroom,
    Portobello
Mushroom, tree
    oyster
Mustard greens

Olives, green
Onions, green
Radicchio
Radishes
Rutabaga
Scallion
Seaweed
Shallots
Sprouts, Brussels
Sprouts, mung
Sprouts, radish
Squash, all types
Water chestnut
Watercress
Zucchini

Avoid

Cabbage,
    Chinese
Cabbage, red
Cabbage, white
Eggplant
Lima beans
Mushroom,
    shiitake

Olives, black
Olives, Greek
Olives, Spanish
Peppers, green
Peppers, jalapeno
Peppers, red
Peppers, yellow

Potatoes, red
Potatoes, sweet
Potatoes, white
Sauerkraut
Tomatoes
Yams
Yucca

Fruits

BLOOD TYPE A	DAILY ▪ ALL ANCESTRAL TYPES	
Food	*Portion*	
All recommended fruits	1 fruit or 3–5 oz.	3–4x

Type As should eat fruits three times a day. Most fruits are allowable, although you should try to emphasize the more alkaline ones, such as berries and plums, which can help to balance the grains that are acid forming in your muscle tissues. Melons are also alkaline, but their high mold counts make them hard for Type As to digest. Cantaloupe and honeydew melons should be avoided altogether, since they have the highest mold counts. Other melons (listed as neutral) can be eaten occasionally.

Type As don't do well on tropical fruits such as mangoes and papaya. Although these fruits contain a digestive enzyme that is good for the other blood types, it doesn't work in the Type A digestive tract. Pineapple, on the other hand, is an excellent digestive aid for Type As.

Oranges also should be avoided, even though they may well be among your favorites. Oranges are a stomach irritant for Type As, and they also interfere with the absorption of important minerals. Lest you get confused, let me clarify that the acid/alkaline reaction happens two different ways—in the stomach and in the muscle tissues. When I say that acidic oranges are a stomach irritant for Type As, I'm talking about the stomach irritation they can cause in the sensitive, alkaline Type A stomach. Although stomach acid is generally low in Type As and could use a boost, oranges irritate the delicate stomach lining. Grapefruit is closely related to oranges and is also an acidic fruit, but it has positive effects on the Type A stomach, exhibiting alkaline tendencies after digestion. Lemons are also excellent for Type As, helping to aid digestion and clear mucus from the system.

Since vitamin C is an important antioxidant, especially for stomach cancer prevention, eat other vitamin C–rich fruits, such as grapefruit or kiwi.

The banana lectin interferes with Type A digestion. I recommend substituting other high-potassium fruits such as apricots, figs, and certain melons.

Highly Beneficial

Apricots	Figs, dried	Pineapple
Blackberries	Figs, fresh	Plums, dark
Blueberries	Grapefruit	Plums, green
Boysenberries	Lemons	Plums, red
Cherries	Limes	Prunes
Cranberries		

Neutral

Apples
Currants, black
Currants, red
Dates
Elderberries
Gooseberries
Grapes, black
Grapes, Concord
Grapes, green
Grapes, red
Guava
Kiwi

Kumquat
Limes
Loganberries
Melon, canang
Melon, casaba
Melon, Christmas
Melon, Crenshaw
Melon, musk
Melon, Spanish
Melon,
   watermelon
Nectarines

Peaches
Pears
Persimmons
Pomegranates
Prickly pears
Raisins
Raspberries
Star fruit,
   carambola
Strawberries

Avoid

Bananas
Coconuts
Mangoes
Melon,
   cantaloupe

Melon, honeydew
Oranges
Papayas
Plantains

Rhubarb
Tangerines

Juices and Fluids

BLOOD TYPE A	DAILY ▪ ALL ANCESTRAL TYPES	
Food	*Portion*	
All recommended juices	8 oz.	4–5x
Lemon and water	8 oz.	1x (in morning)
Water	8 oz.	1–3x

Type As should start every day with a small glass of warm water into which they have squeezed the juice of one-half lemon. This will help you reduce the mucus that has accumulated overnight in the more sluggish Type A digestive tract and stimulate normal elimination.

Alkaline fruit juices, such as black cherry juice concentrate diluted with water, should be consumed in preference to high-sugar juices, which are more acid forming.

Highly Beneficial

Apricot	Grapefruit
Carrot	Pineapple
Celery	Prune
Cherry, black	Water (with lemon)

Neutral

Apple	Grape
Apple cider	Vegetable juice
Cabbage	(corresponding
Cucumber	to highlighted
Cranberry	vegetables)

Avoid

Orange
Papaya
Tomato

Spices

Type As should view spices as more than just flavor enhancers. The right combination of spices can be powerful immune-system boosters. For example, soy-based spices such as tamari, miso, and soy sauce are tremendously beneficial for Type As. If you're concerned about sodium intake, all of these products are available in low-sodium versions.

Blackstrap molasses is a very good source of iron, a mineral that is lacking in the Type A Diet. Kelp is an excellent source of iodine and many other minerals. Vinegar should be avoided because the acids tend to cause stomach lining irritation.

Sugar and chocolate are allowed on the Type A Diet, but only in very small amounts. Use them as you would a condiment. Minimize your use of white processed sugar. Recent studies have shown that the immune system is sluggish for several hours after ingesting it.

Highly Beneficial

Barley malt	Garlic	Soy sauce
Blackstrap molasses	Ginger	Tamari
	Miso	

Neutral

Agar	Corn syrup	Pimiento
Allspice	Cream of tartar	Rice syrup
Almond extract	Cumin	Rosemary
Anise	Curry	Saffron
Arrowroot	Dill	Sage
Basil	Dulse	Salt
Bay leaf	Honey	Savory
Bergamot	Horseradish	Spearmint
Brown rice syrup	Kelp	Sugar, brown
Cardamom	Maple syrup	Sugar, white
Carob	Marjoram	Tamarind
Chervil	Mint	Tapioca
Chives	Mustard (dry)	Tarragon
Chocolate	Nutmeg	Thyme
Cinnamon	Oregano	Turmeric
Cloves	Paprika	Vanilla
Coriander	Parsley	
Cornstarch	Peppermint	

Avoid

Capers	Pepper, peppercorn	Vinegar, apple cider
Gelatin, plain		Vinegar, balsamic
Pepper, black ground	Pepper, red flakes	Vinegar, red wine
Pepper, cayenne	Pepper, white	Vinegar, white
		Wintergreen

Condiments

Condiments are not really recommended for any blood type. Type As in particular should avoid products with pickles or vinegar because of their low levels of stomach acid.

Neutral

Jam (from acceptable
    fruits)
Jelly (from acceptable
    fruits)
Mustard

Salad dressing (low-fat,
    from acceptable
    ingredients)

Avoid

Ketchup
Mayonnaise
Pickles
Pickle relish
Worcestershire sauce

Herbal Teas

The Type A reaction to particular herbal teas is the exact reverse of Type O. While Type Os need to be soothed, Type As need to rev up their immune systems.

Most of your health risk factors as a Type A are related to your sluggish immune system, and certain herbs can have a powerful effect. For example, hawthorn is a cardiovascular tonic; aloe, alfalfa, burdock, and echinacea are immune-system boosters; and green tea possesses important antioxidant effects on the digestive tract, providing protection against cancer.

It is also important for Type As to increase their stomach-acid secretions because they tend to have very low acid levels. Herbs such as ginger and slippery elm increase stomach-acid secretion.

Herbal relaxants, such as chamomile and valerian root, are a perfect fix for stress. The next time you're feeling harried, brew a pot of good tea.

Highly Beneficial

Alfalfa	Ginger	Saint John's
Aloe	Ginseng	Wort
Burdock	Green tea	Slippery elm
Chamomile	Hawthorn	Stone root
Echinacea	Milk thistle	Valerian
Fenugreek	Rose hips	

Neutral

Chickweed	Linden	Shepherd's purse
Coltsfoot	Mulberry	Skullcap
Dandelion	Mullein	Spearmint
Dong quai	Parsley	Strawberry Leaf
Elder	Peppermint	Thyme
Gentian	Raspberry leaf	Vervain
Goldenseal	Sage	White birch
Hops	Sarsaparilla	White oak bark
Horehound	Senna	Yarrow
Licorice root		

Avoid

Catnip	Corn silk	Rhubarb
Cayenne	Red clover	Yellow dock

Miscellaneous Beverages

Red wine is good for Type As because of its positive cardiovascular effects. A glass of red wine every day is believed to lower the risk of heart disease for both men and women.

Coffee may actually be good for Type As. It increases stomach acid and also has the same enzymes found in soy. Alternate coffee and green tea for the best combination of benefits.

All other beverages should be avoided. They don't suit the digestive system of Type As, nor do they support the immune system.

Pure fresh water, of course, should be consumed freely.

Highly Beneficial

Coffee, decaf	Tea, green
Coffee, regular	Wine, red

Neutral

Wine, white

Avoid

Beer	Soda, cola	Tea, black decaf
Liquor, distilled	Soda, diet	Tea, black regular
Seltzer water	Soda, other	

Type A
Supplement Advisory

The role of supplements—be they vitamins, minerals, or herbs—is to add the nutrients that are lacking in your diet or to provide extra protection where you need it. The supplement focus for Type As is:

- Supercharging the immune system
- Supplying cancer-fighting antioxidants
- Preventing infections
- Strengthening the heart

The following recommendations emphasize the supplements that help to meet these goals, and warn against the supplements that can be counterproductive or dangerous for Type As.

Beneficial

VITAMIN B

Type As should be alert to vitamin B_{12} deficiency. Not only is the Type A Diet somewhat lacking in this nutrient, which is found mostly in animal proteins, but Type As tend to have a hard time absorbing the B_{12} they do eat because they lack intrinsic factor in their stomachs. (Intrinsic factor is a substance produced by the lining of the stomach that helps B_{12} be absorbed into the blood.) In elderly Type As, vitamin B_{12} deficiency can cause senile dementia and other neurologic impairments.

Most other B vitamins are adequately contained in the Type A Diet. If, however, you suffer from anemia you may want a small supplement of folic acid. Type A heart patients should ask their doctors about low-dose niacin supplements, as niacin has cholesterol-lowering properties.

Best B-Rich Foods for Type As

whole grains (niacin)	tempeh (B_{12})
	fish
soy sauce (B_{12})	eggs
miso (B_{12})	

VITAMIN C

Type As, who have higher rates of stomach cancer because of low stomach acid, can benefit from taking additional supplements of vitamin C. For example, nitrite, a compound that results from the smoking and curing of meats, could be a particular problem with Type As because its cancer-causing potential is greater in people with lower levels of stomach acid. As an antioxidant, vitamin C is known to block this reaction (although you should still avoid smoked and cured foods). However, don't take this to mean that you should take massive amounts. I have found that Type As do not do sos well on high doses (1,000 mg and up) of vitamin C because it tends to upset their stomachs. Taken over the course of a day, two to four capsules of a 250-mg supplement, preferably derived from rose hips, should cause no digestive problems.

Best C-Rich Foods for Type As

berries	cherries
grapefruit	lemon
pineapple	broccoli

VITAMIN E

There is some evidence that vitamin E serves as a protectant against both cancer and heart disease—two Type A susceptibilities. You may want to take a daily supplement—no more than 400 IU (international units).

Best E-Rich Foods for Type As

vegetable oil
whole grains
peanuts
leafy green vegetables

CALCIUM

As the Type A diet includes some dairy products, the need for calcium supplementation is not so acute as in Type Os, yet a small amount of additional calcium (300- to 600-mg elemental calcium) from middle age onward is advisable.

In my experience, Type As do better on particular calcium products. The worst source of calcium for Type As is the simplest and most readily available: calcium carbonate (often found in antacids). This form requires the highest amount of stomach acid for absorption. In general, Type As tolerate calcium gluconate, do well on calcium citrate, and do best of all on calcium lactate.

Best Calcium-Rich Foods for Type As

yogurt	canned salmon	broccoli
soy milk	with bones	spinach
eggs	sardines with	
goat milk	bones	

IRON

The Type A Diet is naturally low in iron, which is found in the greatest abundance in red meats. Type A women, especially those with heavy menstrual periods, should be especially careful about keeping sufficient iron stores.

If you need iron supplementation, do it under a doctor's supervision, so blood tests can monitor your progress.

In general, use as low a dose as possible, and avoid extended periods of supplementation. Try to avoid crude iron preparations such as ferrous sulfate, which can irritate your stomach. Milder forms of supplementation, such as iron citrate or blackstrap molasses, may be used instead. Floradix, a liquid iron and herb supplement, can be found at most health food stores and is highly assimilable by Type As.

Best Iron-Rich Foods for Type As

whole grains
beans
figs
blackstrap molasses

ZINC [with caution]

I have found that a small amount of zinc supplementation (as little a 3 mg/day) often makes a big difference in protecting children against infections, especially ear infections. Zinc supplementation is a double-edged sword, however. While small, periodic doses enhance immunity, long-term, higher doses depress it and can interfere with the absorption of other minerals. Be careful with zinc! It's completely unregulated and is widely available as a supplement, but you really shouldn't use it without a physician's advice.

Best Zinc-Rich Foods for Type As

eggs
legumes

SELENIUM [with caution]

Selenium, which seems to act as a component of the body's own antioxidant defenses, may be of value to cancer-prone Type As. But check with your physician before taking selenium supplements on your own: Cases of selenium toxicity have been reported in people who have taken excessive supplements.

CHROMIUM [with caution]

Because of a susceptibility to diabetes, Type As with a family history of diabetes may be interested in the fact that chromium enhances the effectiveness of the body's glucose-tolerance factor, which increases the efficiency of insulin. However, we know very little about the long-term effects of chromium supplementation, and I would not advise using it at this time. Type As can best protect themselves from diabetic complications by following the blood type diet.

Herbs/Phytochemicals Recommended for Type As

HAWTHORN *(Crataegus oxyacantha)*. Hawthorn is a great cardiovascular tonic. Type As should definitely add it to their diet regimen if they or members of their family have a history of heart disease. This phytochemical, with exceptional preventive capacities, is found in the Hawthorn tree *(Crataegus oxyacantha)*. It has a number of impressive cardiovascular effects. Hawthorn increases the elasticity of the arteries and strengthens the heart, while also lowering blood pressure and exerting a mild solventlike effect upon the plaques in the arteries.

Officially approved for pharmaceutical use in Germany, the actions of hawthorn are virtually unknown elsewhere. Extracts and tinctures are readily available through naturopathic physicians, health food stores, and pharmacies. I cannot praise this herb too highly. Official German government monographs show the plant to be completely free of any side effects. If I had my way, extracts of hawthorn would be used to fortify breakfast cereals, just as vitamins are.

IMMUNE-ENHANCING HERBS. Because the immune systems of Type As tend to be open to immune-compromising infections, gentle immune-enhancing herbs, such as purple coneflower *(Echinacea purpurea)*, can help ward off colds or flus and may help optimize the immune system's anti-cancer surveillance. Many people take echinacea in liquid or tablet form. It is widely available. The Chinese herb huangki *(Astragalus membranaceous)* is also taken as an immune tonic, but is not as easy to find. In both herbs the active principles are sugars that act as mitogens that stimulate proliferation of white blood cells which act in defense of the immune systems.

CALMING HERBS. Type As can use mild herbal relaxants, such as chamomile and valerian root, as an anti-stress factor. These herbs are available as teas and should be taken frequently. Valerian has a bit of a pungent odor, which actually becomes pleasing once you get used to it. There is a rumor sometimes heard in health food stores that valerian is the natural form of Valium (diazepam), a prescription tranquilizer. This is wrong. Valerian was named for a Roman emperor who had the misfortune to be captured in battle by the Persians. Killed, stuffed, dyed red, and exhibited in a Persian museum, Valerian is fortunate to have had anything named for him.

QUERCETIN. Quercetin is a bioflavonoid found abundantly in vegetables, particularly yellow onions. Quercetin supplements are widely available in health food stores, usually in capsules of 100 to 500 mg. Quercetin is a very powerful antioxidant, many hundreds of times more potent than vitamin E. It can make a powerful addition to Type A cancer-prevention strategies.

MILK THISTLE *(Silybum marianum).* Like quercetin, milk thistle is an effective antioxidant with the additional special property of reaching very high concentrations in the liver and bile ducts. Type As can suffer from disorders of the liver and gallbladder. If your family has any history of liver, pancreas, or gallbladder problems, consider adding a milk thistle supplement (easily found in most health food stores) to your protocol. Cancer patients who are receiving chemotherapy should use a milk thistle supplement to help protect their livers from damage.

BROMELAIN (pineapple enzymes). If you are Type A and suffer from bloating or other signs of poor absorption of protein, take a bromelain supplement. This enzyme has a moderate ability to break down dietary proteins, helping the Type A digestive tract assimilate proteins better.

PRO-BIOTIC SUPPLEMENTS. If the Type A Diet is new for you, you may find that adjusting to a vegetarian diet is uncomfortable and produces excessive gas or bloating. A pro-biotic supplement can counter this effect by supplying the "good" bacteria usually found in the digestive tract. Look for pro-biotic supplements high in "bifidus factor," as this strain of bacteria is best suited to the Type A system.

Avoid

VITAMIN A–BETA CAROTENE

My father always avoided giving beta carotene to his Type A patients, saying that it irritated their blood vessels. I questioned his observation, as it had never been documented. Quite to the contrary, the evidence suggested that beta carotene may prevent artery disease. Yet recently there have been studies suggesting that beta carotene in high doses may act as a pro-oxidant, speeding up damage to the tissues rather than stopping it. Perhaps my father's observation was correct, at least in the case of Type As. If this is so, perhaps Type As may wish to forgo beta carotene supplements and consume high levels of carotenoids in their diet instead.

One caveat: As we age, our ability to assimilate the fat-soluble vitamins may diminish. Elderly Type As might benefit from small supplemental doses of vitamin A (10,000 IU daily) to help counteract the effects of aging upon the immune system.

Best Carotene-Rich Foods for Type As

eggs	spinach
yellow squash	broccoli
carrots	

Type A Stress/Exercise Profile

The ability to reverse the negative effects of stress lives in your blood type. Stress is not in itself a problem; it's how you respond to stress. Each blood type has a distinct, genetically programmed instinct for overcoming stress.

Type As respond to stress with a sharp increase in cortisol and adrenaline, producing anxiety, irritability, and hyperactivity. As the stress signals throb in your immune system, you grow weaker. The heightened sensitivity of your nervous system gradually frays your delicate protective antibodies. You're too weary to fight the infections and bacteria that are waiting to jump in like muggers trailing an intoxicated prey.

If, however, you adopt quieting techniques, such as yoga or meditation, you can achieve great benefits by countering negative stresses with focus and relaxation. Type As do not respond well to continuous confrontation, and need to consider and practice the art of stillness as a calming charm.

If Type As remain in their naturally tense state, stress can produce heart disease and various forms of cancer. Exercises that provide calm and focus are the remedy that pull the Type A from the grip of stress.

Tai chi chuan, the slow-motion, ritualistic pattern of Chinese boxing, and hatha yoga, the timeless Indian stretching system, are calming, centering experiences. Moderate isotonic exercises, such as hiking, swimming, and bicycling, are favored for Type As. When I advise calming exercises, it doesn't mean you can't break a sweat. The key is really your mental engagement in your physical activity.

For example, heavy competitive sports and exercises will only exhaust your nervous energy, make you tense all over again, and leave your immune system open to illness or disease.

The following exercises are recommended for Type As. Pay special attention to the length of the sessions. To achieve a consistent release of tension and revival of energy, you need to perform one or more of these exercises three or four times a week.

EXERCISE	DURATION	FREQUENCY
Tai chi	30–45 min.	3–5x week
Hatha yoga	30 min.	3–5x week
Martial arts	60 min.	2–3x week
Golf	60 min.	2–3x week
Brisk walking	20–40 min.	2–3x week
Swimming	30 min.	3–4x week
Dance	30–45 min.	2–3x week
Aerobics (low impact)	30–45 min.	2–3x week
Stretching	15 min.	3–5x week

Type A Exercise Guidelines

Tai chi chuan, or tai chi, is an exercise that enhances the flexibility of body movement. The slow, graceful, elegant gestures of tai chi chuan routines seem to mask the full-speed hand and foot blows, blocks, and parries they represent. In China, tai chi is practiced daily by groups who gather in public squares to perform the movements in unison. Tai chi can be a very effective relaxation technique, although it takes concentration and patience to master.

Yoga is also good for the Type A stress pattern. It combines inner rectitude with breath control and postures designed to allow for complete concentration without distraction by worldly concerns. Hatha yoga is the most common form of yoga practiced in the West.

If you learn basic yoga postures, you can create a routine best suited to your lifestyle. Many Type As who have adopted yoga relaxation tell me that they will not leave the house until they do their yoga.

However, some patients have told me that they are concerned that adopting yoga practices may conflict with their religious beliefs. They fear that the practice of yoga implies that they have adopted Eastern mysticism. I respond, "If you eat Italian food, does that make you Italian?" Meditation and yoga are what you make of them. Visualize and meditate on those subjects that are relevant to you. The postures are neutral; they are just timeless and proven movements.

SIMPLE YOGA RELAXATION TECHNIQUES

Yoga begins and ends with relaxation. We contract our muscles constantly, but rarely do we think of doing the opposite—letting go and relaxing. We can feel better and be healthier if we regularly release the tensions left behind within the muscles by the stresses and strains of life.

The best position for relaxation is lying on your back. Arrange your arms and legs so that you are completely comfortable in your hips, shoulders, and back. The goal of deep relaxation is to let your body and mind settle down to soothing calmness, in the same way that an agitated pool of water eventually calms to stillness.

Begin with abdominal breathing. As a baby breathes, its abdomen moves, not its chest. However, many of us grow to unconsciously adopt the unnatural and inefficient habit of restrained chest breathing. One of the aims of yoga is to make you aware of the true center of breathing. Observe the pattern of your breathing. Is your breathing fast, shallow, and irregular, or do you tend to hold your breath? Allow your breathing to revert to a more natural pattern—full, deep, regular, and with no constriction. Try to isolate just your lower breathing muscles; see if you can breathe without moving your chest. Breathing exercises are always done smoothly and without any strain. Place one hand on your navel and feel the movement of your breathing. Relax your shoulders.

Start the exercise by breathing out completely. When you inhale, pretend that a heavy weight, such as a large book, is resting on your navel, and that by your inhalation, you are trying to raise this imaginary weight up toward the ceiling.

Then, when you exhale, simply let this imaginary weight press down against your abdomen, helping you to exhale. Exhale more air out than you normally would, as if to "squeeze" more air out of your lungs. This will act as a yoga stretch for the diaphragm and further help release tension in this muscle. Bring your abdominal muscles into play here to assist. When you inhale, direct your breath down so deeply that you are lifting an imaginary heavy weight up toward the ceiling. Try to completely coordinate and isolate the abdominal breath with no chest or rib movement.

Even if you perform more aerobic exercises during the course of your week, try to integrate the relaxing, soothing routines that will help you best manage your Type A stress patterns.

A Final Note:
The Personality Question

Blood Type A was originally adapted to deal with dense population concentrations and the stresses of a more sedentary but intense urban lifestyle. Certain psychological traits would develop in people who must tolerate the demands of a crowded environment.

Probably the most important quality a person must have in that setting is a cooperative nature. The original Type As had to be decent, orderly, and law abiding, and had to exhibit self-control. Communities can't exist if there is no respect for others and their property. Loners do poorly in group settings. If the characteristics of Type Os had not evolved to suit an agrarian society, the result would have been chaos—and ultimately doom. Again, it's thanks to our Type A ancestors that humans survived.

The early Type As had to be clever, sensitive, passionate, and very smart to meet the challenges of a more complex life. But all of these qualities had to exist within a framework. That may be the reason why Type As, even today, tend to have more tightly wired systems. They bottle up their anxiety—because that's what you do when you're trying to get along with others—but when they explode, watch out! The antidotes to this tremendous inner stress are, as we have discussed, the more soothing and contemplative relaxation exercises of yoga and tai chi chuan.

It would seem that Type As are poorly suited for the intense, highly pressured leadership positions at which Type Os excel. That's not to say they can't be leaders. But they instinctively reject the dog-eat-dog manner of contemporary leadership. When Type As get into these positions, they tend to unravel. Former American presidents Lyndon B. Johnson, Richard Nixon, and Jimmy Carter were all Type A. While each man brought an unquestioned brilliance and passion to the job, all of them possessed fatal flaws. When the stress got too great, they became anxious and paranoid, taking everything personally. In the end, it was these Type A responses that forced each of them out of office.

The Type B Program

Lots of Variety

TYPE B: *The Nomad*

- Balanced
- Strong immune system
- Tolerant digestive system
- Most flexible dietary choices
- Dairy eater
- Responds best to stress with creativity
- Requires a balance between physical and mental activity to stay lean and sharp

---

The Type B Diet

Type O and Type A seem to be polar opposites in many respects. But Type B can best be described as idiosyncratic—with utterly unique and sometimes chameleonlike characteristics. In many respects, Type B resembles Type O so much that the two seem related. Then, suddenly, Type B will take on a totally unfamiliar shape—one that is peculiarly its own. You might say that Type B represents a sophisticated refinement in the evolutionary journey, an effort to join together divergent peoples and cultures.

On the whole, the sturdy and alert Type Bs are usually able to resist many of the most severe diseases common to modern life, such as heart disease and cancer. Even when they do contract these diseases, they are more likely to survive them. Yet because Type Bs are somewhat offbeat, their systems seem more prone to exotic immune-system disorders, such as multiple sclerosis, lupus, and chronic fatigue syndrome.

In my experience, a Type B who carefully follows the recommended diet can often bypass severe disease and live a long and healthy life.

The Type B Diet is balanced and wholesome, including a wide variety of foods. In the words of my father, it represents "the best of the animal and vegetable kingdoms." Think of B as standing for balance—the balancing forces of A and O.

The Weight-Loss Factor

For Type Bs, the biggest factors in weight gain are corn, buckwheat, lentils, peanuts, and sesame seeds. Each of these foods has a different lectin, but all of them affect the efficiency of your metabolic process, resulting in fatigue, fluid retention, and hypoglycemia—a severe drop in blood sugar after eating a meal. My patients with hypoglycemia often ask me if they should follow the standard advice of eating several small meals a day in order to keep their blood sugar levels from dropping. I discourage this practice. I find that the major problem is not when they eat, but what they eat. Certain foods trigger a drop in blood sugar—especially for Type Bs. When you eliminate these foods and begin eating the right diet for your type, your blood sugar levels should remain normal after meals. The problem with "grazing"—eating many small meals throughout the day—is that it interferes with your body's natural hunger signals; you may begin to find that you are hungry all the time—not a very helpful situation if you're trying to lose weight.

Type Bs are similar to Type Os in their reaction to the gluten found in wheat germ and whole wheat products. The gluten lectin adds to the problems caused by the other metabolism-slowing foods. When food is not efficiently digested and burned as fuel for the body, it gets stored as fat.

In itself, the wheat gluten doesn't attack Type Bs as severely as it does Type Os. However, when you add wheat to the mix of corn, lentils, buckwheat, and peanuts, the end result is just as damaging. Type Bs who want to lose weight should definitely avoid wheat.

When these foods are avoided, along with others that contain toxic lectins, it has been my experience that Type Bs are very successful in controlling their weight. You don't have any natural physiological barriers to weight loss, such as the thyroid problems that can hamper Type Os. Nor do you suffer from digestive disorders. All you need to do to lose weight is stay on your diet.

Some people are surprised that Type Bs aren't more likely to have problems with weight control, since dairy foods are encouraged on their diet. Of course, if you overeat high-calorie foods, you're going to gain weight! But the moderate consumption of dairy foods actually helps Type Bs achieve a metabolic balance. The real culprits are the particular foods that inhibit the efficient use of energy and promote the storage of calories as fat.

These are the highlights for Type B weight loss:

Foods That Encourage Weight Gain

CORN	*inhibits insulin efficiency*
	hampers metabolic rate
	causes hypoglycemia
LENTILS	*inhibit proper nutrient uptake*
	hamper metabolic efficiency
	cause hypoglycemia
PEANUTS	*hamper metabolic efficiency*
	cause hypoglycemia
	inhibit liver function
SESAME SEEDS	*hamper metabolic efficiency*
	cause hypoglycemia

BUCKWHEAT	*inhibits digestion*
	hampers metabolic efficiency
	causes hypoglycemia
WHEAT	*slows the digestive and metabolic processes*
	causes food to be stored as fat, not
	burned as energy
	inhibits insulin efficiency

Foods That Encourage Weight Loss

GREEN VEGETABLES	*aid efficient metabolism*
MEAT	*aids efficient metabolism*
LIVER	*aids efficient metabolism*
EGGS/LOW-FAT DAIRY PRODUCTS	*aid efficient metabolism*
LICORICE TEA*	*counters hypoglycemia*

*Never take licorice supplements without a doctor's supervision. Licorice tea is okay.

Incorporate these guidelines into the total picture of the Type B Diet, which follows.

Meats and Poultry

BLOOD TYPE B		WEEKLY ▪ IF YOUR ANCESTRY IS		
Food	Portion*	African	Caucasian	Asian
Lean red meats	4–6 oz. (men) 2–5 oz. (women and children)	3–4x	2–3x	2–3x
Poultry	4–6 oz. (men) 2–5 oz. (women and children)	0–2x	0–3x	0–2x

*The portion recommendations are merely guidelines that can help refine your diet according to ancestral propensities.

There appears to be a direct connection among stress, autoimmune disorders, and red meat in the Type B system. That's because your Type B ancestors adapted better to other kinds of meats. (After all, there weren't a lot of steer on the Siberian tundra!) If you are fatigued or suffer from immune deficiencies, you should eat red meat such as lamb, mutton, or rabbit several times a week, in preference to beef or turkey.

In my experience, one of the most difficult adjustments Type Bs must make is giving up chicken. Chicken contains a Blood Type B agglutinating lectin in its muscle tissue. If you're accustomed to eating more poultry than red meat, you can eat other poultry such as turkey or pheasant. Although they are similar to chicken in many respects, neither contains the dangerous lectin.

The news about chicken is troubling to many people because it has become a fundamental part of many ethnic diets. In addition, people have been told to eat chicken instead of beef because it is "healthier." But here is another case where one dietary guideline does not fit all. Chicken may be leaner (although not always) than red meat, but that isn't the issue. The issue is the power of an agglutinating lectin to attack your bloodstream and potentially lead to strokes and immune disorders. So, even though chicken may be a beloved food, I urge you to begin weaning yourself away from it.

Highly Beneficial

Goat	Mutton	Venison
Lamb	Rabbit	

Neutral

Beef	Ostrich	Veal
Buffalo	Pheasant	
Liver	Turkey	

Avoid

Bacon	Grouse	Pork
Chicken	Guinea hen	Quail
Cornish hens	Ham	Squab
Duck	Heart	Squirrel
Goose	Partridge	Turtle

Seafood

BLOOD TYPE B		WEEKLY ■ IF YOUR ANCESTRY IS		
Food	*Portion*	*African*	*Caucasian*	*Asian*
All recommended seafood	4–6 oz.	4–6x	3–5x	3–5x

Type Bs thrive on seafood, especially deep-ocean fish such as cod and salmon, which are rich in nutritious oils. White fish, such as flounder, halibut, and sole, are also excellent sources of high-quality protein for Type Bs. Avoid all shellfish—crab, lobster, shrimp, mussels, etc. They contain lectins that are disruptive to the Type B system. It is interesting to note that many of the original Type Bs were Jewish tribes that forbade the consumption of shellfish. Perhaps this dietary law was an acknowledgment that shellfish are poorly digested by Type Bs.

Highly Beneficial

Cod	Harvest fish	Porgy
Croaker	Mackerel	Sardine
Flounder	Mahimahi	Shad
Grouper	Monkfish	Sole
Haddock	Ocean Perch	Sturgeon
Hake	Pickerel	Sturgeon
Halibut	Pike	eggs (caviar)

Neutral

Abalone	Sailfish	Swordfish
Bluefish	Salmon	Tilefish
Carp	Scallop	Tuna
Catfish	Shark	Weakfish
Herring (fresh)	Silver perch	White perch
Herring (pickled)	Smelt	Whitefish
Rainbow trout	Snapper	Yellow perch
Red snapper	Squid (calamari)	

Avoid

Anchovy	Eel	Sea bass
Barracuda	Frog	Shrimp
Beluga	Lobster	Snail
Bluegill bass	Lox (smoked	Striped bass
Clam	salmon)	Trout, brook
Conch	Mussels	Trout, rainbow
Crab	Octopus	Trout, sea
Crayfish	Oysters	Yellowtail

Dairy and Eggs

BLOOD TYPE B		WEEKLY ■ IF YOUR ANCESTRY IS		
Food	*Portion*	*African*	*Caucasian*	*Asian*
Eggs	1 egg	3–4x	3–4x	5–6x
Cheeses	2 oz.	3–4x	3–5x	2–3x
Yogurt	4–6 oz.	0–4x	2–4x	1–3x
Milk	4–6 oz.	0–3x	4–5x	2–3x

Type B is the only blood type that can fully enjoy a variety of dairy foods. That's because the primary sugar in the Type B antigen is D-galactosamine, the very same sugar present in milk. Dairy foods were first introduced to the human diet during the height of the Type B development, along with the domestication of animals. (By the way, eggs do not contain the lectin that is found in the muscle tissues of chicken.)

However, there are ancestral idiosyncrasies that blur the picture. If you are of Asian descent, you may initially have a problem adapting to dairy foods—not because your system is resistant to them, but because your culture typically has been resistant. Dairy products were first introduced into Asian societies with the invasion of the Mongolian hordes. To the Asian mind, dairy products were the food of the barbarian, and thus not fit to eat. The stigma remains to this day, although there are large numbers of Type Bs in Asia whose soy-based diet is damaging to their systems.

Type Bs of African descent might also have trouble adapting to dairy foods. Type Bs are barely represented in Africa, and many Africans are lactose intolerant.

These intolerances should not be confused with allergies. Allergies are immune responses that cause your blood to produce an antibody to the food. Intolerances are digestive problems you may have with certain foods. Intolerances are caused by migration, cultural assimilation, and other factors—for example, when Type Bs moved into Africa, where dairy foods were not prominent.

What can you do? If you are lactose intolerant, begin using a lactase enzyme preparation, which will make digestion of dairy foods possible. Then, after you have been on your Type B Diet for several weeks, slowly introduce dairy foods, beginning with cultured or soured dairy products, such as yogurt and kefir, which may be tolerated better than fresh milk products, such as ice cream, whole milk, and cream cheese. I've found that lactose-intolerant Type Bs often are able to incorporate dairy foods after they have corrected the overall problems in their diets.

Soy foods often are recommended as dairy substitutes. You may eat soy foods, but they're mostly benign for Type Bs. They don't have the many health benefits for you that they have for Type As. Part of my concern about recommending soy for Type Bs is the danger that people will often substitute them as main courses, instead of eating the meat, fish, and dairy that Type Bs really need for optimum health.

Highly Beneficial

Cottage cheese	Goat cheese	Milk (skim or 2%)
Farmer cheese	Kefir	Mozzarella cheese
Feta cheese	Milk (cow-whole)	Ricotta cheese
	Milk (goat)	Yogurt

Neutral

Brie cheese	Casein cheese	Edam cheese
Butter	Cheddar cheese	Egg, chicken
Buttermilk	Colby cheese	Emmenthal cheese
Camembert cheese	Cream cheese	Ghee

Gouda cheese	Munster cheese	Sherbet
Gruyère cheese	Neufchatel cheese	Swiss cheese
Jarlsberg cheese	Parmesan cheese	Whey
Monterey jack cheese	Provolone cheese	

Avoid

American cheese	Egg, goose	Ice cream
Blue cheese	Egg, quail	String cheese
Egg, duck		

Oils and Fats

BLOOD TYPE B		WEEKLY ▪ IF YOUR ANCESTRY IS		
Food	*Portion*	*African*	*Caucasian*	*Asian*
Oils	1 tablespoon	3–5x	4–6x	5–7x

Introduce olive oil into your diet to encourage proper digestion and healthy elimination. Use at least one tablespoon every other day. Ghee, an Indian preparation of clarified butter, also can be used in cooking. Avoid sesame, sunflower, and corn oils, which contain lectins that are damaging to the Type B digestive tract.

Highly Beneficial

Olive oil

Neutral

Almond oil	Cod liver oil	Linseed (flaxseed) oil
Black currant	Evening primrose	Walnut oil
seed oil	oil	Wheat germ oil

Avoid

Canola oil	Cottonseed oil	Sesame oil
Castor oil	Peanut oil	Soy oil
Coconut oil	Safflower oil	Sunflower oil
Corn oil		

Nuts and Seeds

BLOD TYPE B		WEEKLY ■ IF YOUR ANCESTRY IS		
Food	Portion	African	Caucasian	Asian
Nuts and seeds	6–8 nuts	3–5x	2–5x	2–3x
Nut butters	1 tablespoon	2–3x	2–3x	2–3x

Most nuts and seeds are not advised for Type Bs. Peanuts, sesame seeds, and sunflower seeds, among others, contain lectins that interfere with Type B insulin production.

It might be difficult for Type B Asians to give up sesame seeds and sesame-based products, but in this case, your blood type speaks more definitively than your culture.

High Beneficial

Nuts, walnuts

Neutral

Almond butter
Nuts, almonds
Nuts, Brazil nuts

Nuts, chestnuts
Nuts, hickory
Nuts, litchi

Nuts, macadamia
Nuts, pecans

Avoid

Nuts, cashews
Nuts, filberts
Nuts, pignola
  (pine)
Nuts, pistachio
Peanuts

Peanut butter
Poppy seeds
Pumpkin seeds
Sesame butter
  (tahini)
Sesame seeds

Sunflower butter
Sunflower seeds

Beans and Legumes

BLOOD TYPE B		WEEKLY ▪ IF YOUR ANCESTRY IS		
Food	*Portion*	*African*	*Caucasian*	*Asian*
All recommended beans and legumes	1 cup, dry	3–4x	2–3x	4–5x

Type Bs can eat some beans and legumes, but many beans, such as lentils, garbanzos, pintos, and black-eyed peas, contain lectins that interfere with the production of insulin.

Generally, Type B Asians tolerate beans and legumes better than do other Type Bs because they are culturally accustomed to them. But even Asians should limit their selection of these foods to those that are highly beneficial, and eat them sparingly.

Highly Beneficial

Beans, kidney   Beans, navy
Beans, lima

Neutral

Beans, broad	Beans, jicama	Beans, string
Beans, cannellini	Beans, northern	Beans, tamarind
Beans, copper	Beans, red	Beans, white
Beans, fava	Beans, snap	Peas, green
Beans, green	Beans, soy	Peas, pods

Avoid

Beans, adzuki	Lentils, green	Soy milk
Beans, black	Lentils, red	Soy miso
Beans, garbanzo	Peas, black-eyed	Soy, tempeh
Beans, pinto	Soy cheese	Soy, tofu
Lentils, domestic		

Cereals

BLOOD TYPE B		WEEKLY ▪ IF YOUR ANCESTRY IS		
Food	*Portion*	*African*	*Caucasian*	*Asian*
All cereals	1 cup, dry	2–3x	2–4x	2–4x

When Type B is in good balance—that is, following the fundamental tenets of the diet—wheat may not be a problem. However, wheat is not tolerated well by most Type Bs. Wheat contains a lectin that attaches to the insulin receptors in the fat cells, prohibiting insulin from attaching. The result is reduced insulin efficiency and failure to stimulate fat "burning."

Type Bs also should avoid rye, which contains a lectin that settles in the vascular system, causing blood disorders and potentially strokes. (It is interesting to note that the main victims of vascular disease, sometimes called St. Anthony's fire, are the largely Type B population of eastern European Jews. Rye bread is a popular part of their cultural tradition.)

Corn and buckwheat are major factors in Type B weight gain. More than any other food, they contribute to a sluggish metabolism, insulin irregularity, fluid retention, and fatigue.

Again, for Type Bs the key is balance. Eat a variety of grains and cereals. Rice and oats are excellent choices. I also urge you to try spelt, which is highly beneficial for Type Bs.

Highly Beneficial

Millet	Oatmeal	Rice bran
Oat bran	Rice, puffed	Spelt

Neutral

Cream of rice	Granola
Familia	Grape nuts
Farina	

Avoid

Amaranth
Barley
Buckwheat
Cornflakes
Cornmeal

Cream of wheat
Kamut
Kasha
Rye
Seven-grain

Shredded wheat
Wheat bran
Wheat germ

Breads and Muffins

BLOOD TYPE B		DAILY ▪ IF YOUR ANCESTRY IS		
Food	*Portion*	*African*	*Caucasian*	*Asian*
Breads, crackers	1 slice	0–1x	0–1x	0–1x
Muffins	1 med. muffin	0–1x	0–1x	0–1x

The recommendations here are similar to those for cereals. Avoid wheat, corn, buckwheat, and rye. That still leaves you a wide variety of breads to choose from. Try Essene or Ezekiel bread, found in health food stores. These "live" breads are highly nutritious. Although they are sprouted wheat breads, the problem kernel is destroyed in the sprouting process, and they are perfectly healthful.

Highly Beneficial

Brown Rice
  Bread

Essene Bread
Ezekiel Bread

Millet
Rice Cakes

Neutral

Gluten-free bread
High-protein
  no-wheat bread

Oat bran muffins
Spelt bread

Soy flour bread

Avoid

Bagels, wheat	Multi-grain bread	Wasa bread
Corn muffins	100% rye bread	Wheat bran muffins
Durum wheat	Pumpernickel	Whole wheat
Fin crisp	Rye crisp	bread
Ideal flat bread	Rye vita	

Grains and Pasta

BLOOD TYPE B		WEEKLY ■ IF YOUR ANCESTRY IS		
Food	Portion	African	Caucasian	Asian
Grains	1 cup, dry	3–4x	3–4x	2–3x
Pastas	1 cup, dry	3–4x	3–4x	2–3x

The Type B grain and pasta choices are absolutely consistent with the cereal and bread recommendations. I would, however, advise that you moderate your intake of pasta and rice. You won't need many of these nutrients if you're consuming the meat, seafood, and dairy products advised.

Highly Beneficial

Flour, oat
Flour, rice

Neutral

Flour, graham	Pasta, semolina	Rice, basmati
Flour, spelt	Pasta, spinach	Rice, brown
Flour, white	Quinoa	Rice, white

Avoid

Buckwheat	Couscous	Flour, bulgur
kasha	Flour, barley	wheat

Flour, durum wheat	Flour, rye	Pasta, artichoke
Flour, gluten	Flour, whole wheat	Noodles, soba
		Rice, wild

Vegetables

BLOOD TYPE B	DAILY ▪ ALL ANCESTRAL TYPES	
Food	*Portion*	
Raw	1 cup, prepared	3–5x
Cooked	1 cup, prepared	3–5x

There are many high-quality, nutritious, Type B–friendly vegetables—so take full advantage with three to five servings a day. There is only a handful of vegetables that Type Bs should avoid, but take these guidelines to heart.

Eliminate tomatoes completely from your diet. The tomato is a rare vegetable called a panhemaglutinan. That means it contains lectins that can agglutinate every blood type. While the tomato lectin has little effect on Type O or Type AB, both Type B and Type A suffer strong reactions, usually in the form of irritations of the stomach lining.

Corn is also off your list, as it contains those insulin- and metabolism-upsetting lectins mentioned before. Also avoid olives, since their molds can trigger allergic reactions.

Since Type Bs tend to be more vulnerable to viruses and autoimmune diseases, eat plenty of leafy green vegetables, which contain magnesium, an important antiviral agent. Magnesium also is helpful for Type B children who have eczema.

For the most part, the vegetable world is your kingdom. Unlike other blood types, you can fully enjoy potatoes and yams, cabbages and mushrooms—and many other delicious foods from nature's bounty.

Highly Beneficial

| Beets | Carrots | Collard |
| Beet greens | Cauliflower | greens |

Eggplant
Kale
Lima beans
Mushroom,
    Shiitake
Mustard
    greens
Parsley

Parsnips
Peppers,
    green
Peppers,
    yellow
Peppers,
    Jalapeño

Peppers, red
Potatoes,
    sweet
Sprouts,
    Brussels
Yams

Neutral

Arugula
Asparagus
Bamboo shoots
Bok choy
Celery
Chervil
Chicory
Cucumber
Daikon radish
Dandelion
Dill
Endive
Escarole
Fennel
Fiddlehead ferns
Garlic
Ginger
Horseradish
Kohlrabi

Leek
Lettuce, Bibb
Lettuce, Boston
Lettuce, iceberg
Lettuce, romaine
Lettuce, mesclun
Mushroom,
    abalone
Mushroom,
    silver dollar
Mushroom, enoki
Mushroom,
    Portobello
Mushroom,
    tree oyster
Okra
Onions, green
Onions, red
Onions, Spanish

Onions, yellow
Potatoes, red
Potatoes, white
Radicchio
Rappini
Rutabaga
Scallion
Seaweed
Shallots
Snow peas
Spinach
Sprouts, alfalfa
Squash, all types
Swiss chard
Turnips
Water chestnut
Watercress
Zucchini

Avoid

Artichoke,
    domestic
Artichoke,
    Jerusalem
Avocado
Corn, white

Corn, yellow
Olives, black
Olives, Greek
Olives, green
Olives, Spanish

Pumpkin
Radishes
Sprouts, mung
Sprouts, radish
Tomato

Fruits

BLOOD TYPE B	DAILY ▪ ALL ANCESTRAL TYPES	
Food	*Portion*	
All recommended fruits	1 fruit or 3–5 oz.	3–4x

You'll notice that there are very few fruits a Type B must avoid—and they're pretty uncommon in any case. Most Type Bs won't sorely miss persimmons, pomegranates, or prickly pears in their diets.

Pineapple can be particularly good for Type Bs who are susceptible to bloating—especially if you're not used to eating the dairy foods and meats on your diet. Bromelain, an enzyme in the pineapple, helps you digest your food more easily.

On the whole, you can choose your fruits liberally from the following lists. Type Bs tend to have very balanced digestive systems, with a healthy acid-alkaline level, so you may have some of the fruits that are too acidic for other blood types.

Try to incorporate at least one or two fruits from the highly beneficial list every day to take advantage of their pro-B medicinal qualities.

Highly Beneficial

Bananas	Grapes, green	Plums, green
Cranberries	Grapes, red	Plums, red
Grapes, black	Papaya	
Grapes, Concord	Pineapple	
	Plums, dark	

Neutral

Apples	Boysenberries	Dates
Apricots	Cherries	Elderberries
Blackberries	Currants, black	Figs, dried
Blueberries	Currants, red	Figs, fresh

Gooseberries Melon, cantaloupe Oranges
Grapefruit Melon, casaba Peaches
Guava Melon, Christmas Pears
Kiwi Melon, Crenshaw Plantains
Kumquat Melon, honeydew Prunes
Lemons Melon, musk Raisins
Limes Melon, Spanish Raspberries
Loganberries Melon, watermelon Strawberries
Mangoes Nectarines Tangerines
Melon, canang

Avoid

Avocado Prickly pear
Coconuts Rhubarb
Persimmons Starfruit
Pomegranates (carambola)

Juices and Fluids

BLOOD TYPE B	DAILY ▪ ALL ANCESTRAL TYPES	
Food	*Portion*	
All recommended juices	8 oz.	2–3x
Water	8 oz.	4–7x

Most fruit and vegetable juices are okay for Type Bs. If you'd like a daily juice with built-in immune- and nervous-system boosters designed for Type Bs, try the following beverage first thing every morning. I call it the Membrane Fluidizer Cocktail, but I assure you that it's much more alluring than its name implies.

Mix 1 tablespoon of flaxseed oil, 1 tablespoon of high-quality lecithin granules, and 6 to 8 ounces of fruit juice. Shake and drink. Lecithin is a lipid, found in animals and plants, that contains metabolism- and immune system-enhancing properties. You can find lecithin granules in your local health food store and in some supermarkets.

The Membrane Fluidizer Cocktail provides high levels of choline, serine, and ethanolamine (the phospholipids), which are of great value to Type Bs. You may be surprised to find that it's rather tasty, because the lecithin emulsifies the oil, allowing it to mix with the juice.

Highly Beneficial

Cabbage
Cranberry
Grape

Papaya
Pineapple

Neutral

Apple
Apple cider
Apricot
Carrot
Celery

Cherry, black
Cucumber
Grapefruit
Orange
Prune

Water (with lemon)
Vegetable juice
(corresponding
with highlighted
vegetables)

Avoid

Tomato

Spices

Type Bs do best with warming herbs, such as ginger, horseradish, curry, and cayenne pepper. The exceptions are white and black pepper, which contain problem lectins. On the reverse side, sweet herbs tend to be stomach irritants, so avoid barley malt sweeteners, corn syrup, cornstarch, and cinnamon. The exceptions are white and brown sugar, honey, and molasses, which respond in a neutral way to the Type B digestive system. You may eat these sugars in moderation. You also may eat small quantities of chocolate, but consider it a condiment, not a main course!

Highly Beneficial

Cayenne	Ginger
pepper	Horseradish
Curry	Parsley

Neutral

Agar	Garlic	Saffron
Anise	Honey	Sage
Arrowroot	Kelp	Salt
Basil	Maple syrup	Savory
Bay leaf	Marjoram	Soy sauce
Bergamot	Mint	Spearmint
Brown rice syrup	Miso	Sugar, brown
Capers	Molasses	Sugar, white
Caraway	Mustard (dry)	Tamarind
Cardamom	Nutmeg	Tarragon
Carob	Oregano	Thyme
Chervil	Paprika	Vanilla
Chives	Pepper,	Vinegar, apple cider
Chocolate	peppercorn	Vinegar, balsamic
Clove	Pepper, red	Vinegar, red wine
Coriander	flakes	Vinegar, white
Cream of tartar	Peppermint	Wintergreen
Cumin	Pimiento	
Dill	Rice syrup	
Dulse	Rosemary	

Avoid

Allspice	Gelatin, plain
Almond extract	Pepper, black
Barley malt	ground
Cinnamon	Pepper, white
Cornstarch	Tapioca
Corn syrup	

Condiments

Condiments are basically either neutral or bad for all types. Type Bs can handle just about every common condiment except ketchup (with its dangerous tomato lectins), but common nutritional sense would suggest that you limit your intake of foods that provide no real benefit.

Neutral

Apple butter
Jam (from acceptable fruits)
Jelly (from acceptable fruits)
Pickles, kosher
Pickles, sour
Pickles, sweet
Relish

Mayonnaise
Mustard
Pickles, dill
Salad dressing (low-fat, from
    acceptable ingredients)
Worcestershire sauce

Avoid

Ketchup

Herbal Teas

Type Bs don't reap overwhelming benefits from most herbal teas, and only a few are harmful. Overall, Type Bs play things to a draw. They stay in balance with common-sense teas—ginger to warm, peppermint to soothe the digestive tract, and so on.

Ginseng is highly recommended for Type Bs because it seems to have a positive effect on the nervous system. Be aware, though, that it can act like a stimulant, so drink it early in the day.

Licorice is particularly good for Type Bs. It has antiviral properties that work to reduce your susceptibility to autoimmune diseases. Also, many Type Bs experience a drop in blood sugar after meals (hypoglycemia), and licorice helps regulate blood sugar levels.

More recently, I've discovered that licorice is a fairly powerful elixir for people suffering from chronic fatigue syndrome.

Highly Beneficial

Ginger	Peppermint
Ginseng	Raspberry leaf
Licorice	Rose hips
Licorice root*	Sage
Parsley	

Do not use without your doctor's permission.

Neutral

Alfalfa	Elder	Strawberry leaf
Burdock	Green tea	Thyme
Catnip	Hawthorn	Valerian
Cayenne	Horehound	Vervain
Chamomile	Mulberry	White birch
Chickweed	Saint John's wort	White oak bark
Dandelion	Sarsaparilla	Yarrow
Dong quai	Slippery elm	Yellow dock
Echinacea	Spearmint	

Avoid

Aloe	Hops	Senna
Coltsfoot	Linden	Shepherd's purse
Corn silk	Mullein	Skullcap
Fenugreek	Red clover	
Gentian	Rhubarb	
Goldenseal		

Miscellaneous Beverages

Type Bs do best when they limit their beverages to herbal and green teas, water, and juice. Although beverages like coffee, regular tea, and wine do no real harm, the goal of the Blood Type Diet is to maximize your performance, not to keep it in neutral. If you're a caffeinated coffee or tea drinker, try replacing these beverages with green tea, which has caffeine but also provides some antioxidant benefits.

Highly Beneficial

Tea, green

Neutral

Beer
Coffee, decaf
Coffee, regular
Tea, black decaf

Tea, black regular
Wine, red
Wine, white

Avoid

Liquor, distilled
Seltzer water

Soda, cola
Soda, diet

Soda, other

Type B
Supplement Advisory

The role of supplements—be they vitamins, minerals, or herbs—is to add the nutrients that are lacking in your diet, and to provide extra protection where you need it. The supplement focus for Type Bs is:

- Fine-tuning an already balanced diet
- Improving insulin efficiency
- Strengthening viral immunity
- Improving brain clarity and focus

Type Bs are a special (you might say lucky) case. For the most part, you can avoid major diseases by following your Blood Type Diet. Because your diet is so rich in vitamin A, vitamin B, vitamin E, vitamin C, calcium, and iron, there is no need for supplementation of these vitamins and minerals. So enjoy your unique status—but follow your diet!

The following are the few supplements that can benefit Type Bs.

Beneficial

MAGNESIUM

While the other blood types risk calcium deficiency, Type Bs risk magnesium deficiency. Magnesium is the catalyst for the metabolic machinery in Type Bs. It's the match head—what makes Type Bs metabolize carbohydrates more efficiently. Since you are so efficient in assimilating calcium, you risk creating an imbalance between your levels of calcium and magnesium. Should this occur, you find yourself more at risk for viruses (or otherwise lowered immunity), fatigue, depression, and, potentially, nervous disorders. In these instances, perhaps a trial of magnesium supplementation (300–500 mg) should be considered. Also, many Type B children are plagued with eczema, and magnesium supplementation can often be beneficial.

Any form of magnesium is fine, although more patients report a laxative effect with magnesium citrate than with the other forms. An excessive amount of magnesium could, at least theoretically, upset your body's calcium levels, so be sure that you consume high-calcium foods as well, such as cultured dairy products. The key is balance!

Best Magnesium-Rich Foods for Type Bs

all recommended green vegetables,
   grains, and legumes

Herbs/Phytochemicals
Recommended for Type Bs

LICORICE *(Glycyrrhiza glabra)*. Licorice is a plant widely used by herbalists around the world. It contains at least four benefits—as a treatment for stomach ulcers, as an antiviral agent against the herpes virus, to treat chronic fatigue syndrome, and to combat hypoglycemia.

Licorice is a plant to be respected: Large doses in the wrong person can cause sodium retention and elevated blood pressure. If you are Type B and suffer from hypoglycemia, a condition where the blood sugar drops after a meal, drink a cup or two of licorice tea after meals. If you suffer from chronic fatigue syndrome, I recommend that you use licorice preparations, other than DGL and licorice tea, only under the guidance of a physician. Licorice freely used in its supplemental form can be toxic.

DIGESTIVE ENZYMES. If you are a Type B who is not used to eating meat or dairy foods, you may experience some initial difficulties adapting to your diet. Take a digestive enzyme with your main meals for a while, and you'll adjust more readily to concentrated proteins. Bromelain, an enzyme found in pineapples, is available in supplemental form at many health food stores, usually in the 4x strength.

ADAPTOGENIC HERBS. Adaptogenic herbs increase concentration and memory retention, sometimes a problem for Type Bs with nervous or viral disorders. The best are Siberian ginseng *(Eleutherococcus senticosus)* and *Ginkgo biloba*, both widely available in pharmacies and health food stores. Siberian ginseng has been shown in Russian studies to increase the speed and accuracy of teletype operators. *Ginkgo biloba* is currently the most frequently prescribed drug of any kind in Germany, where more than 5 million people take it daily.

Ginkgo increases the microcirculation to the brain, which is why it is often prescribed to the elderly. It is currently being promoted as a brain stimulant, a pick-me-up for the mind.

LECITHIN. Lecithin, a blood enhancer found principally in soy, allows the cell-surface B antigens to move around more easily and better protect the immune system. Type Bs should seek this benefit from lecithin granules, not soy itself, as soy doesn't have the concentrated effect. Using the Membrane Fluidizer Cocktail that I mentioned in the Type B Diet is a good habit to develop, as it allows you to get an excellent stimulant for your immune system in a rather pleasant way.

Type B Stress/Exercise Profile

The Type B response to stress represents a balance of the nervous mental activity of Type A and the more physically aggressive reactions of Type O. Type Bs temper each of these qualities and so respond with harmony and balance—harnessing the best qualities of the other blood types.

The Type B response to stress is an evolutionary sophistication demanded by a multidimensional environment. Human beings needed the physical endurance required to conquer new lands, as well as the skills and patience to develop those lands. Remember, early Type Bs were represented by both nomads and agrarians.

As a Type B, you confront stress very well for the most part, because you blend more easily into unfamiliar situations. You're less confrontational than Type Os, but more physically charged than Type As. The best way for Type Bs to deal with stress is through organization. You need to exercise your mind, as well as your body to reduce stress.

Type Bs do well with exercises that are neither too aerobically intense nor completely aimed at mental relaxation. The ideal balance for many Type Bs consists of moderate activities that involve other people—such as group hiking, biking excursions, the less aggressive martial arts, tennis, and aerobics classes. You don't do as well when the sport is fiercely competitive—such as squash, football, or basketball.

EXERCISE	DURATION	FREQUENCY
Aerobics	45–60 min.	3x week
Tennis	45–60 min.	3x week
Martial arts	30–60 min.	3x week
Calisthenics	30–45 min.	3x week
Hiking	30–60 min.	3x week
Cycling	45–60 min.	3x week
Swimming	30–45 min.	3x week
Brisk walking	30–60 min.	3x week
Jogging	30–45 min.	3x week
Weight training	30–45 min.	3x week
Golf	60 min.	2x week
Tai chi	45 min.	2x week
Hatha yoga	45 min.	2x week

The most effective exercise schedule for Type B should be three days a week of more intense physical activity and two days a week of relaxation exercises.

Type B
Exercise Guidelines

FOR PHYSICAL EXERCISE

The three components of a high-intensity exercise program are the warm-up period, the aerobic exercise period, and a cool-down period. A warm-up is very important to prevent injuries, because it brings blood to the muscles, readying them for exercise, whether it is walking, running, biking, swimming, or playing a sport. A warm-up should include stretching and flexibility movements to prevent muscle and tendon tears.

The exercise can be divided into two basic types: isometric exercises, in which stress is created against stationary muscles; and isotonic exercises, such as calisthenics, running, or swimming, which produce muscular resistance through a range of movement. Isometric exercises can be used to tone up specific muscles, which can then be further strengthened by active isotonic exercise. Isometrics may be performed by pushing or pulling an immovable object or by contracting or tightening opposing muscles.

To achieve maximum cardiovascular benefits from aerobic exercise, you must elevate your heartbeat to approximately 70 percent of your maximum heart rate. Once that elevated rate is achieved during exercise, continue exercising to maintain that rate for thirty minutes. This regimen should be repeated at least three times each week.

To calculate your maximum heart rate:

1. Subtract your age from 220.
2. Multiply the difference by 70 percent (.70). If you are over sixty years of age, or in poor physical condition, multiply the remainder by 60 percent (.60).
3. Multiply the remainder by 50 percent (.50). For example, a healthy fifty-year-old woman would subtract 50 from 220,

for a maximum heart rate of 170. Multiplying 170 by .70 would give her 119 beats per minute, which is the top level she should strive for. Multiplying 170 by .50 would give her the lowest number in her range.

FOR RELAXATION EXERCISES

Tai chi and yoga are the perfect way to balance the more physical activities of your week.

Tai chi chuan, or tai chi, is an exercise that enhances the flexibility of body movement. The slow, graceful, elegant gestures of tai chi chuan routines hardly resemble the original hand and foot blows, blocks, and parries they represent. In China, tai chi is practiced daily by groups who gather in public squares to perform the movements in unison. Tai chi can be a very effective relaxation technique, although it takes concentration and patience to master.

Yoga combines inner rectitude with breath control and postures designed to allow for complete concentration without distraction by worldly concerns. Hatha yoga is the most common form of yoga practiced in the West.

If you learn basic yoga postures, you can create a routine best suited to your lifestyle. However, some patients have told me that they are concerned that adopting yoga practices may conflict with their religious beliefs. They fear that the practice of yoga implies that they have adopted Eastern mysticism. I respond, "If you eat Italian food, does that make you Italian?" Meditation and yoga are what you make of them. Visualize and meditate on those subjects that are relevant to you. The postures are neutral; they are just timeless and proven movements.

SIMPLE YOGA RELAXATION TECHNIQUES

Yoga begins and ends with relaxation. We contract our muscles constantly, but rarely do we think of doing the opposite—letting go and relaxing. We can feel better and be healthier if we regularly release the tensions left behind within the muscles by the stresses and strains of life.

The best position for relaxation is lying on your back. Arrange your arms and legs so that you are completely comfortable in your hips, shoulders, and back. The goal of deep relaxation is to let your body and mind settle down to soothing calmness, in the same way that an agitated pool of water eventually calms to stillness.

Begin with abdominal breathing. As a baby breathes, its abdomen moves, not its chest. However, many of us grow to unconsciously adopt the unnatural and inefficient habit of restrained chest breathing. One of the aims of yoga is to make you aware of the true center of breathing. Observe the pattern of your breathing. Is your breathing fast, shallow, and irregular, or do you tend to hold your breath? Allow your breathing to revert to a more natural pattern—full, deep, regular, and with no constriction. Try to isolate just your lower breathing muscles; see if you can breathe without moving your chest. Breathing exercises are always done smoothly and without any strain. Place one hand on your navel and feel the movement of your breathing. Relax your shoulders.

Start the exercise by breathing out completely. When you inhale, pretend that a heavy weight, such as a large book, is resting on your navel, and that by your inhalation, you are trying to raise this imaginary weight up toward the ceiling.

Then, when you exhale, simply let this imaginary weight press down against your abdomen, helping you to exhale. Exhale more air out than you normally would, as if to "squeeze" more air out of your lungs. This will act as a yoga stretch for the diaphragm and further help to release tension in this muscle. Bring your abdominal muscles into play here to assist. When you inhale, direct your breath down so deeply that you are lifting an imaginary heavy weight back upward toward the ceiling. Try to completely coordinate and isolate the abdominal breath with no chest or rib movement.

A Final Note:
The Personality Question

Early Type Bs, confronted with new lands, unfamiliar climates, and the intermingling of races, had to be flexible and creative in order to survive. Type Bs required less ordered and harmonious conformity than the settled Type As, as well as less of the hunter's purposefulness that characterized Type Os.

These same characteristics exist in the very cells of Type Bs. Biologically, Type Bs are more flexible than Type Os, Type As, or Type

ABs—less vulnerable to many diseases common to the others. The Type B who lives in harmony—working, exercising and eating in a balanced way—is the essence of a survivor.

In many ways, Type Bs have the best of all possible worlds. They have elements of the mental, more sensitively agitated activity of the Type A, with the sheer physical reactions and aggression of the Type O. Perhaps Type Bs relate more easily to different personality types because they are by genetic nature more in harmony and thus feel less inclined to challenge and confront. They can see others' points of view; they are empathetic.

A notable statistic: While Type B blood constitutes only 9 percent of the United States population, some 30 to 40 percent of all self-made millionaires are Type B!

The Chinese, Japanese, and many other Asian societies are composed of a high number of Type Bs. Chinese medicine—ancient, natural, and complex—places a great emphasis on balancing the physiological and emotional states. Unbridled joy (a desirable state for most Westerners) is viewed by Chinese physicians as being dangerous to the balance of the heart. Balance and harmony; this is a very Type B kind of medicine.

Traditional Jewish populations are primarily Type B, regardless of their geographic locations. Jewish religion and culture represent the blending of mind, soul, and matter. In Jewish tradition, intelligence, peace, and spirituality live side by side with a forceful physicality and readiness for battle. To many people, this seems like a contradiction. It is really the harmonious energies of the Type B in action.

The Type AB Program

A Blending of Traits

TYPE AB: *The Enigma*

- Modern merging of A and B
- Chameleon's response to changing environmental and dietary conditions
- Sensitive digestive tract
- Overly tolerant immune system
- Responds best to stress spiritually, with physical verve and creative energy
- An evolutionary mystery

The Type AB Diet

Blood Type AB is less than a thousand years old, rare (2 to 5 percent of the population), and biologically complex. It doesn't fit comfortably into any of the other categories. Multiple antigens make Type ABs sometimes A-like, sometimes B-like, and sometimes a fusion of both—kind of a blood type centaur.

This multiplicity of qualities can be positive or negative, depending on the circumstances, so the Type AB Diet requires that you read your foods lists very carefully, and familiarize yourself with both the Type A and Type B diets to better understand the parameters of your own diet.

Essentially, most foods that are contraindicated for either Type A or Type B are probably bad for Type AB—although there are some exceptions. Panhemaglutinans, which are lectins capable of agglutinating all of the blood types, seem to be better tolerated by Type ABs, perhaps because the lectins's reaction is diminished by the double A and B antibodies. Tomatoes are an excellent example. Type A and Type B cannot tolerate the lectins, while Type AB eats tomatoes with no discernible effect.

Type ABs are often stronger and more active than the more sedentary Type As. This extra dollop of élan vital may be because their genetic memories still contain fairly recent remnants of their steppe-dwelling Type B ancestors.

The Weight-Loss Factor

When it comes to gaining weight, Type ABs reflect the mixed inheritance of their A and B genes. Sometimes that means special problems. For example, you have Type A's low stomach acid, along with Type B's adaptation to meats. So, although you are genetically programmed for the consumption of meats, you lack enough stomach acid to metabolize them efficiently, and the meat you eat tends to get stored as fat. For weight loss, you should restrict your consumption of meats, eating small amounts that you can supplement with vegetables and tofu.

Your Type B propensities cause the same insulin reaction when you eat kidney or lima beans, corn, buckwheat, or sesame seeds (although your Type A side makes you friendly to lentils and peanuts). Inhibited insulin production causes hypoglycemia, a lowering of blood sugar after meals, and leads to less efficient metabolism of foods.

Type ABs lack the severe reaction of Type Os and Type Bs to wheat gluten. But again, for weight-loss purposes, you should avoid wheat, which tends to make your muscle tissue more acidic. Type ABs utilize calories most efficiently when your tissue is somewhat alkaline.

Foods That Encourage Weight Gain

RED MEAT	*poorly digested*
	stored as fat
	toxifies intestinal tract
KIDNEY BEANS	*inhibit insulin efficiency*
	cause hypoglycemia
	slow metabolic rate
LIMA BEANS	*inhibit insulin efficiency*
	cause hypoglycemia
	slow metabolic rate
SEEDS	*cause hypoglycemia*
CORN	*inhibits insulin efficiency*
BUCKWHEAT	*causes hypoglycemia*
WHEAT	*decreases metabolism*
	inefficient use of calories
	inhibits insulin efficiency

Foods That Encourage Weight Loss

TOFU	*promotes metabolic efficiency*
SEAFOOD	*promotes metabolic efficiency*
DAIRY	*improves insulin production*
GREEN VEGETABLES	*improve metabolic efficiency*
KELP	*improves insulin production*
PINEAPPLE	*aids digestion*
	stimulates intestinal mobility

Use these guidelines along with your entire Type AB diet recommendations.

Meats and Poultry

BLOOD TYPE AB	WEEKLY ▪ IF YOUR ANCESTRY IS			
Food	*Portion**	*African*	*Caucasian*	*Asian*
Lean red meats	4–6 oz. (men) 2–5 oz. (women and children)	1–3x	1–3x	1–3x
Poultry	4–6 oz. (men) 2–5 oz. (women and children)	0–2x	0–2x	0–2x

*The portion recommendations are merely guidelines that can help refine your diet according to ancestral propensities.

When it comes to eating meat and poultry, Type ABs borrow characteristics from both Type A and Type B. Like Type A, you do not produce enough stomach acid to effectively digest too much animal protein. Yet the key for you is portion size and frequency. Type ABs need some meat protein, especially the kinds of meat that represent your B-like heritage—lamb, mutton, rabbit, and turkey, instead of beef. The lectin that irritates the blood and digestive tracts of Type Bs has the same effect on you, so stay away from chicken.

Also avoid all smoked or cured meats. These foods can cause stomach cancer in people with low levels of stomach acid, the trait you share with Type As.

Highly Beneficial

Lamb	Rabbit
Mutton	Turkey

Neutral

Liver	Pheasant
Ostrich	

Avoid

Bacon	Goose	Quail
Beef	Ham	Squab
Buffalo	Heart	Squirrel
Chicken	Partridge	Veal
Cornish hens	Pork	Venison
Duck		

Seafood

BLOOD TYPE AB		WEEKLY ▪ IF YOUR ANCESTRY IS		
Food	*Portion*	*African*	*Caucasian*	*Asian*
All recommended seafood	4–6 oz.	3–5x	3–5x	4–6x

There are a wide variety of seafoods for Type ABs, and it is an excellent source of protein for you. Like Type A, you have trouble digesting the lectins found in sole and flounder. You also share the Type A susceptibility to breast cancer. If you have a family history of breast cancer, introduce snails into your diet. The edible snail, *Helix pomatia*, contains a powerful lectin that specifically agglutinates mutated A-like cells for two of the most common forms of breast cancer. This is a positive kind of agglutination; the snail lectin gets rid of sick cells.

Highly Beneficial

Cod	Pike	Sardine
Grouper	Porgy	Sea trout
Mackerel	Rainbow	Shad
Mahimahi	trout	Snail
Monkfish	Red snapper	Sturgeon
Ocean perch	Sailfish	Tuna
Pickerel		

Neutral

Abalone	Salmon	Swordfish
Bluefish	Scallop	Tilefish
Carp	Shark	Weakfish
Catfish	Silver perch	Whitefish
Caviar	Smelt	White perch
Herring (fresh)	Snapper	Yellow perch
Mussels	Squid (calamari)	

Avoid

Anchovy	Flounder	Octopus
Barracuda	Frog	Oysters
Beluga	Haddock	Sea bass
Bluegill bass	Hake	Shrimp
Clam	Halibut	Sole
Conch	Herring (pickled)	Striped bass
Crab	Lobster	Turtle
Crayfish	Lox (smoked	Yellowtail
Eel	salmon)	

Dairy and Eggs

BLOOD TYPE AB		WEEKLY ▪ IF YOUR ANCESTRY IS		
Food	Portion	African	Caucasian	Asian
Eggs	1 egg	3–5x	3–4x	2–3x
Cheeses	2 oz.	2–3x	3–4x	3–4x
Yogurt	4–6 oz.	2–3x	3–4x	1–3x
Milk	4–6 oz.	1–6x	3–6x	2–5x

For dairy foods, Type ABs can put on the "B" hat. You benefit from dairy foods, especially cultured and soured products—yogurt, kefir, and non-fat sour cream—which are more easily digested.

The primary factor you have to watch out for is excessive mucus production. Like Type As, you already produce a lot of mucus, and you don't need more. Watch for signs of respiratory problems, sinus attacks, or ear infections, which might indicate you should cut back on the dairy foods.

Eggs are a very good source of protein for Type ABs. Although they're very high in cholesterol, and Type ABs (like Type As) have some susceptibility to heart conditions, research has shown that the biggest culprits are not cholesterol-containing foods but rather saturated fats.

However, when you eat eggs, you can increase your protein and lower your cholesterol intake by using two egg whites for every one egg yolk. (Note that the lectin found in the chicken muscle is not present in eggs.)

Highly Beneficial

Cottage cheese	Goat cheese	Ricotta cheese
Farmer cheese	Goat milk	Sour cream (non-fat)
Feta cheese	Kefir	Yogurt
	Mozzarella cheese	

Neutral

Casein	Emmenthal cheese	Munster cheese
Cheddar cheese	Gouda cheese	Neufchatel cheese
Colby cheese	Gruyère cheese	Skim or 2% milk
Cream cheese	Jarlsburg cheese	String cheese
Edam cheese	Monterey jack cheese	Swiss cheese
Egg, chicken		Whey

Avoid

American cheese	Buttermilk	Provolone cheese
Blue cheese	Camembert cheese	Sherbet
Brie	Ice cream	Whole milk
Butter	Parmesan cheese	

Oils and Fats

BLOOD TYPE AB		WEEKLY ■ IF YOUR ANCESTRY IS		
Food	*Portion*	*African*	*Caucasian*	*Asian*
Oils	1 tablespoon	1–5x	4–8x	3–7x

Type ABs should use olive oil rather than animal fats, hydrogenated vegetable fats, or other vegetable oils. Olive oil is a monounsaturated fat that is believed to contribute to lower blood cholesterol. You may also use small amounts of ghee, a semifluid clarified butter popular in India, in your cooking.

Highly Beneficial

Olive oil   Walnut oil

Neutral

Almond oil	Cod liver oil	Peanut oil
Black currant seed oil	Evening primrose oil	Soy oil
		Wheat germ oil
Canola oil	Linseed (flaxseed) oil	

Avoid

Coconut oil	Safflower oil
Corn oil	Sesame oil
Cottonseed oil	Sunflower oil

Nuts and Seeds

BLOOD TYPE AB		WEEKLY ■ IF YOUR ANCESTRY IS		
Food	*Portion*	*African*	*Caucasian*	*Asian*
Nuts and seeds	6–8 nuts	2–5x	2–5x	2–3x
Nut butters	1 tablespoon	3–7x	3–7x	2–4x

Nuts and seeds present a mixed picture for Type ABs. Eat them in small amounts and with caution. Although they can be a good supplementary protein source, all seeds contain the insulin-inhibiting lectins that make them a problem for Type Bs. On the other hand, you share the Type A preference for peanuts, which are powerful immune boosters.

Type ABs also tend to suffer from gallbladder problems, so nut butters are preferable to whole nuts.

Highly Beneficial

Nuts, chestnuts   Peanut butter
Peanuts   Walnuts

Neutral

Almond butter   Nuts, cashews   Nuts, macadamia
Nuts, almonds   Nuts, hickory   Nuts, pignola
Nuts, Brazil   Nuts, litchi   Nuts, pistachio

Avoid

Nuts, filberts   Sesame butter   Sunflower butter
Poppy seeds   (tahini)   Sunflower seeds
Pumpkin seeds   Sesame seeds

Beans and Legumes

BLOOD TYPE AB		WEEKLY ▪ IF YOUR ANCESTRY IS		
Food	*Portion*	*African*	*Caucasian*	*Asian*
All beans and legumes	Cup, dry	3–5x	2–3x	4–6x

Beans and legumes are another mixed bag for Type ABs. For example, lentil beans are an important cancer-fighting food for Type ABs, although they are not advised for Type Bs. In particular, lentils are known to contain cancer-fighting antioxidants. On the other hand, kidney and lima beans, which slow insulin production in Type As, have the same effect in Type ABs.

Highly Beneficial

Beans, navy	Beans, soy	Soy, miso
Beans, pinto	Lentils, green	Soy, tempeh
Beans, red	Soy bean	Soy, tofu

Neutral

Beans, broad	Beans, northern	Beans, jicama
Beans, cannellini	Beans, white	Peas, green
Beans, snap	Lentils, domestic	Peas, pods
Beans, string	Lentils, red	Soy cheese
Beans, tamarind	Beans, green	Soy milk
Beans, copper		

Avoid

Beans, adzuki	Beans, garbanzo	Beans, mung
Beans, black	Beans, kidney	Peas, black-eyed
Beans, fava	Beans, lima	

Cereals

BLOOD TYPE AB		WEEKLY ▪ IF YOUR ANCESTRY IS		
Food	*Portion*	*African*	*Caucasian*	*Asian*
All cereals	1 cup, dry	2–3x	2–3x	2–4x

Guidelines for Type ABs favor both Type A and Type B recommendations. Generally, you do well on grains, even wheat, but need to limit your wheat consumption because the inner kernel of the wheat grain is highly acid forming for Type ABs. Wheat is also not advised if you are trying to lose weight. Type ABs with a pronounced mucus condition caused by asthma or frequent infections should also limit wheat consumption, as wheat causes mucus production. You'll have to experiment for yourself to determine how much wheat you can eat. Here we're not talking about stomach acid, but the acid/alkaline balance in your muscle tissues. Type ABs do best when their tissues are slightly alkaline. While the inner kernel of wheat grain is alkaline in Type Os and Type Bs, it becomes acidic in Type As and Type ABs.

Limit your intake of wheat germ and bran to once a week. Oatmeal, soy flakes, millet, farina, ground rice and soy granules are good Type AB cereals, but you must avoid buckwheat and corn.

Highly Beneficial

Amaranth	Oatmeal	Ryeberry
Millet	Rice bran	Spelt
Oat bran	Rice, puffed	

Neutral

Barley	Granola	Soy flakes
Cream of rice	Grape nuts	Soy granules
Cream of wheat	Seven-grain	Wheat bran
Familia	Shredded wheat	Wheat germ
Farina		

Avoid

Buckwheat	Cornmeal	Kasha
Cornflakes	Kamut	

Breads and Muffins

BLOOD TYPE AB		DAILY • IF YOUR ANCESTRY IS		
Food	Portion	African	Caucasian	Asian
Breads, crackers	1 slice	0–1x	0–1x	0–1x
Muffins	1 muffin	0–1x	0–1x	0–1x

The Type AB guidelines for eating breads and muffins are similar to those for cereals and grains. They are generally favorable foods, but if you produce excessive mucus or are overweight, these conditions make whole wheat inadvisable. Soy and rice flour are good substitutes for you. Be aware that sprouted wheat breads sold commercially often contain small amounts of sprouted wheat and are basically whole wheat breads. Read the ingredient labels. Avoid corn muffins and corn bread. Although Essene and Ezekiel breads (found in health food stores) are sprouted wheat breads, the gluten lectin is destroyed in the sprouting process.

Highly Beneficial

Brown rice bread	Millet	Soy flour bread
Essene bread	Rice cakes	Sprouted wheat bread
Ezekiel bread	100% rye bread	Wasa bread
Fin crisp	Rye crisps	
	Rye vita	

Neutral

Bagels, wheat	Ideal flat bread	Spelt bread
Durum wheat	Matzos, wheat	Wheat bran muffins
Gluten-free bread	Multi-grain bread	Whole wheat bread
High-protein bread	Oat bran muffins	
	Pumpernickel	

Avoid

Corn muffins

Grains and Pasta

BLOOD TYPE AB	WEEKLY ▪ IF YOUR ANCESTRY IS			
Food	Portion	African	Caucasian	Asian
Grains	1 cup, dry	2–3x	3–4x	3–4x
Pasta	1 cup, dry	2–3x	3–4x	3–4x

Type AB benefits from a diet rich in rice rather than pasta, although you may have semolina or spinach pasta once or twice a week. Again, avoid corn and buckwheat in favor of oats and rye. Limit your intake of bran and wheat germ to once a week.

Highly Beneficial

Flour, oat
Flour, rice
Flour, rye
Flour, sprouted
   wheat

Rice, basmati
Rice, brown
Rice, white
Rice, wild

Neutral

Couscous
Flour, bulgur
   wheat
Flour, durum
   wheat
Flour, gluten

Flour, graham
Flour, spelt
Flour, white
Flour, whole
   wheat

Pasta, semolina
Pasta, spinach
Quinoa

Avoid

Buckwheat kasha
Flour, barley
Pasta, artichoke
Soba noodles

Vegetables

BLOOD TYPE AB	DAILY ■ ALL ANCESTRAL TYPES	
Food	*Portion*	
Raw vegetables	1 cup, prepared	3–5x
Cooked or steamed	1 cup, prepared	3–5x

Fresh vegetables are an important source of phytochemicals, the natural substances in foods that have a tonic effect in cancer and heart disease prevention—diseases that afflict Type As and Type ABs more often as a result of weaker immune systems. They should be eaten several times a day. Type ABs have a wide selection—nearly all the vegetables that are good for either Type A or Type B are good for you as well.

The one exception is the panhemaglutinan in tomatoes, which affects all blood types. Since Type ABs have so much blood type material and the lectin isn't specific, you seem able to avoid the ill effects. I've tested Type ABs who were eating a lot of tomatoes, and their Indican Scales were clear.

Type ABs should make tofu a regular part of their diet, in combination with small amounts of meat and dairy. Tofu also has well-acknowledged cancer-fighting benefits.

Like Type Bs, you must avoid fresh corn and all corn-based products.

Highly Beneficial

Beet greens	Dandelion	Parsley
Beets	Eggplant	Parsnips
Broccoli	Garlic	Potatoes,
Cauliflower	Kale	sweet
Celery	Mushroom,	Sprouts,
Collard	maitake	alfalfa
greens	Mustard	Yams
Cucumber	greens	

Neutral

Arugula	Chervil	Horseradish
Asparagus	Chicory	Kohlrabi
Bamboo shoots	Coriander	Leek
Bok choy	Daikon	Lettuce, Bibb
Cabbage, Chinese	Endive	Lettuce, Boston
Cabbage, red	Escarole	Lettuce, iceberg
Cabbage, white	Fennel	Lettuce, mesclun
Caraway	Fiddlehead ferns	Lettuce, romaine
Carrots	Ginger	Mushroom, abalone

Mushroom, Enoki
Mushroom, oyster
Mushroom,
	Portobello
Mushroom,
	shiitake
Mushroom,
	silver dollar
Mushroom, tree
Okra
Olives, Greek
Olives, green

Olives, Spanish
Onions, green
Onions, red
Onions, Spanish
Onions, yellow
Potatoes, red
Potatoes, white
Pumpkin
Radicchio
Rappini
Rutabaga
Scallion

Seaweed
Shallots
Snow peas
Spinach
Sprouts, Brussels
Squash, all types
Swiss chard
Tomato
Turnips
Water chestnut
Watercress
Zucchini

Avoid

Artichoke,
	domestic
Artichoke,
	Jerusalem
Avocado
Corn, white

Corn, yellow
Lima beans
Olives, black
Peppers, green
Peppers, jalapeño
Peppers, red

Peppers, yellow
Radishes
Sprouts, mung
Sprouts, radish

Fruits

BLOOD TYPE AB	DAILY ▪ ALL ANCESTRAL TYPES	
Food	*Portion*	
All recommended fruits	1 fruit or 3–5 oz.	3–4x

Type ABs inherit mostly Type A intolerances and preferences for certain fruits. Emphasize the more alkaline fruits, such as grapes, plums, and berries, which can help to balance the grains that are acid forming in your muscle tissues.

Type ABs don't do particularly well on certain tropical fruits—in particular mangoes and guava. But pineapple is an excellent digestive aid for Type ABs.

Oranges also should be avoided, even though they may well be among your favorites. Oranges are a stomach irritant for Type ABs, and they also interfere with the absorption of important minerals. Lest you get confused, let me reiterate that the acid-alkaline reaction happens two different ways—in the stomach and in the muscle tissues. When I say that acidic oranges are a stomach irritant for Type ABs, I'm talking about the stomach irritation they can cause in the sensitive, alkaline Type AB stomach. Although stomach acid is generally low in Type ABs, the acid contained in oranges irritates the delicate stomach lining. Grapefruit is closely related to oranges and is also an acidic fruit, but it has positive effects on the Type AB stomach, exhibiting alkaline tendencies after digestion. Lemons also are excellent for Type ABs, aiding digestion and clearing mucus from the system.

Since vitamin C is an important antioxidant, especially for stomach cancer prevention, eat other vitamin C–rich fruits, such as grapefruit or kiwi.

The banana lectin interferes with Type AB digestion. I recommend substituting other high-potassium fruits such as apricots, figs, and certain melons.

Highly Beneficial

Blackberries	Grapes,	Lemons
Cherries	Concord	Loganberries
Cranberries	Grapes, green	Pineapples
Figs, dried	Grapes, red	Plums, dark
Figs, fresh	Grapefruit	Plums, green
Gooseberries	Kiwi	Plums, red
Grapes, black		

Neutral

Apples	Boysenberries	Dates
Apricots	Currants, black	Elderberries
Blueberries	Currants, red	Kumquat

Limes	Melon, musk	Pears
Melon, canang	Melon, Spanish	Plantains
Melon, cantaloupe	Melon,	Prunes
Melon, casaba	watermelon	Raisins
Melon, Christmas	Nectarines	Raspberries
Melon, Crenshaw	Papayas	Strawberries
Melon, honeydew	Peaches	Tangerines

Avoid

Bananas	Oranges	Rhubarb
Coconuts	Persimmons	Starfruit
Guava	Pomegranates	(carambola)
Mangoes	Prickly pears	

Juices and Fluids

BLOOD TYPE AB	DAILY ▪ ALL ANCESTRAL TYPES	
Food	*Portion*	
All recommended juices	8 oz.	2–3x
Water	8 oz.	4–7x

Type AB should begin each day by drinking a glass of warm water with the freshly squeezed juice of half a lemon to cleanse the system of mucus accumulated while sleeping. The lemon water also aids elimination. Follow with a diluted glass of grapefruit or papaya juice.

Stress high-alkaline fruits juices such as black cherry, cranberry, or grape.

Highly Beneficial

Cabbage	Cherry, black	Papaya
Carrot	Cranberry	
Celery	Grape	

Neutral

Apple	Pineapple
Apple cider	Prune
Apricot	Water (with lemon)
Cucumber	Vegetable juice (corresponding
Grapefruit	with highlighted vegetables)

Avoid

Orange

Spices

Sea salt and kelp should be used in place of salt. Their sodium content is low—a concern for Type AB—and kelp has immensely positive heart and immune system benefits. It also is useful for weight control. Miso, made from soy, is very good for type ABs, and makes a delicious soup or sauce.

Avoid all pepper and vinegar because they are acidic. Instead of vinegar, use lemon juice with oil and herbs to dress vegetables or salads.

And don't be afraid to use generous amounts of garlic. It's a potent tonic and natural antibiotic, especially for Type ABs.

Sugar and chocolate are allowed in small amounts. Use them as you would condiments.

Highly Beneficial

Curry	Horseradish
Garlic	Parsley

Neutral

Agar	Carob	Cream of tartar
Arrowroot	Chervil	Cumin
Basil	Chive	Dill
Bay leaf	Chocolate	Dulse
Bergamot	Cinnamon	Honey
Brown rice syrup	Clove	Kelp
Cardamom	Coriander	Maple Syrup

Marjoram
Mint
Molasses
Mustard (dry)
Nutmeg
Paprika
Peppermint
Pimiento
Rice syrup
Rosemary

Saffron
Sage
Salt
Savory
Soy sauce
Spearmint
Sugar, brown
Sugar, white
Tamari
Tamarind

Tarragon
Thyme
Turmeric
Vanilla
Vinegar, apple
   cider
Vinegar, balsamic
Vinegar, red wine
Wintergreen

Avoid

Allspice
Almond extract
Anise
Barley malt
Capers
Cornstarch
Corn syrup

Gelatin, plain
   ground
Pepper, black
Pepper, cayenne
Pepper,
   peppercorn

Pepper, red flakes
Pepper, white
Tapioca
Vinegar, white

Condiments

Be sure to avoid all pickled condiments, due to a susceptibility to stomach cancer. Also avoid ketchup, which contains vinegar.

Neutral

Jam (from acceptable fruits)
Jelly (from acceptable fruits)
Mayonnaise
Mustard

Salad dressing (low-fat,
   from acceptable
   ingredients)

Avoid

Ketchup
Pickles, dill
Pickles, kosher
Pickles, sweet

Pickles, sour
Relish
Worcestershire sauce

Herbal Teas

Herbal tea should be employed by Type ABs to rev up the immune system and build protections against cardiovascular disease and cancer. Alfalfa, burdock, chamomile, and echinacea are immune-system boosters. Hawthorn and licorice root are highly recommended for cardiovascular health. Green tea has enormous positive effects on the immune system. Dandelion, burdock root, and strawberry leaf teas will aid your absorption of iron and prevent anemia.

Highly Beneficial

Alfalfa	Ginger	Licorice root*
Burdock	Ginseng	Rose hips
Chamomile	Green tea	Strawberry
Echinacea	Hawthorn	leaf

Do not use without your doctor's permission.

Neutral

Catnip	Mulberry	Spearmint
Cayenne	Parsley	Thyme
Chickweed	Peppermint	Valerian
Dandelion	Raspberry leaf	Vervain
Dong quai	Sage	White birch
Elder	Saint John's wort	White oak bark
Goldenseal	Sarsaparilla	Yarrow
Horehound	Slippery elm	Yellow dock

Avoid

Aloe	Hops	Senna
Coltsfoot	Linden	Shepherd's purse
Corn silk	Mullein	Skullcap
Fenugreek	Red clover	
Gentian	Rhubarb	

Miscellaneous Beverages

Red wine is good for Type ABs because of its positive cardiovascular effects. A glass of red wine every day is believed to lower the risk of heart disease for both men and women.

A cup or two a day of regular or decaffeinated coffee increases your stomach acid and also has the same enzymes found in soy. Alternate coffee and green tea for the best combination of benefits.

Highly Beneficial

Coffee, regular
Coffee, decaf
Tea, green

Neutral

Beer   Wine, red
Seltzer water   Wine, white
Soda, club

Avoid

Liquor, distilled   Soda, diet   Tea, black decaf
Soda, cola   Soda, other   Tea, black regular

Type AB
Supplement Advisory

The role of supplements—be they vitamins, minerals, or herbs—is to add the nutrients that may be lacking in your diet, and to provide extra protection where you need it. The supplement focus for Type ABs is:

- Supercharging the immune system
- Supplying cancer-fighting antioxidants
- Strengthening the heart

Type ABs present a somewhat mixed picture when it comes to supplements. Although you share the vulnerable immune system and disease susceptibilities of Type As, your Type AB diet fortunately provides a rich variety of nutrients with which to fight back.

For example, Type ABs get plenty of vitamin A, vitamin B_{12}, niacin, and vitamin E in their diets, receiving a dietary protection against cancer and heart disease. I would suggest further supplementation only if, for some reason, a Type AB isn't adhering to the diet. Even iron, which is seriously lacking in the Type A vegetarian diet, is readily available in Type AB foods. There are, however, some supplements that can benefit Type ABs.

VITAMIN C

Type ABs, who have higher rates of stomach cancer because of low stomach acid, can benefit from taking additional supplements of vitamin C. For example, nitrite, a compound that results from the smoking and curing of meats, could be a particular problem with Type ABs, because its cancer-causing potential is greater in people with lower levels of stomach acid. As an antioxidant, vitamin C is known to block this reaction (although you should still avoid smoked and cured foods). However, don't take this to mean that you should take massive amounts. I have found that Type ABs do not do as well on high doses (1,000 mg and up) of vitamin C because it tends to upset their stomachs. Taken over the course of a day, two to four capsules of a 250-mg supplement, preferably derived from rose hips, should cause no digestive problems.

Best C-Rich Foods for Type ABs

berries	cherries
grapefruit	lemon
pineapple	broccoli

ZINC (with caution)

I have found that a small amount of zinc supplementation (as little as 3 mg/day) often makes a big difference in protecting Type AB children against infections, especially ear infections. Zinc supplementation is a double-edged sword, however. While small, periodic doses enhance immunity, long-term, higher doses depress it and can interfere with the absorption of other minerals. Be careful with zinc! It's completely unregulated and is widely available as a supplement, but you really shouldn't use it without a physician's advice.

Best Zinc-Rich Foods for Type ABs

recommended meats (especially dark-meat turkey)
eggs
legumes

SELENIUM

Selenium may be of value to Type ABs, as it seems to act as a component of the body's own antioxidant defenses. However, cases of selenium toxicity have been reported in people who have taken excessive supplements. Check with your physician before taking this mineral.

Herbs/Phytochemicals Recommended for Type ABs

HAWTHORN *(Crataegus oxyacantha)*. With a tendency toward heart disease, Type ABs will want to be serious about protecting their cardiovascular system. Following the Type AB diet will substantially reduce the risk, but if you have family members with heart disease or hardening of the arteries, you may want to take your preventive program a step further. A phytochemical with exceptional preventive capacities is found in the hawthorn tree *(Crataegus oxyacantha)*. Hawthorn has a number of impressive antioxidant effects. It increases the elasticity of the arteries and strengthens the heart while also lowering blood pressure and exerting a mild solventlike effect upon the plaques in the arteries. Officially approved for pharmaceutical use in Germany, the actions of hawthorn are virtually unknown elsewhere. Extracts and tinctures are readily available through naturopathic physicians, health food stores, and pharmacies. I cannot praise this herb too highly. Official German government monographs show the plant to be completely free of any side effects. If I had my way, extracts of hawthorn would be used to fortify breakfast cereals, just as vitamins are.

IMMUNE-ENHANCING HERBS. Because the immune systems of Type AB tend to be vulnerable to viruses and infections, gentle immune-enhancing herbs such as purple coneflower *(Echinacea purpurea)* can help ward off colds or flus and may help optimize the immune system's anti-cancer surveillance. Many people take echinacea in liquid or tablet form. It is widely available. The Chinese herb huang-ki *(Astragalus membranaceous)* is also taken as an immune tonic, but is not so easy to find. The active ingredients in both herbs are sugars that act as mitogens to stimulate white blood cell proliferation. The white blood cells, you will remember, defend the immune system.

CALMING HERBS. Type ABs will do well to use mild herbal relaxants such as chamomile and valerian root. These herbs are available as teas and should be taken frequently. Valerian has a bit of a pungent odor, which actually becomes pleasing once you get used to it.

QUERCETIN. Quercetin is a bioflavonoid found abundantly in vegetables, particularly yellow onions. Quercetin supplements are widely available in health food stores, usually in capsules of 100 to 500 mg. Quercetin is a very powerful antioxidant, many hundreds of times more powerful than vitamin E. Quercetin makes a powerful addition to your cancer-prevention strategies.

MILK THISTLE *(Silybum marianum).* Like quercetin, milk thistle is an effective antioxidant with the additional special property of reaching very high concentrations in the liver and bile ducts. Type ABs tend to suffer from digestive disorders, particularly of the liver and gallbladder. If your family has any history of liver, pancreas, or gallbladder problems, add a milk thistle supplement (easily found in most health food stores) to your protocol. Cancer patients who are receiving chemotherapy should use a milk thistle supplement to protect their liver from damage.

BROMELAIN (Pineapple enzymes). If you are Type AB and suffer from bloating or other signs of poor absorption, take a bromelain supplement. This enzyme has a moderate ability to break down dietary proteins, helping the Type AB digestive tracts better assimilate them.

Type AB Stress/Exercise Profile

The heightened sensitivity of the Type AB nervous system gradually frays your delicate protective antibodies. You're too weary to fight the infections and bacteria that are waiting to jump in like muggers trailing an intoxicated prey.

If, however, you adopt quieting techniques, such as yoga or meditation, you can achieve great benefits by countering negative stresses with focus and relaxation. Type ABs do not respond well to continuous confrontation, and need to consider and practice the art of stillness as a calming charm.

If Type ABs remain in their naturally tense state, stress can produce heart disease and various forms of cancer. Exercises that provide calm and focus are the remedy that pull the Type AB from the grip of stress.

Tai chi chuan, the slow-motion, ritualistic pattern of Chinese boxing; and hatha yoga, the timeless Indian stretching system, are calming, centering experiences. Moderate isotonic exercises, such as hiking, swimming, and bicycling, are favored for Type ABs. When I advise calming exercises, it doesn't mean you can't break a sweat. The key is really your mental engagement in your physical activity.

For example, heavy competitive sports and exercises will only exhaust your nervous energy, make you tense all over again, and leave your immune system open to illness or disease.

The following exercises are recommended for Type ABs. Pay special attention to the length of the sessions. To achieve a consistent release of tension and revival of energy, you need to perform one or more of these exercises three or four times a week.

Type AB
Exercise Guidelines

Tai chi chuan, or tai chi, is an exercise that enhances the flexibility of body movement. The slow, graceful, elegant gestures of tai chi chuan routines seem to mask the full-speed hand and foot blows,

EXERCISE	DURATION	FREQUENCY
Aerobics	45–60 min.	3x week
Tai chi	30–45 min.	3–5x week
Hatha yoga	30 min.	3–5x week
Aikido	60 min.	2–3x week
Golf	60 min.	2–3x week
Cycling	60 min.	2–3x week
Brisk walking	20–40 min.	2–3x week
Swimming	30 min.	3–4x week
Dance	30–45 min.	2–3x week
Aerobics (low-impact)	30–45 min.	2–3x week
Hiking	45–60 min.	2–3x week
Stretching	15 min.	every time you exercise

blocks, and parries they represent. In China, tai chi is practiced daily by groups who gather in public squares to perform the movements in unison. Tai chi can be a very effective relaxation technique, although it takes concentration and patience to master.

Yoga is also good for the Type AB stress pattern. It combines inner rectitude with breath control and postures designed to allow for complete concentration without distraction by worldly concerns. Hatha yoga is the most common form of yoga practiced in the West.

If you learn basic yoga postures, you can create a routine best suited to your lifestyle. Many Type ABs who have adopted yoga relaxation tell me that they will not leave the house until they do their yoga.

However, some patients have told me that they are concerned that adopting yoga practices may conflict with their religious beliefs. They fear that the practice of yoga implies that they have adopted Eastern mysticism. I respond, "If you eat Italian food, does that make you Italian?" Meditation and yoga are what you make of them. Visualize and meditate on those subjects that are relevant to you. The postures are neutral; they are just timeless and proven movements.

SIMPLE YOGA RELAXATION TECHNIQUES

Yoga begins and ends with relaxation. We contract our muscles constantly, but rarely do we think of doing the opposite—letting go and relaxing. We can feel better and be healthier if we regularly release the tensions left behind within the muscles by the stresses and strains of life.

The best position for relaxation is lying on your back. Arrange your arms and legs so that you are completely comfortable in your hips, shoulders, and back. The goal of deep relaxation is to let your body and mind settle down to soothing calmness, in the same way that an agitated pool of water eventually calms to stillness.

Begin with abdominal breathing. As a baby breathes, its abdomen moves, not its chest. However, many of us grow to unconsciously adopt the unnatural and inefficient habit of restrained chest breathing. One of the aims of yoga is to make you aware of the true center of breathing. Observe the pattern of your breathing. Is your breathing fast, shallow, and irregular, or do you tend to hold your breath? Allow your breathing to revert to a more natural pattern—full, deep, regular, and with no constriction. Try to isolate just your lower breathing muscles; see if you can breathe without moving your chest. Breathing exercises are always done smoothly and without any strain. Place one hand on your navel and feel the movement of your breathing. Relax your shoulders.

Start the exercise by breathing out completely. When you inhale, pretend that a heavy weight, such as a large book, is resting on your navel, and that by your inhalation, you are trying to raise this imaginary weight up toward the ceiling. Then, when you exhale, simply let this imaginary weight press down against your abdomen, helping you to exhale. Exhale more air out than you normally would, as if to "squeeze" more air out of your lungs. This will act as a yoga stretch for the diaphragm and help to further release tension in this muscle. Bring your abdominal muscles into play here to assist. When you inhale, direct your breath down so deeply that you are lifting an imaginary heavy weight back upward toward the ceiling. Try to completely coordinate and isolate the abdominal breath with no chest or rib movement.

Even if you perform more aerobic exercises during the course of your week, try to integrate the relaxing, soothing routines that will help you best manage your Type AB stress patterns.

A Final Note:
The Personality Question

Type AB followers of blood type–personality analysis love to boast that Jesus Christ was Type AB. Their evidence comes from blood tests conducted on the Shroud of Turin. It's a provocative idea, although I have my doubts, since Jesus was supposed to have lived a good one thousand years before the emergence of Type AB.

But that's Type AB for you. They don't always sweat the details. Type AB is a merging of the edgy, sensitive Type A with the more balanced and centered Type B. The result is a spiritual, somewhat flaky nature that embraces all aspects of life without being particularly aware of the consequences. These characteristics are clearly evident in Type AB blood. The Type AB immune system is the best friend to nearly every virus and disease on the planet. If Type O has high-tech security gates on its immune system, Type AB doesn't even have a lock on its door.

Naturally, these qualities make Type ABs very appealing and popular. It's easy to like people who welcome you with open arms, don't hold grudges when you disappoint them, and always say the most diplomatic thing in every situation. Not surprisingly, many healers and spiritual teachers are Type AB.

The problem is, since Type ABs' immune systems are so indiscriminate, you begin to suspect that they have no loyalty to any one group. Benedict Arnold, our nation's most famous traitor, was said to be Type AB.

On the positive side, Type ABs are considered some of the most captivating and interesting of the blood types. But their natural charisma can often lead to heartache. John F. Kennedy and Marilyn Monroe were Type ABs, and though long gone, both remain prominent. There was a public connection to them so intense that it haunts the American psyche to this day. But for all their luster, their charisma exacted a heavy toll.

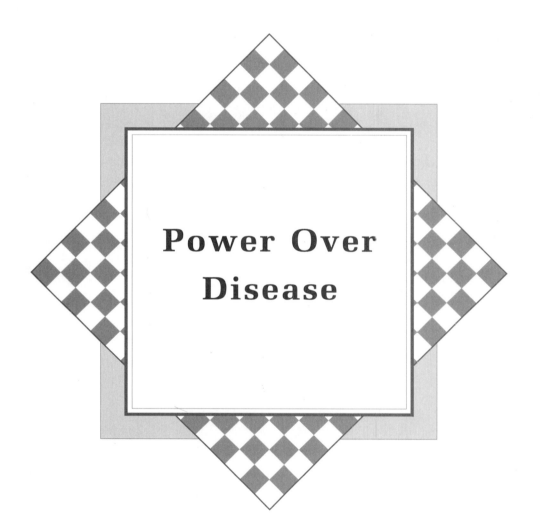

PART III

Power Over Disease

Medications and You

Choose Wisely

BY NOW YOU ARE AWARE OF THE STRONG LINK BETWEEN your blood type and your health. I hope you are also beginning to see that you can exert meaningful control, even when you have a susceptibility to a certain condition. Your Blood Type Plan is the cornerstone to a lifetime of health.

In the next chapters, we will talk in more detail about the specific medical issues that concern everyone, and how you can use your blood type information to make the best choices for your health. We begin with the drugs and treatments that are commonplace in modern life.

Drugs have been used as medicine for thousands of years. When a shaman or witch doctor brewed a potion, that potion had not only medical authority, but spiritual power. Although the infusion was often malodorous and vile, it contained magic, and the patient would gladly drink the bitter brew in hope of a cure.

Not that much has changed.

Today physicians overprescribe medications, and we overuse them. It's a serious problem. Yet unlike other naturopaths who reject the entire modern pharmacopoeia, I believe we must take a more reasoned and flexible point of view. Most medical preparations are designed to be effective on a broad range of the population, and should be used to treat the most severe and potentially dangerous conditions.

But let us also keep medication in perspective: All drugs are poisons. The good drugs that have been discovered over the centuries are selective poisons. Many others are broader, less selective poisons. An excellent example of the latter is the diffuse arsenal of drugs used by oncologists for chemotherapy. In the process of destroying cancerous cells, many of these drugs indiscriminately attack healthy cells as well. (It is not my intention to vilify oncologists. This is just the state of the art.)

The good news is that chemotherapy sometimes works. The bad news is that sometimes chemotherapy works, but the patient dies of complications related to the treatment. It's a terrible conundrum.

Modern science has presented the medical community with a bewildering array of medications, and all of them are being prescribed by well-meaning physicians worldwide. But have we been careful enough in our use of antibiotics and vaccines? How do you know which medications are best for you, for your family, for your children?

Again, blood type holds the answer.

Over-the-Counter Medications

There is a wide range of over-the-counter (OTC) medications designed for every common ailment—from headaches to aching joints to congestion to indigestion. On the face of it, these seem to be inexpensive, convenient, and effective remedies.

As a naturopathic physician, I try to avoid prescribing OTC medications whenever I can. In most cases, there are natural alternatives that work just as well or better. In addition, there are dangers inherent in using many OTC preparations, including:

- Aspirin's blood-thinning properties can be trouble for Type Os, who already have thin blood. Furthermore, they can mask the symptoms of a serious infection or illness.
- Antihistamines can raise blood pressure—a particular danger for Types A and AB. They can also cause sleeplessness and exacerbate prostate problems.
- Habitual use of laxatives actually can cause constipation, disrupting the natural process of elimination. They also can

be harmful for people with Crohn's disease—primarily a Type O problem.

■ Cough, throat, and chest remedies often have side effects, including high blood pressure, drowsiness, and dizziness.

Before you take an OTC remedy to treat a headache, cramps, or any other malady, investigate the possible causes of your problem. Often, it relates to your diet or stress. For example, you might ask:

■ Is my headache a result of stress?
■ Is my stomach discomfort caused by eating foods that are indigestible for my blood type?
■ Are my sinus problems the result of mucus caused by eating too many mucus-generating foods? Or by eating histamine-releasing foods (such as wheat for Type O)?
■ Is my flu virus the result of immune-system weaknesses?
■ Is my congestion or bronchitis caused by an overproduction of mucus in my respiratory passages?
■ Is my toothache caused by an infection that requires immediate medical treatment?
■ Is my overreliance on commercial laxatives interfering with natural elimination and causing diarrhea?

I urge you to seek medical attention if your symptoms are chronic or particularly severe. Pain, weakness, coughs, fever, congestion, and diarrhea all can be signs of deeper problems. You might cover them up with medications, but you won't be addressing the root cause.

For occasional aches, pains and irregularities, the following remedies are excellent natural replacements for OTC drugs. They're available in many forms from your local health food store or natural nutrition center—including teas, compresses, liquid tinctures, extracts, powders, and capsules.

To make your own herbal tea, boil water and steep the natural herbs for about five minutes.

Please note the key indicating special considerations for each blood type.

Key

●	Type O avoid
■	Type A avoid
▼	Type B avoid
†	Type AB avoid
★	Special note for all blood types

Headache

chamomile

damiana ●

feverfew

valerian

white willow bark (salix)

Sinusitus

fenugreek ▼ †

thyme

Arthritis

alfalfa ●

boswella

calcium

epsom salt bath

rosemary tea soak

Earache

garlic-mullein-olive oil ear drops

Toothache

crushed garlic gum
  massage

oil of cloves gum
  massage

Indigestion, Heartburn

bladderwrack

bromelain (from pineapple)

gentian ● †

ginger

goldenseal

peppermint

Cramps, Gas

chamomile tea
fennel tea
ginger

peppermint tea
probiotic supplement
   with bifidus factor

Nausea

cayenne ■
ginger

licorice root tea

Flu

arabino galactan
echinacea
garlic

goldenseal
rose hip tea

Fever

catnip ■
feverfew

vervain
white willow bark

Cough

coltsfoot ● ▼
horehound

linden ▼

Sore Throat

fenugreek tea gargle ▼
goldenseal root and sage tea gargle

stone root

Congestion

licorice tea
mullein ▼

nettle
vervain

Constipation

aloe vera juice ● ▼ †
fiber ★★
larch tree bark (ARA-6) ★

psyllium
slippery elm

Diarrhea

blueberries

elderberries

L. acidophilus (yogurt culture)

raspberry leaf

Menstrual Cramps

Jamaican dogwood

★ Currently under patent, substance of larch tree bark in a powdered form is available from my office under the name ARA-6. It has been tested to be an excellent natural immune system booster. Furthermore, a substance in larch tree bark, called butyrate, is a safe and effective natural source of fiber for all blood types.

★★ Natural fiber is available in many fruits, vegetables, and grains. Be sure to check your blood type food list before you choose a fiber source.

Vaccines: The Blood Type Sensitivities

Vaccination is an emotionally charged issue in both the conventional and alternative medical communities. From the more orthodox viewpoint, vaccination represents the first line of defense in preventive medicine. Increasing emphasis is being placed on mandatory universal vaccination by the federal, state, and local levels of government. What are the consequences of such a strategy?

Vaccines have been of unquestioned benefit to mankind, saving hundreds of thousands of lives and preventing needless suffering. In the rare circumstances where there have been problems, the vaccines have sometimes reacted badly with a particularly hypersensitive individual. Our knowledge of the immune system does not yet reveal if vaccines have more profound resonances, possibly lowering some of our innate immunities to cancer. Yet many public health officials and medical scientists behave as though it is somehow unpatriotic to question whether every new vaccine must be injected into the collective national bloodstream.

Meanwhile, the public remains confused. Parents want to know which vaccines, if any, their children should be exposed to. The elderly, the hypersensitive, pregnant women, and others worry about the effects of vaccinations. It shouldn't surprise you that there is no single answer for everyone. Your reaction to vaccines has a lot to do with your blood type.

Type O Vaccine Sensitivities

With all vaccines, parents of Type O children should be alert to any sign of inflammation, such as fever or joint pain, since the Type O immune system is prone to these reactions.

Avoid the injectable form of polio vaccine for Type O children, and opt instead for the oral preparation. Since Type Os have hyperactive immune systems, they do best with a less potent form of the vaccine.

Recently vaccinated Type O children should be watched carefully for a couple of days to ensure that there are no complications. Don't give them acetaminophen, the most commonly prescribed over-the-counter medication for vaccination-related problems (found in Tylenol). In my experience, Type O children seem to react poorly to this drug. A natural remedy that will work for Type Os is available at most health food stores. It is an herb called feverfew, derived from the common chrysanthemum flower (*Chrysanthemum parthenium*). In liquid tincture form, feverfew can be given to a child every few hours. Four to eight drops of the tincture in a glass of juice is sufficient to achieve a positive effect.

If you are a pregnant woman with Type O blood, the flu vaccine holds special dangers, especially if the father of your baby is a Type A or Type AB. The flu vaccine could boost the presence of anti-A antibodies in your system, which could attack and damage your fetus.

Type A and Type AB Vaccine Sensitivities

Type A and Type AB children respond well to vaccines. A full vaccination program—including the whooping cough vaccine—should produce few side effects.

In contrast to Type O, Type A and Type AB children should take the injectable form of the polio vaccine because their digestive mucus does not react well to the oral polio vaccine.

Type B Vaccine Sensitivities

Type B children sometimes have severe neurological reactions to vaccinations. Parents should be acutely aware of any signal indicating a complication, be it an alteration in your child's walking or crawling gait, or a personality change of some kind. If you intend to vaccinate your Type B child, it is imperative that you make sure he or she is first completely healthy—free of colds, flu, or ear infections. Like Type Os, Type B children should use the oral form of polio vaccine.

Why do Type Bs tend to react so badly to vaccines? Type Bs produce an enormous number of B antigens in their nervous system. I believe a cross-reaction occurs in the Type B immune system when a vaccine is introduced that causes the body to turn and attack its own tissues. It may be the vaccine itself that causes this cross-reaction. Or perhaps it's one of the chemicals used to enhance the vaccine's effectiveness. It might even be the culture medium used to grow the vaccine. We just don't know yet.

Pregnant Type B women should also avoid the flu vaccine, especially if the father of the child is of Type A or Type AB blood. The flu vaccine could increase your production of anti-A antibodies, which could interfere with the healthy development of the fetus.

The Pros and Cons of Antibiotic Therapy

If your physician or your child's pediatrician often prescribes antibiotics for simple colds and flu, I have one piece of advice: Find another doctor.

The constant misuse of antibiotics is a leading factor in our growing inability to eradicate disease. The overuse of such wonder drugs promotes the development of progressively more resistant pathogens, which require ever stronger antibiotics to treat. Far more powerful than any of the antibiotics currently being manufactured is the natural prescription of proper diet, proper rest, and stress reduction.

Typically, there is a lag between the time you develop an infection and the time your body's immune system responds. It's like dialing the 911 emergency number; you know they aren't going to be at your door the second they answer your call. Antibiotics may get to an infection faster, but they hang up the phone on your body's own 911 emergency number—the immune system. Antibiotics basically cut off immune response; your body's responsibility for fighting an infection has been taken over by medication.

We race to treat fever with antibiotics, yet fever is generally a good sign. It indicates that your body's metabolic rate has kicked into overdrive, burning out invaders by making the environment as inhospitable to infectious organisms as it possibly can.

In my own practice I have discovered that a majority of people can eliminate an infection without the use of an antibiotic. Did you know that antibiotics only reduce the level of infection? Your body's immune system is still required to finish the battle. When you allow your body to go to war on its own terms, without antibiotic intervention, it develops not only a memory of specific antibodies to the current infection and any similar to it, but also the ability to fight more effectively the next time it is challenged or attacked.

A number of people are allergic to various antibiotics, but as a rule they produce few serious medical conditions. Very often, however, continued and heavy use of antibiotics destroys not only the infection, but all of the good bacteria in the digestive tract. Many people experience diarrhea, and quite often women become subject to recurring and persistent yeast infections. Supplements of a friendly digestive bacteria, *L. acidophilus*, may be taken in either tablets or yogurt to restore the proper balance of bacteria in the digestive tract.

There are, of course, times when an appropriate antibiotic is needed and should be used. If you are given an antibiotic, take a supplement of bromelain to ensure that your antibiotic spreads rapidly and penetrates tissue more readily. Pineapples contain this enzyme, so you may drink pineapple juice or take bromelain tablets when you're on a course of antibiotics.

Parents of sick children on antibiotics should set the alarm clock for three or four A.M. to administer an extra dose during the child's sleep cycle. This ensures a more rapid concentration of the drug to fight the infection.

Once more: If you need antibiotics, take them. If an infection becomes protracted, you certainly should consider using an antibiotic. I just think the body's immune system should be allowed to do what it's been created for—to resist.

Type O Antibiotic Sensitivities

Type Os should avoid penicillin-class antibiotics. The Type O immune system is more allergically sensitive to this class of drugs.

Also avoid sulfa-class drugs such as Bactrim. They can cause skin rashes in Type Os.

Try to avoid macrolide-class antibiotics. Erythromycin and the newer macrolides Biaxin and Zithromax can aggravate bleeding tendencies in Type Os. Be especially wary of this problem if you are currently taking blood-thinning medications such as Coumadin or Warferin.

Type A Antibiotic Sensitivities

Carbacephem-class antibiotics such as Lorabid seem to work well for Type As. There are very few side effects. Most Type As respond well to penicillin-class and sulfa-class antibiotics. These are preferable to tetracycline or the newer macrolide-class antibiotics.

If a macrolide-class antibiotic is prescribed for a Type A, Erythromycin is preferred over Zithromax or Clarythromycin. Both of these antibiotics can cause digestive problems and interfere with iron metabolism in the Type A system.

Type AB and Type B Antibiotic Sensitivities

Avoid quinolone-class antibiotics such as Floxin and Cipro if you can. If you must use them, take them (as Europeans do) in smaller doses than prescribed. Be aware of any sign of a nervous system disorder when taking a course of antibiotics, such as blurred vision, confusion, dizziness, or insomnia. Type AB and Type B should immediately discontinue the use of such medication and contact their physicians.

Antibiotic Therapy at the Dentist

It is standard practice for dentists to use antibiotics as a preventive measure against infection. Patients with mitral valve prolapse, a heart condition, are always given a course of antibiotics to guard against any possibility of bacterial infection and subsequent valve damage.

However, a recent study in the British medical journal *Lancet* found no benefit to a course of antibiotics for the majority of patients prior to invasive dental procedures. However, if you are a non-secretor (see the back of this book), you are at much greater risk than a secretor for infections following dental surgery. There are many more instances of streptococcal bacteria causing endocarditis (an inflammation of the lining of the heart muscle) and rheumatic fever in non-secretors, because they produce much lower levels of protective antibodies in the mucous membranes of the mouth and throat. Secretors, on the other hand, have higher levels of these IgA antibodies, which trap bacteria and destroy them before they can gain access to the bloodstream.

Non-secretors should always undertake preventive antibiotic therapy prior to any invasive dental procedure—from deep cleaning to oral surgery.

If you are Type O you may wish to opt out of antibiotic therapy, unless there is deep-rooted infection or the promise of heavy bleeding. Instead, try herbal medications with anti-strep activity, such as goldenseal (*Hydrastis canadensis*).

Type A, Type B, and Type AB may wish to discuss alternative therapies with their dentist or physician if they respond poorly to antibiotics.

Many dentists will refuse to treat a patient who declines the prophylactic use of antibiotics. If you are a healthy individual with no prior history of infections, you might want to consider going elsewhere for your dental work.

Surgery: Better Recovery

Any invasive procedure is a shock to your system. Never take it lightly, even if it is a minor surgery. Tune up your immune system in advance, no matter what your blood type.

Vitamins A and C have a profound effect on wound healing and minimize the formation of scar tissue. Every blood type can benefit from supplementation before surgery. Start taking vitamins A and C at least four or five days prior to surgery, and continue for at least a week afterward. All of my patients who have followed this recommendation report that both they and their surgeons were astonished at the rapidity of their recovery.

RECOMMENDED SURGICAL SUPPLEMENTATION PROTOCOL

Blood Type	Daily Vitamin C	Daily Vitamin A
Type O	2000 mg	30,000 IU
Type A	500 mg	10,000 IU
Type AB, Type B	1000 mg	20,000 IU

Type O Surgical Cautions

Type Os often experience greater blood loss than other blood types during and after surgery because they have lower levels of serum clotting factors. Make sure that you have plenty of vitamin K in your system before surgery; it is essential to clot formation. Kale, spinach, and collard greens contain ample amounts of this vitamin, although you might want to supplement your diet with liquid chlorophyll. Chlorophyll supplements are available at any health food store.

Type Os with a history of phlebitis or who are on a course of blood thinners should consult with their physicians as to any supplementation recommendations. (It's worth noting that the thinner blood of Type Os does not necessarily protect against blood clots. Phlebitis often starts as an inflammatory condition of the veins that affects blood flow.)

Type Os can also boost their immune systems and metabolism with strong physical activity. If it is realistic for you to pursue this prior to surgery, exercise will allow your body to deal with the stress of surgery much more effectively and heal more rapidly.

Type B Surgical Cautions

Type Bs are fortunate in that they are less likely to experience post-surgical complications. The vitamin protocol should be followed as already indicated.

Type Bs who are suffering from a weakened condition may also want to use immune-boosting herbal teas prior to surgery. Burdock root *(Arctium lappa)* and purple coneflower *(Echinacea purpurea)* are excellent immune boosters. A few cups of tea taken every day over a number of weeks can be a positive stimulant for your immune system.

Type A and Type AB Surgical Cautions

Type A and Type AB are both more prone to postsurgical bacterial infections. These infections can become a major stumbling block to recovery and can exacerbate an already difficult situation. I strongly suggest that Type A and Type AB adopt a blood-building, immune system–enhancing protocol of additional vitamin supplementation a week or two prior to surgery. Vitamin B$_{12}$, folic acid, and supplemental iron should all be taken daily along with the already suggested levels of vitamins A and C. The concentration of vitamins you need to achieve is difficult to squeeze out of the Type A and Type AB diets, so supplementation is best.

Floradix is a liquid iron and herb source that is both gentle on the digestive tract and highly assimilable. I highly recommend its use for iron supplementation since iron is usually an irritant to the digestive tracts of Type As and Type ABs. Floradix is found in most health food stores.

Avail yourself of the two excellent immune-enhancing herbal teas, burdock root and echinacea. Drink a few cups daily of these herbal teas at least a couple of weeks prior to surgery.

More than the other blood types, Type As and Type ABs often experience profound physical, mental, and emotional stress because of the trauma of surgery. Relaxation techniques, such as meditation and visualization, can be of tremendous benefit to the more highly strung Type A and Type AB patient. By practicing these techniques, you can have a profound influence upon your own healing process. Some anesthesiologists will work with patients on visualizations while the patient is under anesthesia. I urge you to ask your doctor about this. It's a perfect method for Type As.

After the Surgery

Calendula succus (marigold) is used to help the wound heal and keep it clean. A solution of this homeopathic herb—a form of the marigold flower—is a wonderful healer for all cuts and scrapes in general. The juice has mild antibiotic properties and can be left on after application. Be sure you buy the juice, or *succus*, and not the *calendula* tincture, which has a high alcohol content. The tincture will really sting if you try to clean a wound with it.

As your incision heals and the stitches or staples are removed, a topical vitamin E preparation will minimize scar tissue formation and skin tightening. Many people just snip open a vitamin E capsule and smear it on, but oral supplements aren't formulated for use as skin healers. Use a topical cream or lotion blended for just this purpose.

Listen to Your Blood Type

There are many vitamins and herbal supplements that aid the body in both defending and healing itself. The recommended surgical supplementation is just the minimum you should do to protect and strengthen yourself.

Each of the Blood Type Diets contains pertinent information that allows you to make reasoned choices about what you should and should not allow yourself to eat and drink. All of these choices can have a profound effect on your health and the quality of your life.

By making knowledgeable choices about what is best for your body, you will be able to dramatically affect the course of both your treatment and recovery from surgery. This not only grants you greater control over your present circumstances, but enables you to ensure your future health.

Parents whose children are of vaccination age . . . people who have viral infections . . . those facing surgery—everyone can achieve benefits from an awareness of the blood type connection. It makes sense. It also solves the puzzle of why some people do very well with conventional treatments, while others suffer complications and pain. I urge you to put yourself in the position of being someone who does well.

Stay Disease Free

*How Blood Type
Affects Your Risks*

*E*VERYONE WHO GETS SICK WANTS TO KNOW "WHY ME?"
Even with our enormous technological arsenal, we often have no
certain answer to that question.

It has become clear, however, that there are individuals who are
more prone to certain diseases because of their blood type. Perhaps
this is the missing link—the way we can understand the cellular causes
of disease, and devise ways to combat and eliminate it more effectively.

Why Some People Are Susceptible . . . and Some Are Not

Can you remember being young and having a close friend who
wanted you to do something that you were reluctant to do? Take a
puff of a forbidden cigarette? Sneak a drink of whiskey from your
father's liquor cabinet? Did you take that puff? Drink that whiskey?

If you did, you exhibited your susceptibility—your lack of resistance—to the suggestion of a friend.

Susceptibility, or lack of resistance, is the basic issue with most
disease. Many microbes have the ability to mimic antigens that are

■ ■ ■ ■

considered friendly by the security force of a particular blood type. These clever mimics bypass the security guards and gain entry. Once in the system, they quickly overwhelm it and take control.

Don't you ever wonder why one person stays perfectly healthy while everyone else is falling prey to the latest cold or flu? It is because the healthy person's blood type is not susceptible to those particular invaders.

The Blood Type Connection

There are many causal factors for disease that are clearly influenced by blood type. For instance, Type As with a family history of cardiovascular disease should examine their diets very carefully. Red meats and saturated fats of all kinds are poor choices for a digestive tract ill suited to their processing, which results in higher levels of both triglycerides and cholesterol in Type As. The friendly Type A immune system is also more prone to cancer, since it has a hard time recognizing foes.

Type Os, as I've said, are very sensitive to the agglutinating lectin found in whole wheat. This lectin interacts with the lining of the Type O intestinal tract and produces additional inflammation. If you're Type O and suffer from Crohn's disease, colitis, or irritable bowel syndrome, wheat acts like a poison in your system. Although the Type O immune system is generally hardy, it is also limited. Original Type Os had fewer microbes to conquer, and the blood type does not adapt easily to the complex viruses prevalent today.

The disease profiles of Type Bs are independent of Type O and Type A by virtue of the idiosyncratic B antigens. They tend to be susceptible to slow-moving, sometimes bizarre viral diseases that don't manifest themselves for many years—such as multiple sclerosis and rare neurological ailments—sometimes triggered by the lectins in foods such as chicken and corn.

Type ABs have the most complex disease profile, since they possess both A-like and B-like antigens. Most of their disease susceptibilities are A-like, so if you had to categorize them you would say they were more A than B.

The blood type connection between good health and disease is a potent tool in our search for the best way to treat the body as it is meant to be treated.

Still, I must add a caveat, lest you think that I am proposing a magic formula. There are many factors in every individual life that contribute to disease. It would be overly simplistic and certainly foolish to suggest that blood type is the sole determining factor. If a Type O, a Type A, a Type B, and a Type AB each drank a cup of arsenic, each of them would die. By the same token, if four people of different blood types were all heavy smokers, they would all be susceptible to lung cancer.

The blood type information is not a panacea, but a meaningful refinement that will enable you to function at your peak.

Let's turn to the most common and troubling diseases and conditions for which we can identify a blood type relationship. Some blood type–disease relationships are more clearly defined than others. We are still learning. But every day blood type is revealed as a dominating factor—the previously missing link in our quest for health.

Categories

- Aging Diseases
- Allergies
- Asthma and Hay Fever
- Autoimmune Disorders
- Blood Disorders
- Cardiovascular Disease
- Diabetes
- Digestive Illnesses
- Infections
- Skin Disorders
- Women/Reproduction

Aging Diseases

All people age, no matter what their blood type. But why do we age—and can we slow down the process? These questions have fascinated us for as long as we can remember. The promise of a Fountain of Youth has appeared in every century. Today, with our sophisticated medical technology and our increased knowledge of the factors that contribute to aging, we are closer to an answer.

But there's another question: Why do individual aging patterns differ so greatly? Why does the fifty-year-old runner, lean and seemingly fit, drop dead of a heart attack, while the eighty-nine-year-old woman who has never broken a sweat in her life, remains hale and hardy? Why do some people develop Alzheimer's disease or dementia, while others do not? At what age does physical deterioration become inevitable?

We understand some pieces of the puzzle. Genetics play a role; unique variations in chromosomes contribute to susceptibilities that cause deterioration more rapidly in one person than in another. But these studies are incomplete.

I have discovered, however, a critical link between blood type and aging—specifically, a correlation between the agglutinating action of lectins and the two biggest physiological associations with aging—kidney failure and brain deterioration.

As we age we experience a gradual drop in kidney function so that by the time the average person reaches age seventy-two, his or her kidneys are operating at only 25 percent of their capacity.

Your kidney function is a reflection of the volume of blood that gets cleaned and recirculated into your bloodstream. This filtering system is very delicate—large enough for the various fluid elements of blood to go through, but small enough to prevent whole cells from passing through.

Consider the way the agglutinating actions of lectins gum up the works. Because the kidneys play a central role in the filtration of blood, the actions of many lectins can, over time, upset the delicate process. Those lectins that find their way into the bloodstream end up agglutinating and lodging in the kidneys. The process is similar to having a clogged drain. Over time, the filtration system ceases to function. As more and more agglutination occurs, less and less blood is able to be cleaned. It is a slow process, but ultimately deadly. Kidney failure is one of the leading causes of physical deterioration in the elderly.

The second large physiological association with aging occurs in the brain. Here lectins play an equally destructive role. Scientists have observed that the difference between an old brain and a young brain is that in an old brain many elements of neurons get tangled up. This tangling, which leads to dementia and overall deterioration (and might even be a factor in Alzheimer's disease), occurs very gradually over the decades of adult life.

How do lectins reach the brain? Remember, lectins come in all shapes and sizes; some are small enough to pass the blood-brain barrier. Once they reach the brain they begin to agglutinate the blood cells, gradually interfering with neuron activity. The process occurs over many decades, but eventually the neurons get tangled enough to have an effect on brain function.

It is clear to me that by reducing or eliminating the most harmful lectins from your diet, you can maintain healthier kidneys and brain function for a longer period of time. That is why some very old people remain mentally sharp and physically active.

A third way that lectins contribute to aging is their effects on our hormonal functions. It is well documented that as people age, they have more trouble absorbing and metabolizing nutrients. That's one reason why elderly people often become malnourished, even when they are eating their normal diets. Dietary guidelines normally call for added supplementation for the elderly. But if agglutinating lectins are not overwhelming the system and interfering with hormonal activity, it is likely that elderly people can absorb nutrients as effectively as when they were younger.

I am not proposing that the Blood Type Solution is the Fountain of Youth! It is not a formula for reversing the effects of aging that have already occurred. But you can reduce cellular damage by reducing your lectin intake at any age. Most of all, your Blood Type Plan is designed to be age sparing—enabling you to slow down the process of aging during your entire adult life.

Allergies

Food Allergies

In my opinion, no area of alternative medicine is as shot full of humbug as the concept of food allergy. Complex and expensive tests are conducted on practically every patient, resulting in a list of foods to which that person is "allergic."

My own patients habitually term any reaction to something they've eaten a "food allergy," although most of the time it is not an allergy they are describing, but rather a food intolerance. If you have a problem with lactose in milk, for example, you are not allergic to it; you lack an enzyme to break it down. You are lactose intolerant, not lactose allergic. This intolerance does not necessarily mean you'll get sick if you drink milk. Type Bs who are lactose intolerant, for example, are often able to introduce milk products into their diets gradually. There are also products that add the lactose enzyme to milk products, making them more palatable for the intolerant.

A food allergy is a very different type of reaction that occurs, not in the digestive tract, but in the immune system. Your immune system literally creates an antibody to a food. The reaction is swift and harsh—rashes, swelling, cramps, or other specific symptoms that indicate your body is struggling to rid itself of the poisonous food.

Not everything in nature is perfectly cut and dried. Occasionally I'll come across a person who is allergic to a food that is on his Blood Type Diet. The solution: Simply remove the offending food. The main point is that you have more to fear from the hidden lectins entering your system than you do from food allergies. You may not feel sick when you eat the food, but it is affecting your system nonetheless. Type As should also be aware that if they produce excessive mucus, it may appear to be an allergy when they should actually be avoiding mucus-producing foods.

Asthma and Hay Fever

Type Os win the allergy sweepstakes hands down! They are more likely to be asthma sufferers, and even hay fever, the bane of so many, appears to be specific to Type O blood. A wide range of pollens contain lectins that stimulate the release of the powerful histamines, and *boom!* Itching, sneezing, runny nose, wheezing, coughing, red, watery eyes—all allergy symptoms.

Many food lectins, especially wheat, interact with IgE (immunoglobin-E) antibodies found in the blood. These antibodies stimulate white blood cells called basophiles to release not only histamines, but other powerful chemical allergens called kinins. These can cause severe allergic reactions, swelling the tissues of the throat and constricting the lungs.

Asthma and hay fever sufferers really do best when they follow the diet recommended for their blood type. For example, Type Os who eliminate wheat often relieve many of their symptomatic behaviors, such as sneezing, respiratory problems, snoring, or persistent digestive disorders.

Type As have a different problem. Instead of environmental reactions, they often develop stress-related asthma as a result of their intense stress profiles (see the Type A Plan). When Type As suffer from excessive production of mucus caused by poor dietary choices, it makes the stress-related asthma worse. Type As, as you will remember, naturally produce copious amounts of mucus, and when they eat foods that are mucus producing (such as dairy), they suffer from too much mucus, which can exacerbate respiratory problems. In this case, when Type As are careful to avoid mucus-producing foods, and when the causes of the stress are addressed positively, their asthmatic condition always improves or is eliminated.

By design, Type Bs are not prone to developing allergies. They have a high allergy threshold, unless they eat the wrong foods. For example, the B-poisoning chicken and corn lectins will trigger allergies in even the most resistant Type Bs.

Type ABs seem to have the least problem with allergies, probably because their immune systems are the most environmentally friendly. The combination of A-like and B-like antigens gives Type ABs a double dose of antigens with which to deal with environmental intrusion.

Autoimmune Disorders

Autoimmune disorders are immune-system breakdowns. Your immune defenses develop what amounts to severe amnesia; they no longer recognize themselves. The result is that they run amok, making autoantibodies, which attack their own tissues. These warlike autoantibodies think they are protecting their turf, but in reality they are destroying their own organs and inciting inflammatory responses.

Examples of autoimmune disease include rheumatoid arthritis, lupus nephritis, chronic fatigue syndrome/Epstein-Barr, multiple sclerosis, and amyotrophic lateral sclerosis (Lou Gehrig's disease).

Arthritis

Type Os are the predominant sufferers of the autoimmune disorder arthritis. Type O immune systems are environmentally intolerant, and there are many foods—grains and potatoes among them—whose lectins produce inflammatory reactions in their joints.

My father observed many years ago that Type Os tended to develop a gritty sort of arthritis, a chronic deterioration of the bone cartilage. This is the kind of arthritic condition called osteoarthritis, typically found in the elderly. Type As tend to develop a puffy arthritis, which is the more acute rheumatoid form of the disease—a painful and debilitating breakdown of multiple joints.

In my own practice, most of my patients who suffer from rheumatoid arthritis are Type As. The anomaly of Type As, with their immunologically tolerant systems, developing this form of arthritis may be related to A-specific lectins. Laboratory animals injected with A-specific lectins developed inflammation and joint destruction that was indistinguishable from rheumatoid arthritis.

Just as likely, there is a stress connection. Some studies show that people with rheumatoid arthritis tend to be more high strung and less emotionally hardy. When they have poor coping mechanisms for life stress, the disease progresses more rapidly. This makes some sense in light of what we know about the stress factor, and about Type As who are inherently high strung. Type As with rheumatoid arthritis should certainly incorporate daily relaxation techniques, as well as calming exercises.

Chronic Fatigue Syndrome

In recent years, I have treated many people who suffered from the baffling disease called chronic fatigue syndrome (CFS). The primary symptom is great tiredness. Other more advanced symptoms include painful muscles and joints, persistent sore throats, digestive problems, allergies, and chemical sensitivities.

The most important thing I've learned from my research and clinical work is that CFS may not be an autoimmune disease at all, but rather a liver disease. (I place it in this section because that's where people are accustomed to looking for it.)

Although CFS masquerades as a virus or autoimmune disease, the root cause is more likely a problem of poor metabolism in the liver. In other words, the liver is unable to detoxify chemicals. To my reasoning, only this sort of liver problem could produce immunological effects as well as effects characteristic of other systems, such as digestive or musculoskeletal.

I've found that Type O CFS patients in particular do very well on licorice and potassium supplements, in addition to the Type O Diet. Licorice has many effects in the body, but in the liver it really shines. The bile ducts (where detoxification occurs) become more efficient, with greater protection against chemical damage. This preliminary removal of stress to the liver seems to positively influence the adrenals and blood sugar, increasing energy and producing a feeling of well-being. The blood type–specific exercise activities seem to serve also as a valuable guide to help return to appropriate forms of physical activity. (NOTE: Please do not use licorice without a physician's supervision.)

CASE HISTORY: CHRONIC FATIGUE SYNDROME
from Dr. John Prentice, Everett, Washington
Karen, 44: Type B

My colleague Dr. John Prentice tried the Blood Type Plan for the first time on a patient with severe CFS. He wasn't totally convinced it would work, but all efforts to help his very sick patient had failed, and he contacted me when he heard of the work I was doing with CFS patients.

Karen was a tough case. She had suffered terrible fatigue for her entire adult life, and had needed twelve hours of sleep every night since she was a teenager. She would steal naps when she could. For the past seven years her exhaustion prevented her from holding a job. In addition, her neck, shoulders, and back were constantly in pain, and she suffered debilitating headaches. Recently, Karen had started experiencing terrible anxiety attacks, with heart palpitations so severe she would call 911. It felt as if her circulation were shutting down, along with her whole body.

Karen was a wealthy woman, but most of her inheritance was spent on making the rounds to doctors. She had been to more than fifty doctors, both conventional and alternative, before she came to Dr. Prentice.

Dr. Prentice started Karen on a program of strict adherence to the Type B Diet, supplements, and exercise regimen. Both he and Karen were astonished to see that within only a week she had a tremendous increase in energy. Within a few weeks, most of her symptoms were resolved.

Dr. Prentice tells me that today Karen is a new person. "It's like clockwork," he says. "When she eats 'off' her diet, her body reminds her with severe symptoms, so she sticks with it closely." He shared a letter she had written to him: "I have a whole new life. All my symptoms are practically gone and I hold two jobs, having great energy fourteen hours a day consistently. I believe the diet is key to this tremendous change. I am extremely active and feel like nothing can stop me. Thank you so very much!"

Multiple Sclerosis, Lou Gehrig's Disease

Both multiple sclerosis and Lou Gehrig's disease (amyotrophic lateral sclerosis) are seen in very high frequency in Blood Type B. It's an example of the Type B tendency to contract unusual slow-growing viral and neurological disorders. The Type B association may explain why many Jews, with high numbers of Type B blood, suffer from these diseases more than other groups. Some researchers believe that multiple sclerosis and Lou Gehrig's disease are caused by a virus, contracted in youth, that has a B-like appearance. The virus cannot be combatted by the Type B immune system since it can't produce anti-B antibodies. The virus grows slowly and without symptoms until twenty or more years after it has entered the system.

Type ABs also are at risk for these B-like diseases, since their bodies do not produce anti-B antibodies. Type O and Type A seem to be relatively immune by virtue of their strong anti-B antibodies.

CASE HISTORY: AUTOIMMUNE DISORDER
Joan, 55: Type O

Joan, a middle-aged dentist's wife, was a classic example of the ravages of autoimmune disorders. She suffered from severe symptoms of chronic fatigue/Epstein-Barr, arthritis, and tremendous discomfort caused by gas and bloating. Joan's digestive system was so disrupted that practically everything she ate caused bouts of diarrhea. By the time she arrived in my office, she had been struggling with these conditions for more than a year. Needless to say, she was terribly weakened and in great pain. She was also very discouraged. Since autoimmune disorders can be hard to pin down, many people (even some physicians) don't believe chronic fatigue sufferers are really sick. Imagine the humiliation and frustration of feeling deathly ill but having people tell you it's all in your head!

Worse still, Joan's doctors had experimented with a number of drug therapies, including steroids, which made her even sicker and contributed to her bloating. She had also been told to adopt a diet high in grains and vegetables, and to limit or eliminate red meat—exactly the opposite of what this Type O should have been doing.

As severe as Joan's symptoms were, the treatment was fairly simple—a detoxification program, the Type O diet, and a regimen of nutritional supplements. Within two weeks, Joan experienced significant improvement. By the six-month mark, she was feeling "normal" again. To this day, Joan's energy level is good, her digestion is healthy, and her arthritis flares up only when she indulges in the rare sandwich or ice cream.

CASE HISTORY: LUPUS
From Dr. Thomas Kruzel, N.D., Gresham, Oregon
Marcia, 30: Type A

My colleague Dr. Kruzel was interested in trying the blood type treatments, but he was initially skeptical. It was a case of lupus nephritis that showed him the true value of serotyping for the treatment of disease.

Marcia, a frail young woman suffering from lupus, was carried into Dr. Kruzel's office by her brother after being discharged from the hospital's intensive-care unit. She had suffered kidney failure from circulating immune complexes related to her disease. Marcia had been on shunt dialysis for several weeks and was scheduled for renal transplantation within the next six months.

Dr. Kruzel took her history and learned that Marcia's diet was very high in dairy, wheat, and red meat—all dangerous foods for a Type A person in her condition. He placed her on a strict vegetarian diet along with hydrotherapy and homeopathic preparations. Within two weeks, Marcia's condition had improved and her need for dialysis had decreased. Remarkably, within a two-month period, Marcia was taken completely off dialysis and her previously scheduled kidney transplant was canceled. Three years later, she is still doing well.

Blood Disorders

It should come as no surprise that blood-related illnesses, such as anemia and clotting disorders, are blood type specific.

Pernicious Anemia

Type As constitute the greatest number of pernicious anemia sufferers, but the condition has nothing to do with the vegetarian Type A Diet. Pernicious anemia is the result of a vitamin B_{12} deficiency, and Type As have the most difficulty absorbing B_{12} from the foods they eat. Type ABs also have a tendency toward pernicious anemia, although not as great as Type As.

The reason for the deficiency is that the body's use of B_{12} requires high levels of stomach acid and the presence of intrinsic factor, a chemical produced by the lining of the stomach that is responsible for B_{12}'s assimilation. Type As and Type ABs have lower levels of intrinsic factor than the other blood types, and they don't produce that much stomach acid. For this reason, most Type As and Type ABs who suffer from pernicious anemia respond best when vitamin B_{12} is administered by injection. By eliminating the need for the digestive process to assimilate this vital and potent nutrient, it is made available to the body in a more highly concentrated way. This is a case where dietary solutions alone don't work, although Type As and Type ABs are able to absorb Floradix, a liquid iron and herb supplement.

Type O and Type B tend not to suffer from anemia; they have high acid contents in their stomachs and sufficient levels of intrinsic factor.

CASE HISTORY: ANEMIA
From Jonathan V. Wright, M.D., Kent, Washington
Carol, 35: Type O

The blood type diets have begun to make their way into conventional medicine, as I have shared them with my M.D. colleagues. Dr. Wright was one who successfully used the diet to treat a woman with chronically low blood levels of iron. Carol had tried every available form of iron supplement with no success. Dr. Wright tried a number of other treatments without success. The only thing that worked at all was injectable iron, but it was only a temporary solution. Her iron levels would inevitably drop again.

I had spoken to Dr. Wright on an earlier occasion about my work with lectins and blood types, and he called me for more details. He decided to try the Type O Diet for Carol. After eliminating the incompatible lectins, which may have been damaging her red blood cells, and adhering to a high animal protein diet, Carol's blood iron levels started to rise, and previously ineffective supplementation started to help. Dr. Wright and I agreed that the agglutination of the intestinal tract by the incompatible food lectins prevented the iron from assimilating.

Clotting Disorders

Type Os face the biggest problems when it comes to blood clotting. Most often, Type Os lack sufficient quantities of the various blood-clotting factors. This can have severe consequences, especially during surgery, or in situations where there is blood loss. Type O women, for example, tend to lose significantly more blood after childbirth than women of other blood types.

Type Os with a history of bleeding disorders and stroke should emphasize foods containing chlorophyll to help modify their clotting factors. Chlorophyll is found in almost all green vegetables, and also can be taken as a supplement.

Type A and Type AB don't suffer clotting disorders, but their thicker blood can work to their disadvantage in other ways. Thicker blood is more likely to deposit plaque in the arteries—one reason why Type A and Type AB are more prone to cardiovascular disease. Type A and Type AB women might have problems with heavy clotting during their menstrual periods if they don't keep their diets under control.

Type Bs tend not to suffer from clotting disorders or thick blood. As long as they follow the Type B Diet, their balanced systems work efficiently.

Cardiovascular Disease

Cardiovascular disease is epidemic in Western societies, with many factors to blame, including diet, lack of exercise, smoking, and stress.

Is there a connection between your blood type and your susceptibility to cardiovascular disease? When the famous Framingham [Massachusetts] Heart Study examined the connection between blood type and heart disease, it found no clear-cut blood type distinction as to who gets heart disease. It did, however, discover a strong connection between blood type and who survives heart disease. The study found that Type O heart patients between the ages of thirty-nine and seventy-two had a much higher rate of survival than Type A heart patients in the same age group. This was especially true for men between the ages of fifty and fifty-nine.

Although the Framingham Heart Study did not explore this subject in real depth, it does appear that the same factors involved in surviving heart disease also offer some protection against getting it in the first place. Given these factors, clearly there is a greater risk for Type As and Type ABs. Let's examine them.

The most significant factor is cholesterol, the primary causal factor in coronary artery disease. Most of the cholesterol in our bodies is produced in our livers, but there is an enzyme called phosphatase manufactured in the small intestine that is responsible for the absorption of dietary fats. High-alkaline phosphatase levels, which speed the absorption and metabolism of fats, lead to low serum cholesterol levels. Type O blood normally has the highest natural levels of this enzyme. In Type B, Type AB, and Type A, the alkaline phosphatase enzyme is seen in ever-declining levels, with Type B having the highest level after Type O.

Another factor in Type Os' high survival rate is blood-clotting factors. As we discussed earlier, Type Os have fewer clotting factors in their blood. This defect in Type O blood may actually work to their advantage, as this essentially thinner blood is less likely to deposit plaque that will clog the arterial flow. On the other hand, Type A, and to a slightly lesser extent, Type AB, have a consistently higher level of serum cholesterol and triglycerides (blood fats) than do Type O and Type B blood.

CASE HISTORY: HEART DISEASE
Wilma, 52: Type O

Wilma was a fifty-two-year-old Lebanese woman with advanced cardiovascular disease. When I first examined her, she had recently come out of the hospital after receiving a balloon angioplasty, a procedure used to treat clogged coronary arteries. She told me that her cholesterol had been over 350 at the time of the original diagnosis (normal is 200 to 220), and three of her arteries had blockages of over 80 percent.

Since Wilma was Type O, her illness was a bit of a surprise, considering that Type Os normally have a lower-than-average incidence of heart disease. She was also quite a bit younger than most women who present with such severe blockages; women tend not to develop heart disease until long after menopause. (Remember, though, there are always exceptions. Susceptibilities are not certainties!)

Wilma had always eaten the traditional Lebanese diet, including lots of olive oil, fish, and grains, which most doctors feel is beneficial for the circulatory system. However, five years earlier, at the age of forty-seven, she began to experience pain in her neck and arms. Heart disease didn't even occur to her! She assumed the pain was arthritis, and was stunned when her doctor diagnosed her problem as angina pectoris, pain caused from an inadequate blood and oxygen supply to the heart muscle.

After her angioplasty, Wilma's cardiologist advised her to begin taking the cholesterol-lowering drug Mevacor. A well-read health consumer, Wilma worried about long-term problems with drug therapy, and she wanted to try a natural approach before opting for the drug. That's when she came to me.

Since Wilma was Type O, I suggested that she add lean red meat to her diet. In light of her condition, she was understandably nervous about eating foods that are usually restricted in people with high cholesterol or heart disease. She immediately consulted her cardiologist, who was—no surprise—appalled at the idea. Again, he urged her to take Mevacor. But Wilma was serious about avoiding drug therapy, so she decided to follow the Type O Diet for three months and do a cholesterol check at that time.

Wilma confirmed many of my theories about susceptibility to high cholesterol. Often, through heredity or by other mechanisms, people have high levels of cholesterol in their blood in spite of a severely restricted diet. Usually they have some defect in the manipulation of the internal cholesterol metabolism. My suspicion is that when Type Os eat a lot of certain carbohydrates (usually wheat products), it modifies the effectiveness of their insulin, resulting in its becoming more potent and longer lasting. From the increased insulin activity, the body stores more fat in the tissues and elevates the triglyceride stores.

In addition to advising Wilma to increase the percentage of red meats in her diet, I also helped her find substitutes for the large amounts of wheat she was consuming, and prescribed an extract of hawthorn (an herb used as a tonic for the heart and arteries) and a low dose of the B vitamin, niacin, which helps reduce cholesterol levels.

Wilma was an executive secretary with a stressful job and she did very little exercise. She was intrigued when I described the relationship between stress and physical activity in people with Type O blood, as well as the relationship between stress and heart disease. She had never been a regular exerciser, so hardly knew where to begin. I started her on a walking program to gradually increase her aerobic fitness. After a couple of weeks, Wilma reported that walking was a godsend; she'd never felt better.

Within six months Wilma's cholesterol plummeted, without medication, to 187, where it stabilized. She was elated to have cholesterol in the normal range. It had seemed impossible.

The naturopath intern working in my office was astounded and perplexed. All conventional evidence indicates that people with high cholesterol should avoid red meats, yet Wilma flourished. Blood type was the missing link.

CASE HISTORY: DANGEROUSLY HIGH CHOLESTEROL
John, 23: Type O

John, a recent college graduate, had a skyrocketing cholesterol level, high triglycerides, and high blood sugar. These were very unusual symptoms in a young man—especially since he was Type O. As there was a strong family history of heart disease, naturally his parents were alarmed. After extensive workups at Yale by consulting cardiologists, John was told that his genetic predisposition was so overwhelming that even cholesterol-reducing medication would be useless. In effect, John was told that he was destined to develop coronary artery disease—sooner, rather than later.

In the office, John seemed depressed and lethargic. He complained of severe fatigue. "I used to love to work out," he said, "but now I just don't have the energy." John also suffered from frequent sore throats and swollen glands. His past history revealed mononucleosis and two separate incidences of Lyme disease.

John had been following a vegetarian diet prescribed by his cardiologist for some time. He admitted, however, that he was feeling worse on this diet, not better.

After only a few weeks on the Type O Diet, however, the results were amazing. Within five months, John's serum cholesterol, triglycerides, and blood sugar all dropped to normal levels. A repeat blood profile after three months revealed similar results.

If John continued to follow the Type O Diet, exercise regularly, and take nutritional supplements, there was a good chance that he would beat the odds of his genetic inheritance.

High Blood Pressure

Constantly at work within us is the dynamic force of our beating hearts, rhythmically pumping blood through our bodies. The process is normally so smooth that we rarely think much about it. That's why high blood pressure (or hypertension) is called the silent killer. It's possible to have dangerously high blood pressure and be entirely unaware of it.

When blood pressure is taken, two numbers are read. The systolic reading (the number on top) measures the pressure within the arteries as your heart beats out blood. The diastolic reading (the number on the bottom) measures the pressure present within the arteries as your heart rests between beats.

Normal systolic pressure is 120, and normal diastolic pressure is 80—or 120 over 80 (120/80). High blood pressure (or hypertension) is 140/90 under age forty, and 160/95 over age forty.

Depending on the severity and duration, high blood pressure left untreated opens the door to a host of problems, including heart attacks and strokes.

Little is known about the blood type–related risk factors for hypertension. However, hypertension often occurs in conjunction with heart disease, so Type A and Type AB should be particularly vigilant.

Hypertension carries the same risk factors as cardiovascular disease. Smokers, diabetics, post-menopausal women, the obese, the sedentary, and people in stressful positions should pay extra attention to the details of their blood type program—especially to the diet and exercise recommendations.

CASE HISTORY: HYPERTENSION
Bill, 54: Type A

Bill was a middle-aged bond trader with high blood pressure. When I first saw him in my office in March 1991, his blood pressure was an almost explosive 150/105 to 135/95. It didn't take me long to find clues to these numbers in his incredibly stressful life, which included a partnership in a high-powered firm and a host of domestic problems. Against his doctor's urging, Bill had discontinued his blood pressure medication because it made him dizzy and constipated. He wanted to try a more natural therapy, but it had to be done immediately.

I placed Bill on a Type A Diet—a huge adjustment for this burly Italian-American. And I immediately began to address Bill's stress with the exercise regimen designed for Type As. He was initially embarrassed about doing yoga and relaxation exercises, but was soon converted when he saw how much calmer and more positive he felt.

At his first visit, Bill also confided that he had a special problem of a different nature. He and his partners were in the process of negotiating their office health plan, and if his hypertension were detected at his insurance physical, his firm would have to pay a much higher premium. Using the stress-reduction techniques, the Type A Diet, and several botanicals, Bill was able to sail through his insurance physical.

Diabetes

The Blood Type Diets can be effective in the treatment of Type I (childhood) diabetes, and in both the treatment and prevention of Type II (adult) diabetes.

Blood Type A and Type B are more prone to Type I diabetes, caused by a lack of insulin, the hormone manufactured by the pancreas responsible for allowing glucose to enter the cells of the body. The cause of insulin deprivation is the destruction of the beta cells of the pancreas, which are the sole cells capable of producing insulin.

Although there is currently no effective natural-treatment alternative for injectable insulin-replacement therapy in Type I diabetics, one important natural remedy to consider using is quercetin, an antioxidant derived from plants. Quercetin has been shown to help prevent many of the complications stemming from lifelong diabetes, such as cataracts, neuropathy, and cardiovascular problems. Talk with a nutritionist who is skilled in the use of phytochemicals if you plan on using any natural medicine for diabetes; you may have to readjust your insulin dosage.

Type II diabetics typically have high levels of insulin in their bloodstreams, but their tissues lack sensitivity to insulin. This condition develops over time and is usually the result of a poor diet.

Type II diabetes is often observed in Type Os who have eaten dairy, wheat, and corn products for many years, and in Type As who eat a lot of meat and dairy foods. Type II diabetics are usually overweight and often have high cholesterol and elevated blood pressure—signs of a lifetime of poor food choices and lack of exercise. In this respect, any blood type can develop Type II diabetes.

The only real treatment for Type II diabetes is diet and exercise. Your Blood Type Diet and exercise regimen will achieve results if you stick to the guidelines. A high-potency vitamin B complex can also help to counter insulin intolerance. Again, check with a physician and nutritionist before using any substance to treat your diabetes. You might have to adjust the dosage of your diabetic medication.

Digestive Illnesses

Constipation

Constipation occurs when the stools are unusually hard or a person's bowel patterns have changed and become less frequent. Most chronic constipation is caused by poor bowel habits and irregular meals, with a diet low in bulk and water content. Some other causes are a habitual use of laxatives, a rushed and stressful daily schedule, and travel that requires abrupt adjustments of eating and sleeping patterns. Lack of physical exercise, acute illness, painful rectal conditions, and some medications also may cause constipation.

Every blood type is susceptible to constipation given the circumstances. Constipation is not so much a disease as a warning flare that something is not right with your digestive system. You'll find most of the clues in your diet.

Are you eating enough foods on your diet that are high in fiber content? Are you drinking enough fluids—in particular, water and juices? Are you exercising regularly?

Many people simply take a laxative when they're constipated. But that doesn't solve the natural systemic causes of constipation. The long-term solution is in the diet. However, Type A, Type B, and Type AB can supplement their diets with fibrous unprocessed bran. Type Os, in addition to eating plenty of the fibrous fruits and vegetables on their diets, can take a supplement of butyrate, a natural bulk-forming agent as a substitute for bran which is not advised for them.

Crohn's Disease and Colitis

These are depleting, enervating diseases that add the elements of uncertainty, pain, blood loss, and suffering to the process of elimination. Many food lectins can cause digestive irritation by attaching to the mucous membranes of the digestive tract. As many of the food lectins are blood type specific, it is possible for each blood type to develop the same problem from different foods.

In Type As and Type ABs, Crohn's disease and colitis often involve a major stress component. If you have Type A or Type AB blood and suffer from inflammatory bowel disease, pay careful attention to your stress patterns and refer to the discussion of stress in your Blood Type Plan.

Type Os tend to develop the more ulcerative form of colitis that causes bleeding with elimination. This is probably due to the lack of adequate clotting factors in their blood. Type As, Type ABs, and Type Bs tend to develop more of a mucous colitis, which is not as bloody. In either case, follow the diet for your blood type. You will be able to avoid many of the food lectins that can aggravate the condition, and you may find your symptoms easing.

CASE HISTORY: IRRITABLE BOWEL SYNDROME
Virginia, 26: Type O

I first examined Virginia, a twenty-six-year-old woman with chronic bowel trouble, three years ago, after she had received extensive treatment from a variety of conventional gastroenterologists. Her problems included chronic irritable bowel syndrome with painful constipation alternating with an unpredictable, almost explosive diarrhea that made it difficult for her to leave the house. She also suffered from fatigue and low-grade chronic anemia. Her previous doctors conducted an enormous amount of testing (to the tune of $27,000!) and could only suggest anti-spasmodic drugs and a daily dose of fiber. Food allergy testing was inconclusive. Virginia was a vegetarian who followed a strict macrobiotic diet, and I immediately detected the foods in her diet that were causing her suffering. The absence of meat in her diet was a primary factor. She also was unable to properly digest the grains and pasta she was eating as a main course.

Since Virginia was Type O, I suggested a high-protein diet, including lean red meats, fish and poultry, and fresh fruits and vegetables. As the digestive tract of Type O does not tolerate most grains very well, I suggested that she avoid whole wheat altogether and severely limit her consumption of other grains.

Initially, Virginia was resistant to the idea of making these dietary changes. She was a vegetarian and she believed that her current diet was truly healthier. But I urged her to look again. "How has this diet helped you, Virginia?" I asked. "You seem to be pretty sick."

Eventually, I convinced her to try it my way for a limited period of time. In eight weeks Virginia returned looking hale and hardy, with a ruddy complexion. She boasted that her bowel problems were 90 percent better. Blood tests showed a complete resolution of her anemia, and she said her energy levels were almost back to normal. A second follow-up visit one month later resulted in Virginia's being discharged from my care, completely free of bowel problems.

CASE HISTORY: CROHN'S DISEASE
Yehuda, 50: Type O

I first saw Yehuda, a middle-aged Jewish man, in July 1992 for active Crohn's disease. By that point he had already had several bowel surgeries to remove sections that were obstructing his small intestine. I put Yehuda on a wheat-free diet, with an emphasis on lean meats and boiled vegetables. I also gave him a high-powered extract of licorice and the fatty acid butyrate.

Yehuda's compliance was exemplary, a testament to the concerns both he and his family had for his health. For example, his wife, the daughter of a baker, baked him a special wheat-free bread. Yehuda took his supplements, including the licorice, very seriously, as he took everything else.

From the start, Yehuda consistently improved. To this day he continues to be asymptomatic, although he must still be careful about using certain grains and dairy products, as they bother his digestion.

He never required additional surgery, even though his gastroenterologist had earlier said it was inevitable.

Sarah, 35: Type B

Sarah was a thirty-five-year-old woman of eastern European ancestry. She first came to my office in June 1993 for treatment of Crohn's disease. She had already had several surgeries to remove scarred tissue from the bowel, was anemic, and suffered from chronic diarrhea.

I prescribed a basic Type B diet, instructing that Sarah remove chicken and other lectin-containing foods specific for Type B. I also used supplemental licorice and fatty acids as part of her protocol.

Sarah was very cooperative. Within four months, most of her digestive symptoms, including the diarrhea, were eliminated. As she wanted to have more children, Sarah recently had surgery to remove scar tissue from her bowel that had attached to her uterus. Her surgeon told her that there was no sign of active Crohn's disease anywhere in her abdominal cavity.

Food Poisoning

Anyone can get food poisoning. But certain blood types are naturally more susceptible because of their tendency toward a weakened immune system. In particular, Type A and Type AB are more likely to fall prey to salmonella food poisoning, which is usually the result of leaving food uncovered and unrefrigerated for long periods of time. Furthermore, the bacteria will be harder for Type A and Type AB to get rid of once they've found a home in their systems.

Type Bs, who are generally more susceptible to inflammatory diseases, are more likely to be severely affected when they eat food that is contaminated with the shigella organism, a bacteria found on plants that causes dysentery.

Gastritis

Many people confuse gastritis with ulcers, but it is exactly the opposite. Ulcers are produced by hyperacidity—more common for Type O and Type B. Gastritis is caused by very low stomach acid content—common for Type A and Type AB. Gastritis occurs when the stomach acid gets so low that it no longer functions as a microbial barrier. Without adequate levels of acid, microbes will live in the stomach and cause serious inflammation.

The best course of action that Type A and Type AB can take is to stress the more acidic food choices in their Blood Type Diets.

Stomach and Duodenal Ulcers

It has been known since the early 1950s that peptic ulcer of the stomach is more common in Blood Type O, with the highest occurrence in Type O non-secretors. Type Os also have a higher rate of bleeding and perforation, which was not shown to be different between secretors and non-secretors. One reason is that Type Os have higher stomach-acid levels and an ulcer-producing enzyme called pepsinogen.

More recent research has uncovered another reason why Type Os are prone to ulcers. In December 1993, researchers at Washington University School of Medicine in St. Louis reported in the *Journal of Science* that people with Type O blood are a favorite target for the bacteria now known to cause ulcers. This bacteria, *H. pylori*, was found to be able to attach itself to the Type O antigen lining the stomach, and then work its way into the lining. As we've seen, the Type O antigen is the sugar fucose. The researchers found an inhibitor in breast milk, which apparently blocked the attachment of the bacteria to the stomach surface. No doubt this is one of the many fucose sugars found in human breast milk.

The common seaweed bladder wrack is an inhibitor of *H. pylori*. The content of fucose in bladder wrack is so great that it factors into its Latin name—*Fucus vesiculosis*. If you are Type O and suffer from ulcers or want to prevent them, using bladder wrack will make the ulcer-causing bacteria, *H. pylori*, slide off your stomach lining.

CASE HISTORY: CHRONIC STOMACH ULCERS
Peter, 34: Type O

I first met Peter in April 1992. He had suffered from stomach ulcers since he was a child, and had used every conventional ulcer medication available, with little result. I began by prescribing the basic high-protein Type O Diet, stressing that he avoid the whole wheat products that had always been a major part of his diet. I also prescribed a supplement of bladder wrack, and a combination medicine of licorice and bismuth.

Within six weeks Peter had made considerable progress. On a follow-up visit to his gastroenterologist, he was "scoped" and heard the encouraging news that 60 percent of his stomach lining now appeared normal. A second examination in June 1993 showed complete resolution of Peter's stomach ulcers.

Infections

Many bacteria prefer specific blood types. In fact, one study showed that over 50 percent of 282 bacteria carried antigens of one blood type or another.

It has been observed that viral infections in general seem to be more frequent in Type Os because they do not possess any antigens. These infections are less frequent and milder in Type A, Type B and Type AB.

Acquired Immune Deficiency Syndrome (AIDS)

I have treated many people who were HIV positive or had full-blown AIDS, and I have yet to find a clear-cut connection between blood type and susceptibility to HIV. Having said that, let's look at how the information in this book can be used to help people hold their own against the virus.

While all the blood types appear to be equally susceptible to AIDS, given the exposure, there are variations in their susceptibility to the opportunistic infections (such as pneumonia and tuberculosis) to which their weakened immune systems fall prey.

If you are HIV positive or have AIDS, modify your diet to encompass the suggestions that are specific to your blood type. For example, if you are Type O, begin to increase the amount of animal proteins in your diet and develop a physical training program. Following the blood type program will help to fully mobilize and optimize your immune functions by stressing the highest-value foods for your particular needs. Be careful to limit your fat intake, choosing lean cuts of meat, because bowel parasites, common in people with AIDS, interfere with fat digestion and lead to diarrhea. Also avoid foods such as wheat that contain lectins that could further compromise your immune system and bloodstream.

Since many of the opportunistic infections cause nausea, diarrhea, and mouth sores, AIDS is often a wasting disease. Type As will need to work a little harder to be sure that their calorie intake is high, since many Type A foods are calorically low. Rigorously eliminate any foods, such as meat or dairy, that can cause digestive problems. Your immune system is already naturally sensitive; don't give the lectins a chance to get in and weaken you further. Meanwhile, increase your portions of "good" Type A foods, such as tofu and seafood.

Type Bs should avoid the obvious problem foods, such as chicken, corn, and buckwheat. But you should also eliminate nuts, which are hard to digest, and reduce the amount of wheat products in your diet. If you are lactose intolerant, avoid dairy foods; even if you're not, dairy can be a digestive irritant for immune-compromised Type Bs. This is a case where the disease is contraindicative of the favored food.

Type ABs should limit their intake of lectin-rich beans and legumes, and eliminate nuts from their diets. Your primary protein source should be fish, and there is a wide variety available to Type ABs. Occasional servings of meat and dairy are okay, but watch the fat. And limit your wheat consumption.

In general, whatever your blood type, you want to avoid lectins that could damage the cells of your immune system and bloodstream. These cells cannot be as easily replaced, the way they are in a healthy body. This cell-sparing aspect of the Blood Type Diets makes them invaluable to the person with AIDS who has anemia or low T-helper cells.

The Blood Type Diets add a powerful rook to your chessboard, helping preserve your precious immune cells from unnecessary damage. This can be a critical difference, especially as there are no really successful treatments for HIV infection.

Case History: AIDS
Arnold, 46: Type AB

Arnold was a middle-aged businessman with AIDS. He was married and believed he had been infected with HIV twelve years earlier. When I first saw him, Arnold's T-cell count, the barometer of the virus's destruction, was 6, with normal being 650 to 1,700. He had a skin condition called molluscum, which is often seen in end-stage AIDS, and he was painfully thin from months of diarrhea and nausea.

Arnold decided to come to a naturopath as a desperate, last-ditch effort to stay alive. I could see in his face that he didn't really believe this would work, either, and I couldn't promise him dramatic results because I didn't really know what to expect.

My first goal was to prevent any lectins that were toxic to the Type AB immune system from entering his body. Along with that, it was urgent that I halt Arnold's wasting so he would be strong enough to fight the infection.

I began by tailoring the Type AB Diet to the special needs raised by AIDS. This included the elimination of all poultry except turkey, the introduction of low-fat organic meats, seafood several times a week, rice, lots of vegetables and fruit. I reduced most of the beans and legumes, and eliminated butter, cream, processed cheese, corn, and buckwheat. In addition, I prescribed immune-boosting herbs, in tablet and tea form, including alfalfa, burdock, echinacea, ginseng, and ginger.

Within three months, Arnold's molluscum cleared up and he was back in the gym. To this day he continues to be asymptomatic, even though his T-cells have not increased. He works and leads a fairly active life. The physicians at the infectious disease center of his hospital are amazed. This is a man without an immune system!

Case History: AIDS
Susan, 27: Type O

After learning that her husband was HIV-positive, Susan was tested. She was frantic when she learned that she had HIV. Lab tests revealed a very low T-cell count. Susan begged me to help her; she didn't want to die, and she was afraid to take AZT or any other drug specified for HIV.

We began with a Type O Diet, along with nutritional supplements and regular exercise, instructing Susan to follow the program closely.

A few months later, Susan called to report that her T-cell count was in the 800s. She has been symptom free ever since.

Since there is at present no cure for HIV or AIDS, we can't gauge how long Susan will continue to do well. But I believe that the more we discover about the mysteries of the immune system, the closer we'll come to making AIDS a disease to live with, rather than a disease to die from.

Bronchitis and Pneumonia

In general, Type A and Type AB have more bronchial infections than Type O and Type B. This may result from improper diets that produce excessive mucus in their respiratory passages. This mucus facilitates the growth of blood type-mimicking bacteria, such as the A-like pneumococcus bacteria in Type A and Type AB, and the B-like hemophilus bacteria in Type B and Type AB. (Since Type AB has both A-like and B-like characteristics, the risk is double.)

The Blood Type Diets seem to substantially reduce the incidences of bronchitis and pneumonia for all blood types. However, we are just beginning to discover some other blood type connections that are not so easily remedied. For example, it appears that Type A children born to Type A fathers and Type O mothers die more frequently of broncho-pneumonia in early life. It is thought that some form of sensitization occurs at birth between the Type A infant and the mother's anti-A antibodies that inhibits the infant's ability to fight the pneumococcus bacteria. There is no solid data yet to confirm the reason this occurs, but information of this kind can spark research interest in a potential vaccine. We'll have to gather much more data before we can make a valid scientific conclusion.

Candidiasis (Common Yeast Infection)

Although the candidiasis organism shows no preference for blood type, I have noticed that Type A and Type AB have a tougher time eradicating a severe yeast overgrowth once the organism finds a home in their tolerant systems. Candidiasis becomes like the unwanted guest who won't leave. Type A and Type AB also develop more yeast infections after antibiotic usage, which makes sense, because antibiotics destroy their already weakened defense systems.

Type Os, on the other hand, develop more of an allergic-type hypersensitivity to the candidiasis organism, especially if they eat too many grains. This has been the basis of a theory called the yeast syndrome and a variety of candida diets. These diets stress high protein intake and the avoidance of grains, but they tend to be generalized across blood types, when it is only Type Os who appear to have this yeast sensitivity. If you're Type A or Type AB, yeast avoidance won't do anything to prevent yeast infections, and you'll only further compromise your immune system.

In general, Type Bs are less prone to this organism, as long as they follow the Type B Diet. If you are a Type B who has a history of candidiasis, cut down on your wheat consumption.

Cholera

A report from Peru recently published in the *Lancet* attributed the severity of a recent epidemic of cholera, an infection characterized by extreme diarrhea with severe fluid and mineral depletion, to the high incidence of Type Os in the Peruvian population. Historically, the susceptibility of Type Os to cholera was probably responsible for the decimation of the population of many of the ancient cities, leaving as survivors the more cholera-resistant Type As.

Common Cold and Flu

There are hundreds of different strains of cold virus, and it would be impossible to see blood type specificity in all of them. However, studies of British military recruits showed a slightly lower overall incidence of cold viruses in recruits who were Type A, which is consistent with our findings that Blood Type A was developed to resist these common viruses. Viruses also have less impact on Type AB. The A antigen, carried by both Type A and Type AB, blocks the attachment of various strains of flu to the membranes of the throat and respiratory passages.

Influenza, a more serious virus, also strikes Type O and Type B in preference to Type A and Type AB. In its early stages, influenza may have many of the symptoms of a common cold. However, the flu causes dehydration, muscle pains, and serious weakness.

The symptoms of a common cold or flu are miserable, but they are actually a sign that your immune system is trying hard to fight off the offending virus. While your immune system is doing its job, there are measures you can take that will make coexistence on the battlefield more comfortable:

1. Maintain general good health with adequate rest and exercise, along with learning to cope with the stresses of life. Stress is a major factor in the depletion of immune system resources. This may protect you from frequent infections and may even shorten the duration of the colds and flus you do get.
2. Follow the basic dietary protocol for your blood type. It will optimize your immune response and help shorten the course of your cold or flu.
3. Take vitamin C (250 to 500 mg), or increase the sources of vitamin C in your diet. Many people feel that taking small doses of the herb echinacea helps prevent colds, or at least helps shorten their duration.
4. Increase the humidity in your room with a vaporizer or humidifier to prevent a dry throat and nasal tissue.
5. If your throat is sore, gargle with salt water. One-half teaspoon of ordinary table salt and a tall glass of comfortably warm water provides a soothing and cleansing rinse. Another good gargle, especially if you are prone to tonsilitis, is a tea of equal parts goldenseal root *(Hydrastis canadensis)* and sage. Gargle with this mixture every few hours.
6. If your nose is runny or stuffy, use an antihistamine to reduce the reaction of tissues to the infecting virus and relieve nasal congestion. Be especially careful with Ephedra-type antihistamines, such as those found in health food stores and in some over-the-counter decongestants. These can raise the blood pressure, keep you awake at night, and complicate prostate problems in men.

7. Antibiotics are not effective against viruses, so if someone offers you leftover antibiotics, or if you have some around the house, don't take them.

Skin Disorders

To date, there is little blood type-specific information available on skin disorders. We do know, however, that conditions such as dermatitis and psoriasis usually result from allergic chemicals acting within the blood. It is worth noting again that many of the common food lectins specific for one blood type or another can interact with the blood and digestive tissues, causing the liberation of histamines and other inflammatory chemicals.

Allergic skin reactions to chemicals or abrasives show the highest incidences in Type A and Type AB. Psoriasis is found more frequently in Type Os. My own experience is that many Type Os who develop psoriasis are eating diets too high in grains or dairy products.

CASE HISTORY: PSORIASIS
From Anne Marie Lambert, N.D., Honolulu, Hawaii
Mariel, 66: Type O

My colleague Dr. Lambert used my blood type protocol to treat a complicated case of psoriasis in an older woman.

Mariel went to see Dr. Lambert in March 1994. Her symptoms included severe shortness of breath, difficulty walking, with limited range of motion in all joints, psoriasis lesions covering 70 percent of her skin surface, and burning pain throughout her body, especially in her muscles and joints. Her medical history was a catalog of constant medical problems: vaginal/bladder/bowel repairs (1944–45), appendectomy (1949), hysterectomy (1974), history of ovarian cysts, psoriasis (1978), hospitalization for pneumonia (1987), psoriatic arthritis (1991), and osteoporosis (1992).

Mariel told Dr. Lambert that her typical diet was high in dairy, wheat, corn, nuts and processed foods, with a high sugar and fat content. She said that she craved sweets, nuts, and bananas. This was a terrible diet for almost anyone, but it was anathema to some-one of Mariel's blood type.

Dr. Lambert immediately started Mariel on a moderated Type O Diet, which initially excluded red meat and nuts, with additional vitamins and minerals. Within two months, there was a marked decrease in swelling of Mariel's joints, improved breathing, and her psoriatic lesions were healing. By June, Mariel's psoriasis covered only 20 percent of her body, and the lesions were nearly healed. There was a marked improvement in her breathing, her pain had lessened by half, and the range of motion in her joints continued to improve. By July, Mariel's psoriasis was no longer evident, there was only slight swelling in the joint spaces, and her breathing was no longer labored.

At a follow-up visit to Dr. Lambert on October 10, 1994, Mariel's breathing had improved, and she had no new lesions on her skin.

Mariel had been to numerous medical professionals since she became ill. She had tried all types of conventional as well as alternative therapies, including food plans specifically designed for psoriatic arthritis and asthma. Although these diets were well intended, none of them was specifically tailored to ensure compatibility with Mariel's blood. The Type O Diet was able to provide nutrition without causing health problems from foods that were incompatible with Mariel's blood. With the exception of some minor pain relief from Chinese herbs, none of the other treatments had been successful. Mariel considered her progress a miracle!

Women/Reproduction

Pregnancy and Infertility

Many of the disorders related to pregnancy result from some form of blood type incompatibility—either between the mother and the fetus, or between the mother and the father. Unfortunately, we have only initial studies on this phenomenon, and have little idea about its ultimate implications. I suggest that you read this section in the spirit of information gathering, not hysteria. Sometimes a little bit of knowledge can be dangerous unless you keep it in perspective.

TOXEMIA OF PREGNANCY

As early as 1905 it was proposed that some form of blood type sensitization resulted in pregnancy toxemia—a poisoning of the blood that can occur in late pregnancy and cause grave illness and even death. In a later study, an excess of Type O women were found to suffer from toxemia, resulting possibly from a reaction to a Type A or Type B fetus.

BIRTH DEFECTS

Blood type incompatibility, which may occur between a Type O mother and a Type A father, has been implicated in several common birth defects, including hydatiform mole, choriocarcinoma, spinal bifida, and anencephaly. Several studies imply that these disorders appear to be maternal ABO incompatibility with fetal nervous and blood tissue.

HEMOLYTIC DISEASE OF THE NEWBORN

Hemolytic (blood-destroying) disease of the newborn is the primary condition related to the positive/negative aspect of your blood (see the back of this book). It is a condition that afflicts only the offspring of Rh– women, so if you are O, A, B, or AB positive, it doesn't concern you.

Some fifty years ago, researchers discovered that Rh– women who were missing an antigen and who were carrying Rh+ babies had a unique situation. The Rh+ babies carried the Rh antigen on their blood cells. As is not the case with the major blood type system where the antibodies to other blood types develop from birth, Rh– people do not make an antibody to the Rh antigen unless they are first sensitized. This sensitization usually occurs when blood is exchanged between the mother and infant during birth, so the mother's immune system does not have enough time to react to the first baby, and that baby suffers no consequences. However, should a subsequent conception result in another Rh+ baby, the mother, now sensitized, will produce antibodies to the baby's blood type, potentially causing birth defects and even infant death. Fortunately, there is a vaccine for this condition which is given to Rh– women after the birth of their first child, and after every subsequent birth.

It shouldn't arise as a problem, but it's best to know your Rh status so you can be certain that the vaccine is administered.

INFERTILITY AND HABITUAL MISCARRIAGE

For forty years, scientists have been studying the reasons why childlessness seems more common among Type A, Type B, and Type AB women than Type O women. Many researchers have suggested that infertility and habitual abortion may be the result of antibodies in a woman's vaginal secretions reacting with blood type antigens on her husband's sperm. A 1975 study of 288 miscarried fetuses showed a predominance of Type A, Type B and Type AB fetuses, which may have been the result of incompatibility with Type O mothers and their anti-A and anti-B antibodies.

A large sample of families showed that the rate of miscarriages were highest when the mother and father were ABO incompatible, as with a Type O mother and a Type A father. In Caucasian and African mothers, Type B fetuses incompatible with the mother's Type O or Type A blood were more frequently found among miscarriages.

This link to infertility is not yet fully established. In my own practice, I find that there are many reasons for fertility problems, including food allergies, poor diet, obesity, and stress.

CASE HISTORY: REPEATED MISCARRIAGE
Lana, 42: Type A

Lana came to my office in September 1993 after a long history of repeated miscarriages. She told me she'd heard about me from someone she had been talking with in the waiting room of her fertility doctor. Lana was desperate. In the previous ten years she'd had over twenty miscarriages, and she was just about to give up on trying to start a family. I suggested that she try the Blood Type A Diet. For the next year, Lana followed the Blood Type Diet assiduously, also taking several botanical preparations to strengthen the muscular tone of her uterus. At the end of the year, she became pregnant. She was thrilled, but also very nervous. Now, in addition to her previous miscarriages, Lana was worried about her age and the possibility of the fetus having Down's syndrome. Her obstetrician recommended amniocentesis, which is common for women over age forty, but I advised against it because the procedure carries a risk of miscarriage. After talking with her husband, Lana decided to forgo the amniocentesis, accepting the possibility of a birth defect. In January 1995, she delivered a perfectly healthy baby boy.

CASE HISTORY: INFERTILITY
Nieves, 44: Type B

Nieves, a forty-four-year-old South American massage therapist, first came to see me in 1991 for a variety of digestive problems. Within one year of beginning the Type B Diet, most of her digestive complaints were resolved.

One day Nieves shyly announced to me that she was pregnant. Although she had not told me before, she now said that she and her husband had tried for many years to conceive a child, but had finally given up hope. She believed that the Type B Diet was responsible for restoring her fertility. Approximately nine months later, Nieves delivered a healthy baby girl. She was named Nasha, meaning "gift from God."

NOTE: SEX RATIOS

In both European and non-European populations, the rate of male offspring is higher in Type O babies born to Type O mothers. This is also true if both the baby and mother are Type B. The opposite is true of Type A babies born to Type A mothers, where female offspring are more frequent.

Menopause and Menstrual Problems

Menopause affects every midlife woman regardless of her blood type. A decrease in estrogen and progesterone, the two basic female hormones, causes profound mental and physical problems for many women, including hot flashes, loss of libido, depression, hair loss, and skin changes.

The decline in female hormones also creates a risk for cardiovascular disease, as it appears that estrogen provides protection to the heart and lowers cholesterol levels. Osteoporosis, a thinning of the bones that leads to frailty and even death, is another outcome of estrogen deficiency.

With our newfound understanding of the risks associated with hormone depletion, many doctors prescribe hormone-replacement therapy, involving high doses of estrogen and sometimes progesterone. Many women are concerned about conventional estrogen-replacement therapy because some studies show a greater risk of breast cancer in women who use these hormones—primarily when there is a family history of breast cancer. The question of whether or not to take these synthetic hormones is a dilemma.

Knowing your blood type may help you to resolve the conflict and decide which approach is best for your own personal needs.

If you are Type O or Type B and entering menopause, begin to exercise in a manner recommended for your blood type, and in a way appropriate to your current fitness and lifestyle. Eat a high-protein diet. Conventional estrogen replacement generally works reasonably well for Type O and Type B women, unless you have high-risk factors for breast cancer.

If you are Type A or Type AB, you should avoid using conventional estrogen replacement, because of your unusually high susceptibility to breast cancer. Instead, use the newly available phytoestrogens, which are estrogen- and progesterone-like preparations derived from plants, principally soybeans, alfalfa, and yams. Many of these preparations are available as a cream that can be applied to the skin several times a day. Plant phytoestrogens are typically high in the estrogen fraction called estriol, whereas chemical estrogens are based on estradiol. The medical literature conclusively shows that supplementation with estriol inhibits the occurrence of breast cancer.

Phytoestrogens lack the potency of the chemical estrogens, but they are definitely effective against many of the troubling symptoms of menopause, including hot flashes and vaginal dryness. Because they are only weak estrogens, they will not suppress any estrogen production by the body, unlike the chemical estrogen. For the woman who is not taking any estrogen supplementation because of a family history of breast cancer, phytoestrogens are a godsend. Talk to your gynecologist about using these preparations. If you have no special risk factors for breast cancer, the stronger chemical estrogen is more effective for reducing heart disease and osteoporosis, in addition to the symptoms of menopause.

It is interesting that in Japan, where the typical diet is high in phytoestrogens, there is no concise Japanese word for menopause. Undoubtedly the widespread use of soy products, which contain the phytoestrogens genestein and diaziden, serves to modulate the severe symptoms of menopause.

CASE HISTORY: MENSTRUAL PROBLEMS
Patty, 45: Type O

Patty was a forty-five-year-old African-American woman with a variety of problems, including arthritis, high blood pressure, and severe premenstrual syndrome with heavy bleeding. I first met Patty in December 1994, when she came to my office accompanied by her husband. At the time, she was being treated by one drug or another for her ailments. I learned that Patty had been consuming a basically vegetarian diet, so it was no surprise that she was also anemic. I recommended that she begin exercising, adopt the Type O high-protein diet, and prescribed a course of botanical medicines.

Within two months, Patty made an astounding turnabout. Arthritis: cured. Hypertension: under control. PMS: last two periods, all symptoms gone. Menstrual flow: normal.

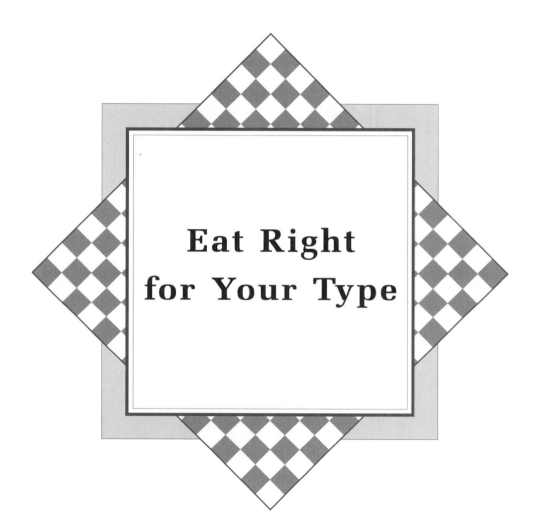

PART IV

Eat Right
for Your Type

Getting Started

From Theory to Table

ONE OF THE MAIN REASONS PEOPLE GET TURNED OFF TO diets is that the plans are so often cloaked in righteousness. There's a "my way or the highway" tone to them that leaves people jittery and afraid to diverge even the tiniest bit for fear of falling off their imaginary wagon.

I believe that the right dietary program is one that you grow into, not one that you jump into all in one day. It should feel comfortable and right, not like a straitjacket. That's one of the reasons I stay away from rigid calorie counts or complicated equations to determine the percentage of protein, fat, and carbohydrates in your diet. The portion sizes are likewise just broad recommendations. There will always be individual variations according to your height, weight, age, physical condition, and the availability of food. It is not my goal to strangle you with a diet. In order for you to truly eat the way nature intended, it has to feel natural. That can take time— and it certainly involves some flexibility.

If you have tried other diet plans—and most of you have—you're probably used to the feeling that something terrible will happen if you "go off" your diet. I can't tell you how many times people have contacted me in desperation because they have encountered a situation that is completely incompatible with the Blood Type Diet. I once had a woman call me, frantic, because she was going to her best friend's wedding and was worried about what would happen if she ate a piece of wedding cake. My answer was, "Well, I suppose you'll enjoy it." This is typical of the terrible anxiety people feel about food. Since anxiety is very bad for digestion, I don't encourage it. The fact is, if you're generally healthy, you can be flexible when the occasion demands it. Chances are, armies of lectins won't march in and destroy your fortress. I am a Type A who happens to love tofu. I've eaten it all my life. But about once every year or so I get a terrible craving for my wife Martha's stuffed cabbage with ground meat. And I don't feel guilty about the indulgence.

The point is, it's great if you are truly committed to the Blood Type Diet. But life is too short to worry about the pinch of cinnamon that's the eighth ingredient in your favorite recipe.

If You're New to the Blood Type Diet

You may be eager to dive right into the diet that fits your blood type. But before you sweep your kitchen clean of any and all offending foods and go on a Highly Beneficial binge, take some time to learn what this diet is all about. The best way to introduce yourself to the Blood Type Diet is to follow these steps over a period of time:

1. Read the beginning chapters of this book thoroughly and don't just skip to the section about your own blood type. You can't understand the Type B factors unless you also understand the historical context—the evolutionary process that has contributed to the role blood type plays in every person's diet. And that's true for Types O, A, and AB, too. I know that people often follow diets that seem arbitrary to them. They're told, "Eat this, don't eat that," and they follow it to the letter. Maybe they get results; maybe they don't. But in the long run, nobody will abide by a method that doesn't live in their head and heart.

2. Begin by adding foods to your diet from the Highly Beneficial list. Take a look at the foods that have a positive medicinal effect on your blood type. Start incorporating into your diet foods you are not already eating.

3. Start exercising for your blood type. Exercise is a critical component of the Blood Type Diet. Briefly, the recommendations are: Type

O—intense physical exercise such as aerobics or jogging; Type A—calming, tension-relieving exercises such as yoga, walking, and Tai Chi; Type B—moderate activities such as hiking, cycling, and martial arts; and Type AB—the same calming exercises as Type A. It has been demonstrated that the combination of eating Highly Beneficial foods and doing the appropriate exercise makes a very big difference for beginners.

4. Begin to eliminate foods from your Avoid list. Start looking for natural replacements for your Avoid foods. For example, a Type A who is accustomed to eating meat can start by replacing meat with fish and substituting chicken for beef or lamb. Your goal should be to gradually replace the Avoid items with Highly Beneficial and Neutral foods. When you read the descriptions of the interactions between certain foods and your blood type, you'll discover that some food lectins are particularly potent. Try to eliminate these first.

At the Market

You don't have to be a food scientist or carry a gram counter or calculator when you go to the market. Simply focus on selecting the freshest foods in their most natural state. And use your knowledge of basic nutritional principles. Here are a few tips:

Avoid heavily fatted meats. Free-range poultry and meats have been raised without the excessive use of antibiotics and other chemicals, and they're recommended for the Blood Type Diet. *Free range* means just that—that animals haven't been penned in. Once you try free-range meat or poultry, you'll see the difference. The flesh is leaner, the color and texture are richer, and there is very little fat. It's possible to raise red meats that have fat and cholesterol levels that are closer to those of the leaner poultry, but the meat may be less tender and flavorful by modern standards. The giant agribusinesses are still locked into the traditional notion that consumers want rich, high-fat meats. Our ancestors consumed rather lean game or domestic animals that grazed on alfalfa and other grasses. Today's meats are corn-fed, kept healthy with antibiotics, and prized for the tenderness of their meat and the marbling of their fat. Fortunately, some

Blood Type-Priority Checklist

There are many reasons why people are not able to follow their Blood Type Diet completely. I am often asked, "If I could do just two or three things to make a difference in my diet, what would they be?" Here are some suggestions. They might also be helpful for those who are just getting started.

TYPE O: Begin eating small portions of lean red meat three to four times a week. Eliminate wheat.

TYPE A: Replace meat with vegetable protein, supplemented with fish. Add more beans and grains to your diet.

TYPE B: Start eating dairy foods several times a week and eliminate chicken.

TYPE AB: Make seafood, tofu, and small quantities of meat, such as lamb and turkey, your staples. Avoid chicken, corn, and most beans.

ALL BLOOD TYPES: Eat organic meat, poultry, vegetables, and fruit. If you can't afford to do that, start with meat and poultry, and wash your vegetables and fruit thoroughly. Exercise right for your blood type.

---

businesses are beginning to respond to the growing demand for lean, organic meat. If your market hasn't caught on to the trend, be sure to let the manager know.

Fresh fish is fairly simple to identify. Look at the eyes. If they are clear and reflective, the fish is probably fresh. Pull the gills out from back of the head. They should be bright red or dark pink. If the skin is slimy to the touch, or the fish has any kind of off odor or fishy smell, it is not fresh.

Try to avoid the canned-foods aisles. Commercially canned foods are subjected to high heat and pressure, and they lose a great deal of their vitamin content, especially the antioxidants, such as vitamin C. They do retain the vitamins that are not heat sensitive, such as vitamin A. Canned foods are usually lower in fiber and higher in salt. The salt is added to boost the flavor lost during production. Few of the natural enzymes remain; for the most part, they're destroyed by the canning process.

Other than fresh, frozen foods are your best bet, since freezing doesn't alter the nutritional content of the food very much. The quality and variety of frozen foods have improved greatly in just the last few years. New processing methods and new freezing methods allow foods to be kept as close to fresh as possible. Whole lines of organic and vegetarian foods are now being offered commercially, making it easier than ever before to bring a wide variety of items to the consumer's table that might have been difficult to find before. Still, I'm an old-fashioned guy. My favorite foods are still fresh foods!

Stay Smart About Safety

According to a March 10, 1998, *New York Times* report, the federal government is being urged by health officials to undertake new and comprehensive efforts to detect cases of illness caused by contaminated foods and to prevent future outbreaks.

The National Center for Health Statistics reported that food-borne illnesses are among the leading reasons for emergency-room visits each year. As an example, it was estimated that in a one-year period between 1996 and 1997, the state of Minnesota's 4.4 million residents suffered 6.1 million diarrheal illnesses.

Although there are no firm numbers regarding the consumption of unsafe foods, botulism, staphylococcus, and toxoplasmosis are among the more common examples of fish-related contamination. Viral hepatitis, caused by fecal contamination, unsafe mercury levels, and high levels of PCBs are potential hazards of eating foods from polluted water supplies. As with any animal product, bacterial and parasitic contamination are always possible. Alarmingly, fish is not subject to the same level of federal inspection as meat and poultry. Rather, a voluntary program of inspection is maintained by wholesale distributors and processors. It wasn't until 1991 that the Food and Drug Administration created a unit to monitor the safety of seafood!

Although the United States has long been touted as having the world's safest and least expensive food supply, it is becoming less so. A tremendous amount of our nation's food supply pours in from countries without even the minimal safeguards we employ to ensure food safety. An increasing number of food-borne illnesses, in fact, closely resemble what was once considered classic traveler's diarrhea. In other words, Montezuma's Revenge no longer requires luggage, merely a trip to the local supermarket.

Don't assume that you can relax your guard when you shop in a health-food store. Many health-food stores, especially the smaller ones, do not have the rapid turnover of a busy greengrocer or supermarket. Check the "sell by" dates on every package.

Know Your Organics

Commercial markets are stocking organic produce on a regular basis, a fairly recent innovation. Most of the organic produce and fruits are from California, a state with specific laws concerning the use of the word *organic*. In some markets, organic vegetables and fruits are displayed side by side with the nonorganic produce. In many instances, they're priced identically! I suspect that market demand will continue to push more and more vegetable and fruit growers back to the organic methods of cultivation. The cost of commercial fertilizers and pesticides will eventually make the nonorganic produce more expensive to grow. Despite the old pro and con arguments about the use of pesticides, it simply comes down to this piece of common sense: No amount of pesticides, however small, has ever been discovered to be beneficial to the human body. Conversely, it is best to remember that organic fruits and vegetables bruise easily and spoil rapidly. Many areas of the world couldn't sustain sufficient levels of food production at this point without using pesticides. That's the paradox.

Pragmatically, a good rule of thumb is to purchase organic vegetables in preference to nonorganic vegetables if they're not exorbitantly priced. They taste better and are healthier for you. However, if you don't have a lot of money to spend and can't find reasonably priced organic produce, improvise. Fresh, high-quality nonorganic produce will be fine. The important thing is to eat plenty of fruits and vegetables. Organic or commercial, the valuable nutrients are there for the eating.

Make Your Kitchen
Blood-Type Friendly

You'll find it easier and more convenient to stock your kitchen with the staples that are right for your type. If you have more than one blood type in your household, mark your bins and containers accordingly.

In the Kitchen

Preparing Fish and Meats

Most of the nutritional value of food can be lost by improper preparation. This is especially true of high-protein animal foods such as meats and fish. I ask those of my patients who eat meat as part of their Blood Type Diet to take a couple of extra steps before cooking any meats. First, I ask them to remove any excess skin or fat from the meat. Second, boil water in a pot large enough to hold the meat, turn off the heat, and just let the meat soak in the water three to five minutes. I know this sounds distressing. Won't the meat be ruined? Actually, this won't alter the flavor or texture, but it will remove any chemicals that have resulted from the oxidation of the meat's surface. It will also kill any bacteria that may have developed from improper handling. A caution, however: If the piece of meat you're treating is at all suspect in terms of freshness, placing it in the hot water won't make it any more edible. If meat is spoiled or tainted in any way, discard it. The same treatment should be given to fish.

Frying, Smoking, Curing, Pickling

Fried, smoked, cured, or pickled meats or fish should be avoided by all blood types. Although many cultures favor the flavors produced by deep frying, dangerous carcinogens are produced in the process. The effects of eating fried foods on the heart and cardiovascular system are well documented.

Smoked or cured meats and fish, such as cold cuts, hot dogs, ham, and bacon as well as smoked salmon and pickled herring, contain undesirable levels of nitrates and nitrites as well as high levels of sodium. Nitrates have been linked to stomach cancer, a disease which Type Os, Type As, and Type ABs are prone to: Type O because of high stomach-acid levels, and Type A and Type AB because of their low stomach acid.

Stir-Frying

Stir-frying is a lot healthier than deep frying. Certainly less oil is used. The concept of stir-frying involves cooking food at a high temperature in a searingly hot pan. This quickly seals in the foods' flavors in a crisply textured manner. Meat, fish, tofu, and vegetables can be stir fried using a deep, cone-shaped wok, designed to concentrate the heat in a small area at its base. This allows small amounts of food to be cooked there and then moved to the cooler upper edges of the pan. Cook the meats and vegetables that require a longer time first, then move them to the upper edges of the pan. Then add the vegetables that require less cooking to the base of the wok. The idea is to keep all of the food hot and cooking, but at different times and at different degrees. Skillful stir-frying can add a lot of taste and enjoyment to a few vegetables and a little meat, fish, or tofu.

Broiling, Poaching, Parboiling, and Baking

Broiling generates some carcinogenic materials, but it is generally healthier than frying. If meats are lean and the cooking time is limited to simply "browning" the surface, it should not cause any problems. Baking, poaching, and parboiling are safe methods of cooking that are usually best used for foods such as fish filets or eggs, which require only a short amount of time to cook thoroughly.

Steaming

Steaming is the most delicious way I know to prepare a host of vegetables. It's a quick and effective method of cooking that keeps the nutrients in the food. Boiling leaves most of the nutrients in the water. A simple steamer basket can be purchased at most supermarkets and at almost any hardware or department store. The basket sits inside a large pot filled with a shallow amount of water below the level of the basket. Add vegetables, cover, and heat. Crisp broccoli takes about five or six minutes; Brussels sprouts a while longer. The most important thing to remember about steaming is that all of the nutrients in the vegetable find their way to you. None of the flavor or goodness of the food is lost in the cooking process. The food has merely been made more assimilable.

Pots, Pans, Utensils

It can be dangerous to use the wrong kind of pot or pan for cooking. Never use decorative-type pots and pans for cooking, such as copper or pewter pans. Some are made of a mixture of lead and silver, toxic metals that can leach into the food during the cooking process. Also be especially careful with ceramic pots. Make sure the glazes and paints are free of lead. Porcelain, Corning-type glassware, and enameled surfaces are fine for cooking.

Cast-iron skillets, which allow small amounts of iron to get into the food, are generally safe, and probably provided an important source of iron in the old days. Make sure that any rust or corrosion that has built up on the surface of the pan is thoroughly removed with an abrasive, such as steel wool.

Aluminum cookware is very inexpensive and still commonly used and sold. I believe there's a real potential health problem with using aluminum for cooking. Aluminum is not easily removed from the body, and the one characteristic common to all people who suffer from Alzheimer's disease is that they have an inordinately high accu-

TOOL	ALTERNATIVES	USES	ADVANTAGES
Set of mixing bowls			
Small & large colanders			
Blender	Food processor		
Bread machine (2-lb.)			
Food processor	Blender	Drinks Sauces Dressings	

mulation of aluminum in their brain tissue. Aluminum is a soft metal that is easily transferred to food by spoons and ladles made of harder metals. Aluminum also reacts with acids in the foods, which can result in the binding and loss of vitamin C content.

Stainless steel is your safest choice for pots and pans. The metal is hard and virtually inert. In other words, none of it will transfer to your food during the cooking process. Some stainless-steel cookware is "aluminum-clad" on the bottom to create a surface that acts as a heat conductor. This is fine, as the aluminum is bonded to the outside of the pot and cannot react with the food inside. Most Teflon-coated cooking surfaces eventually become scratched unless you are careful about washing and drying. If you do use Teflon-coated cookware, always use soft plastic tools when cooking to avoid scratching the surface. Some of the latest Teflon-like surfaces are harder and therefore much safer.

At the Table

There's more to eating than the food you put into your system. The digestive process is truly holistic. You might be surprised about the elements that have a practical impact on the way your body utilizes foods. To make the most of your meal, heed the following:

1. Don't drink with your meal.

The first time Martha visited my father's house before we were married, she was surprised to find no water glasses on the table. My father discovered many years ago that consuming liquids with food dilutes the digestive juices. You'll notice that we include beverages with the blood type menus. However, try to drink them separately from the meal itself. For example, have a glass of wine a half hour before dinner and drink your tea or coffee a half hour after dinner.

2. Leave your tension at the door.

According to a Roman proverb, the secret to healing is "Dr. Diet, Dr. Quiet, and Dr. Happy." If you eat when you're nervous or tense, your stress hormones produce too many digestive juices, which leads to heartburn and acid stomach. The dinner hour is not the time to discuss Johnny's failing report card.

3. Stop talking.

In addition to the obvious connection between talking and stress, there's a very practical reason why meals should be silent. When you talk, you tend to swallow large amounts of air, and that causes gas. Talking also interferes with the chewing process, and food must be well chewed in order to be digested properly. The old parental reminder "Don't talk with your mouth full" is a good rule of thumb, and not just for etiquette reasons.

4. Chew your food.

People who bolt down their food as if they're in some kind of contest deprive themselves of one of life's greatest pleasures—eating and enjoying the flavors, aromas, colors, and textures of their food. The importance of mastication—using your teeth, lips, gums, and mouth to thoroughly chew and break down whatever it is that you're eating—can't be emphasized enough. Because the secretion of gastric juices is initiated by the sense of taste, chewing thoroughly and keeping the food in your mouth long enough to fully extract its full

> ## Understanding Food Combining
>
> When you can, try to keep meats and seafood away from dense starches, such as potatoes and grains. Combining starches and proteins is a favorite of many people, especially in the form of sandwiches, which are a quick, convenient, and portable meal. It's okay to eat sandwiches sometimes—we even offer some delicious and healthy variations in this book.
>
> The word *sandwich* originated with Lord Sandwich, an English noble who asked that his meat be placed between two pieces of bread, so that he could remain at the gambling table. Are you using this sort of thinking to decide what to eat? Stuffing a sandwich down your throat during a fifteen-minute lunch break almost guarantees a feeling of lethargy. It's also a quick path to gas, bloating, and other intestinal problems. Paying attention to which foods you eat together is important, as proteins and carbohydrates digest at different rates.

flavor helps prepare the stomach for proper digestion. This is also why foods should be eaten in their natural state. Digestive enzymes react only on the surface of food particles, not on their interior, so the rate of digestion depends upon the total surface area exposed to gastric and intestinal secretions. The more you chew the food, the greater the surface area, and the more effective the digestion throughout the gastrointestinal tract. This, in turn, increases the ease with which food is passed from the stomach to the small intestines and other areas of the body, thereby placing less strain on the digestive system.

If your diet includes meats and seafood, you must take the time to thoroughly chew them, even up to thirty times per bite. Because starches such as bread, potatoes, and fruit begin the process of digestion right in the mouth, they need to be thoroughly chewed to facilitate that breakdown. In addition to expediting proper digestion, thorough chewing also eases elimination because it warms the food, and this accelerates the catalytic activities of the enzymes. Swallowing cold foods whole slows the digestive process by inhibiting the proper secretion of enzymes.

The recipes and menus that we have developed for you reinforce the philosophy that eating well is a restorative, energizing, and almost mystical experience. Let's all eat in happiness and good health.

A Few Words About the Recipes That Follow

The recipes in the following chapters are delicious, healthy, imaginative, and right for your blood type. For those who fear that the Blood Type Diet will deprive them of the pure pleasure of eating wonderful foods, these recipes will put their minds at ease. They've been prepared by professional chefs Martine Lloyd Warner and Gabrielle Sindorf. Treat the recipes as suggestions, and invent your own variations.

Each recipe is keyed to blood type. Refer to the box at the top of each recipe. Read the key this way:

- Highly Beneficial indicates that the primary ingredients are Highly Beneficial for your type. Minor ingredients may be either Highly Beneficial or Neutral. There are no Avoid ingredients.
- Neutral indicates that the primary ingredients are Neutral for your type. Minor ingredients may be either Neutral or Highly Beneficial. There are no Avoid ingredients.
- Avoid indicates that there are ingredients in the recipe that your type should avoid.

HIGHLY BENEFICIAL		NEUTRAL		AVOID	

The recipes in this section include every food category on your blood type list. There is truly something for everyone.

Meat and Poultry

Quick Main Dishes

THE MOST DELICIOUS—AND HEALTHY—WAY TO EAT MEAT is very lean (trimmed of visible fat), and cooked simply, alone or with vegetables. When you don't have time to cook an elaborate meal, meat is also quick and easy. These recipes include both everyday and special-occasion meals that recapture what we all loved so much about meat and poultry in simpler times.

Try to find an organic source. Most commercially produced meats and poultry are raised on feed that is laced with chemical residues from pesticides, herbicides, and fertilizers. The animals are also fed hormones to increase their rate of growth. There is an enormous effort taking place to produce healthy, relatively pure food, but those efforts need the support of consumers. The greater the demand for organic meat and poultry, the greater the quantity available and the lower the prices.

BEEF BRISKET

HIGHLY BENEFICIAL	O	NEUTRAL	B	AVOID	A, AB

A warming fall and winter dinner. Try adding six yellow onions, the size of your fist, for the last hour of cooking. They add a pleasant savory flavor.

2 tablespoons olive oil
2- to 3-lb. brisket
1 onion, diced
2 cups red wine
4 cloves garlic, crushed and
    peeled

1 teaspoon dried thyme
3 bay leaves
2 cups boiling water
salt

- Heat oil in a heavy casserole pan over low heat. Add brisket and brown on both sides.
- Add onion and cook several minutes, until golden.
- Add wine and bring to a boil. Reduce heat and simmer 20 minutes.
- Add garlic, thyme, bay leaves, and boiling water and bring to a boil again.
- Reduce heat and simmer 3 hours, turning meat once or twice, until done. Add salt to taste. Brisket needs plenty of time to get tender. *Serves 8.*

CHICKEN PAPRIKA

HIGHLY BENEFICIAL	AB	NEUTRAL	A, B	AVOID	O

This satisfying recipe is perfect for cooler weather. Type B and Type AB should substitute turkey for the chicken in this recipe.

2 tablespoons olive oil
1 large yellow onion, diced
paprika
1 chicken, cut into 8 pieces
1 to 2 cups water or chicken
    (turkey) stock

salt
spelt flour
8 oz. sour cream (if too rich,
    try substituting some
    drained yogurt)

- Heat oil in a large skillet and sauté onion until golden. Sprinkle paprika liberally over onion and stir to cook paprika; do not scorch.
- Push onions to side of pan and add chicken. Allow chicken to color on one side, then turn and spoon onions over top of chicken. Allow to color on other side.
- When chicken parts are a rich red color, add water or stock and bring to a boil. Add salt to taste, reduce heat, and simmer 45 minutes, or until chicken is thoroughly cooked.
- Transfer chicken and sauce to a bowl and add 2 to 3 tablespoons flour to the skillet. Slowly pour the liquid from chicken back into the skillet, stirring constantly until thickened.
- Add sour cream or yogurt and stir. Return chicken or turkey to pan and heat thoroughly. Do not boil.
- Serve over noodles or rice.   *Serves 4 to 8.*

ITALIAN CHICKEN

HIGHLY BENEFICIAL		NEUTRAL	O, A	AVOID	B, AB

An uncomplicated chicken dish that is simple to prepare. It lends itself to risotto or pilaf as an accompaniment, and a salad of mixed greens.

3 tablespoons olive oil
1 chicken, cut into 8 pieces
6 to 8 cloves garlic, crushed and peeled
½ teaspoon chopped fresh rosemary

salt
pepper
water or chicken stock

- Heat 1 tablespoon oil in a heavy skillet over low heat. Add chicken pieces and cook several minutes. When they begin to color, add remaining 2 tablespoons oil and garlic.
- Turn chicken in the oil. Sprinkle with rosemary, salt, and pepper. Add ½ cup to 1 cup water or stock, and let it come to a boil, then reduce heat and cover skillet.

- Cook chicken 35 to 45 minutes, checking frequently to make sure there's still liquid in the pan. Add water as needed in small amounts (1 to 2 tablespoons). Chicken will fall away from the bone.
- Transfer chicken to dinner plates and deglaze the pan with a few tablespoons of water or wine, pouring pan liquid over chicken as sauce. *Serves 4 to 8.*

BRAISED RABBIT

HIGHLY BENEFICIAL	B, AB	NEUTRAL	O	AVOID	A

Rabbit has a taste very similar to that of chicken and can be cooked in many of the same ways. This method omits the traditional marinade, necessary for the gamier-tasting hare, resulting in tender, moist meat.

2 tablespoons olive oil
1 rabbit, cut into about 12
   pieces
2 tablespoons butter
   (Type AB use olive oil)
1 large carrot, diced

4 cloves garlic, chopped
1 stalk celery, finely sliced
1 medium onion, diced
1½ cups white wine
water
salt

- Heat oil in a heavy skillet over low heat. Add rabbit pieces and cook until nicely browned. Transfer rabbit to platter.
- Add butter or olive oil to pan. When melted, add carrot, garlic, celery, and onion, and sauté, turning, until golden.
- Pushing aside the vegetables, return rabbit to skillet. Spoon vegetables over the pieces and add wine.
- Cook for a few moments, then add 1 cup water, or enough to braise the rabbit, and bring to a boil.
- Cover skillet, reduce heat, and check to make sure that there is always enough braising liquid in the pan. Salt to taste. Cook rabbit for at least 90 minutes, or until very tender.
- Serve with rice. *Serves 3 to 4.*

SIMPLE SESAME CHICKEN

HIGHLY BENEFICIAL			NEUTRAL	O, A	AVOID	B, AB

When you need a good meal but don't have a lot of preparation time, try this simple and delicious recipe. Serve it with rice or spelt noodles and a salad of tossed greens.

8 chicken pieces or breasts on bone	3 to 4 cloves garlic, crushed and peeled
2 tablespoons soy sauce or tamari sauce	¼ cup sesame seeds

- Preheat oven to 375 degrees F.
- Put chicken pieces in a baking dish. Sprinkle each piece with soy sauce. Rub with crushed garlic.
- Sprinkle sesame seeds over top and bake 50 minutes, or until done. *Serves 4 to 8.*

GRILLED CURRIED LEG OF LAMB

HIGHLY BENEFICIAL	O, B, AB	NEUTRAL		AVOID	A

Other than the fact that lamb is highly beneficial for three of the four blood types, with the exception of Type A, it has other advantages as well. The meat is tremendously flavorful and also very lean. Even a leg of lamb, once it has been boned and trimmed, is an affordable meat. The serving portions are generous. One leg of lamb can easily serve a family of four for two meals.

This simple but elegant grilled dinner can be made even easier if you grill your vegetables at the same time. Try summer squashes, peppers, eggplant, sweet potatoes, onions . . . whatever your particular Blood Type Diet allows. Use plenty of olive oil and tend closely.

2 tablespoons curry powder
2 tablespoons ground cumin
1 tablespoon salt
2 tablespoons kelp powder

1 tablespoon five-spice
powder
1 leg of lamb, boned and
butterflied

- Combine spices and rub them dry all over leg of lamb. Let sit 1 hour.
- Prepare grill.
- Grill lamb 20 minutes on each side for medium rare; 25 to 30 minutes for well done.
- Remove lamb from grill and let stand 10 minutes, then slice thinly. *Serves 4.*

BROILED LAMB CHOPS

HIGHLY BENEFICIAL	O, B, AB	NEUTRAL		AVOID	A

Lamb chops are very quick and easy to prepare. In fact, the simpler the treatment, the better. Rib chops are fattier and have less meat, but are quite tasty. Loin chops are often smaller, less fatty, and have more meat.

2 to 3 lamb chops per
person
1 large clove garlic, peeled
and cut

1 tablespoon dry rub of fresh
rosemary and salt per
serving
olive oil

- Preheat broiler. Adjust broiler pan so that the chops are 3 to 4 inches from heat source.
- Remove excess fat from the chops, and place in a flame-proof pan. Rub meat with cut garlic cloves, then the herb mix. Pour a few teaspoons of olive oil over chops, and turn them once to coat both sides with oil.
- Place in broiler and cook 5 to 7 minutes on each side, or until meat is well browned. Turn chops and replace under broiler, browning other side as well.
- Serve with mashed sweet potatoes and braised greens.

TURKEY BURGERS

HIGHLY BENEFICIAL	AB	NEUTRAL	O, A, B	AVOID	

Turkey is usually quite lean, so how can it make a good burger? Eggs, onions, and bread add the necessary moisture to make these light and delicious. If you're concerned as to who would eat them, surprise. Children love them!

1 lb. ground turkey
2 slices of spelt or Ezekiel
  bread
1 tablespoon olive oil
1 medium onion, finely
  chopped

2 eggs
handful of chopped fresh
  parsley
pinch of salt
olive oil for frying

- Place ground turkey in a large bowl and shred the bread over the meat.

- In a skillet, heat oil over medium heat. Add onion and sauté until soft and golden; add to bowl.

- Beat eggs in a small bowl until light and pour into bowl with turkey. Add chopped parsley and salt.

- With your hands, mix the ingredients gently but completely, using a very light touch. Do not condense the mixture; keep it fluffy.

- When ingredients are well mixed, shape them into 5 or 6 patties and cook in olive oil over medium heat until brown, about 5 minutes. Turn and continue to cook another 5 minutes.

- Cover pan, reduce heat, and let them steam just a little, until the juices run clear. This also keeps the turkey burgers moist.
  Serves 5 to 6.

GRILLED LOIN LAMB CHOPS

HIGHLY BENEFICIAL	O, B, AB	NEUTRAL		AVOID	A

These grilled chops are an easy outdoor meal. The marinade would also work for a butterflied leg of lamb.

6 to 8 double-loin chops or 1   Tamari-Mustard Marinade
leg of lamb, butterflied

- Marinate lamb in tamari-mustard marinade 1 to 2 hours.
- Prepare grill.
- Grill lamb over medium heat 15 minutes on each side for chops, or 30 to 35 minutes on each side for boneless leg. Let sit 10 minutes before serving. *Serves 6 to 8.*

TAMARI-MUSTARD MARINADE

Brush this on chicken parts before you grill them or bake them in the oven. It is also very good on tuna steaks.

¼ cup tamari sauce
2 tablespoons Dijon mustard
    or dry mustard
1 tablespoon honey
2 cloves garlic, minced
zest and juice of 1 lemon

1 tablespoon ground ginger
1 tablespoon ground cumin
2 tablespoons olive oil
    (Type O may use sesame
    oil, if desired)

- Mix all ingredients together and store, tightly covered, in refrigerator. *Makes about ¾ cup marinade.*

CHICKEN OREGANO

HIGHLY BENEFICIAL		NEUTRAL	O, A	AVOID	B, AB

A perfect dinner when you're in a rush. It's also ideal "picnic" chicken, served warm or cold.

1 cup spelt bread crumbs
   made from heels of bread
¼ cup grated pecorino romano
3 tablespoons dried oregano
   or ¼ cup chopped fresh

2 tablespoons kelp powder
8 chicken pieces or breasts on
   bone

- Preheat oven to 375 degrees F.
- Combine all ingredients, except chicken.
- Roll each piece of chicken in the seasoning mix. Put pieces in baking dish and bake 50 minutes or until done. *Serves 4 to 8.*

PEANUT OR ALMOND CHICKEN

HIGHLY BENEFICIAL		NEUTRAL	O, A	AVOID	B, AB

This is a delectable cold chicken dish that can serve either as an entrée or an hors d'oeuvre. Type O should use almonds, and Type A, peanuts.

2 lbs. boneless chicken
   breasts
2 cups unsalted, dry-roasted
   peanuts or almonds

Pineapple Chutney-Yogurt
   Sauce (see page 373)
shredded lettuce (optional)

- Poach, then cool and drain the chicken breasts. Cut into finger-length pieces; set aside.
- Toast nuts by placing them in a skillet over medium heat and stirring them around for a few minutes. Watch carefully to make sure they don't scorch.

- When cool, place nuts in the bowl of a food processor or in a blender, and pulse until they are finely chopped.
- Dip the chicken in the sauce, then roll each piece in the nuts. Carefully arrange on a serving tray or on a bed of lettuce. *Serves 6 to 8.*

OLD-FASHIONED YANKEE POT ROAST

HIGHLY BENEFICIAL	O	NEUTRAL	B	AVOID	A, AB

This is the kind of dinner to prepare when you'll be home for a good part of the day. Long, slow simmering is the best method for cooking this particular cut of meat. This is also a good dish to make a day ahead, refrigerate overnight, and serve the following night. Once the pot has had a chance to chill, the fat hardens and can easily be skimmed off. Prepare some spelt noodles and serve with the pot roast for a great, comforting meal on a chilly fall or winter night.

There's a choice of stock for this recipe, but please avoid bouillon cubes with MSG. Read the labels. If you need to use water, that's okay; just add more vegetables to the pot: zucchini or other squash, leeks, and garlic. By using water and the extra vegetables, you're making the stock as you go.

¼ cup canola or olive oil for browning
3- to 4-lb. chuck roast from the shoulder
4 cups stock (chicken, beef, or vegetable) or water
1 sprig each fresh rosemary, marjoram, thyme

1 bay leaf
2 large carrots
2 stalks celery
1 large onion
1 sweet potato

- In a large pot, heat oil over medium to high heat for 1 minute. Add meat and brown on both sides.
- Add the stock, herbs and salt, and bring to a boil. Reduce heat and simmer 1 to 1½ hours.

- Peel and cut vegetables into smaller pieces, and add to the pot. Cook another 45 to 60 minutes.
- Check meat for tenderness. If necessary, continue to cook an additional 20 to 30 minutes, or until done. Drain off pan juices before serving.   *Serves 4 to 6—and makes great leftovers.*

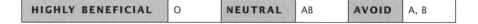

GREAT MEAT LOAF

HIGHLY BENEFICIAL	O	NEUTRAL	AB	AVOID	A, B

The key to a light and fluffy meat loaf depends on the quality of the ingredients and a minimum of handling. This recipe is a protein-packed main course, which, leftover, makes great sandwiches.

1 egg
1 cup soy milk or chicken
  stock
3 slices of stale bread (Ezekiel
  or spelt)
1 lb. ground organic beef

1 lb. ground free-range
  turkey
2 tablespoons kelp powder
1 tablespoon ground cumin
2 tablespoons tamari sauce
3 tablespoons tomato paste

- In a large bowl, beat egg and mix in the soy milk or chicken stock.
- Cut stale bread into cubes and soak in egg and milk mixture until soggy.
- Add remaining ingredients and mix together in the bowl.
- Preheat oven to 375 degrees F.
- Form meat into a 10 × 5 × 5-inch loaf, and bake on a sheet pan 1 hour and 15 minutes, or until juices run clear. Let sit 10 minutes before serving.
- Cut into 1-inch-thick slices and serve with spelt noodles.   *Serves 4.*

SKEWERED LAMB KABOBS

HIGHLY BENEFICIAL	O, B, AB	NEUTRAL		AVOID	A

Lamb is so delicious marinated and then grilled on an open fire. This recipe is a good way to make use of the other half of the leg of lamb used in Indian Lamb Stew with Spinach, page 311.

2 lbs. lamb cubes, cut from the leg

Tamari-Lime Marinade (see next page)

■ Combine lamb and marinade and leave in the refrigerator anywhere from a couple of hours to a couple of days.
■ When you're ready to grill, choose from the following list of vegetables:

TYPES O AND B

2 red peppers, cut into 2-inch squares
1 large onion, quartered

1 zucchini, cut into 1-inch-thick slices

TYPE AB

1 eggplant, cut into 2-inch squares

1 large onion, quartered
12 mushrooms, left whole

■ Prepare grill.
■ On long stainless-steel skewers, alternate vegetables and lamb, using about 4 pieces of meat per skewer. The more vegetables, the better.
■ Grill over medium to high heat about 20 minutes, turning frequently.
■ Serve over rice or with spelt pita.
■ For Type B and Type AB, serve the shish kabob with either Cucumber-Yogurt Sauce, page 372, or Pineapple Chutney-Yogurt Sauce, page 373. *Serves 4.*

TAMARI-LIME MARINADE

3 tablespoons Garlic-Shallot Mixture (see page 375)	2 tablespoons tamari sauce
¼ cup olive oil	juice of 1 lime
	1 tablespoon ground cumin

- Mix all ingredients together. This marinade can be used by every blood type.

TURKEY CUTLETS

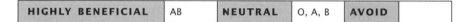

HIGHLY BENEFICIAL	AB	NEUTRAL	O, A, B	AVOID	

A nice change from a large roast is the presliced turkey breast meat that can be cooked in a matter of minutes. This is a good choice for a small family or for singles on a night when time is short. Leftover cutlets also make quick and easy sandwiches.

2 tablespoons olive oil	¼ cup spelt bread crumbs
1 package turkey cutlets (about 1 pound)	squeeze of lemon juice
	salt

- In a large skillet, heat oil over medium-high heat until very hot but not smoking.
- Dredge each cutlet in bread crumbs and slip into pan, being careful not to overcrowd. Do two batches if necessary.
- Cook 4 to 5 minutes on each side or until nicely browned, turning only once. Serve with a squeeze of lemon. Salt to taste. *Serves 4.*

Fish and Seafood

The Wonders of Rivers, Lakes, and Oceans

*E*VERY BLOOD TYPE CAN SAMPLE THE WONDERS OF THE rivers, lakes, and sea. Seafood, by which we mean crustaceans, such as shrimp and lobster; and mollusks, such as scallops, clams, and oysters, is a little trickier. While all fish and seafood are rich sources of protein and other nutrients, they are blood type-specific. Check your lists.

Many fish run seasonally, and they are much better eating when you buy them at the height of their availability. Imported fish generally has been frozen, and so differs markedly in texture from fresh fish. Fish also harbor parasites, some species more than others. Always cook fish thoroughly.

Short, simple cooking procedures seem to bring out the best qualities in fish. Overcooking makes it tough and dry. Fish can lose its delicate freshness and nutritional benefits very quickly.

SHRIMP KABOBS

HIGHLY BENEFICIAL		NEUTRAL	O	AVOID	A, B, AB

juice of 1 lemon

¼ cup olive oil

3 cloves garlic, crushed and peeled

2 tablespoons chopped fresh parsley

1 stalk lemongrass, bottom third only, peeled and chopped

1-inch piece fresh ginger, peeled and chopped or grated

1 lb. large shrimp, cleaned and deveined

- Combine all ingredients, except shrimp, in a medium bowl.
- Add the shrimp and marinate, turning to coat thoroughly, at least 4 hours. The longer you marinate, the better. Overnight would be best.
- Prepare grill.
- Place 4 to 6 shrimp on each skewer and grill over high heat 3 minutes on each side. *Serves 2.*

BROILED SALMON WITH LEMONGRASS

HIGHLY BENEFICIAL	O, A	NEUTRAL	AB	AVOID	B

3 stalks lemongrass, bottom third only, finely chopped

3 tablespoons soy sauce

2 tablespoons peeled and coarsely grated ginger

2 plum tomatoes (Type O only)

2 tablespoons fresh cilantro, chopped finely

juice of 1 lemon

2 scallions, thinly sliced

4 to 6 salmon fillets or steaks, 1 to 1½ pounds

- Combine all ingredients, except salmon.
- Put salmon on large platter and pour marinade over the whole fillet. Let marinate approximately 2 hours.
- Preheat broiler.
- Remove salmon from marinade and broil 15 minutes for medium, 20 minutes for well done.   *Serves 4 to 6.*

SAUTÉED GROUPER

HIGHLY BENEFICIAL	A, B, AB	NEUTRAL	O	AVOID	

This is a fish dish that will delight the kids. It's easy and beats frozen fish sticks by a country mile.

3 tablespoons olive oil
1- to 1½-lb. fresh grouper, trimmed of bones and cut into finger-sized pieces

¼ cup quinoa flour
salt

- In a large cast-iron skillet, heat oil over medium heat.
- Roll grouper in the flour, shaking off excess. Slip each piece into the hot oil, being careful not to overcrowd the pan.
- Cook in small batches, adding more oil to the pan if necessary. Make sure the oil is very hot before adding the fish.
- Turn once when nicely browned on one side, then cook another 3 to 4 minutes. Test for doneness.
- Pat off excess oil on a paper towel and serve.   *Serves 3 to 4.*

SWORDFISH WITH CHERRY TOMATOES, RED ONION, AND BASIL

HIGHLY BENEFICIAL	O	NEUTRAL	AB	AVOID	A, B

This is a colorful and moist swordfish dish. You can use the same preparation for halibut, mako shark, and any other dense, steaklike fish.

2 tablespoons olive oil
2 cloves garlic, crushed and
   peeled
1 lb. swordfish
water
1 small red onion, chopped

1 cup yellow or red cherry
   tomatoes, halved
½ cup fresh basil, chopped
splash of white wine
   (optional)

- Heat oil over low heat. Add garlic and sauté gently.
- Add swordfish, distributing the garlic around it. Add ½ cup water. Cover pan and steam swordfish 7 to 10 minutes. Turn fish and steam another 2 to 3 minutes.
- Add onion and halved tomatoes. Steam 5 more minutes. The onion and tomatoes should be soft.
- Add basil and cook another moment.
- Arrange the swordfish and all the vegetables on a plate, using the vegetables as a sauce for the fish.
- If desired, deglaze pan with a splash of wine, pour over fish, and serve.   *Serves 2.*

INDONESIAN BROILED SWORDFISH

HIGHLY BENEFICIAL	O	NEUTRAL	A, B, AB	AVOID	

This is an easy Asian-inspired dish. Serve it with steamed rice and a fruit salad for a light, healthful meal.

3 tablespoons tamari sauce
2 cloves garlic, minced
2 tablespoons olive oil
1 tablespoon honey
1 tablespoon tahini (ground sesame seeds)

juice of 1 lemon
1 tablespoon ground cumin
1 tablespoon chopped fresh cilantro
2 lbs. swordfish

> TYPE B: Replace tahini with 1 tablespoon almond butter.
>
> TYPE AB: Replace tahini with 1 tablespoon peanut butter or almond butter.

- Combine all ingredients, except swordfish.
- Put swordfish on large platter and pour marinade over it. Turn fish once.
- Allow to marinate at least 1 hour. Turn again.
- Preheat broiler and place fish as close to heat source as possible.
- Broil 5 to 8 minutes on each side, depending on the thickness of the steak. Make sure the interior of the fish is properly cooked. *Serves 4.*

PETER'S SNAILS

HIGHLY BENEFICIAL	A, AB	NEUTRAL	O	AVOID	B

Most snail—or escargot—recipes rely on lots of butter and garlic. You never have a chance to taste the real flavor of the snails. It's an experience not to be duplicated. This is a favorite recipe among the Type As in the D'Adamo household. You can even use canned snails. Since snails have tremendous healing properties for As and ABs, make this simple dish a regular part of your diet.

¼ cup olive oil
2 tablespoons garlic, peeled, chopped, and pressed

12 escargot
parsley flakes

- Preheat broiler.
- Combine oil and garlic in a small bowl and mash into a paste using back of spoon.
- Arrange escargot on a broiling sheet and brush them with garlic paste.
- Broil about 10 minutes. When they're almost done, sprinkle them with fresh parsley flakes and broil another minute.   *Serves 2.*

BROILED SALMON STEAKS

HIGHLY BENEFICIAL	O, A	NEUTRAL	B, AB	AVOID	

This is quick and easy for a mixed-blood type family.

4 salmon steaks
1 tablespoon Garlic-Shallot Mixture (see page 375)
2 tablespoons olive oil
juice of 1 lemon

salt
3 tablespoons chopped fresh dill (optional)
lemon wedges (optional)

- Preheat broiler.
- Rub steaks with Garlic-Shallot Mixture, oil, lemon, and salt.
- Cook fish as close to heat source as possible about 4 to 8 minutes on each side. Test for doneness by prodding with a fork to see if the flesh separates easily.
- Salmon steaks can be served hot or cold, and dressed with fresh chopped dill and a wedge or two of lemon.   *Serves 4.*

SAUTÉED MONKFISH

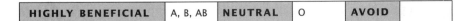

HIGHLY BENEFICIAL	A, B, AB	NEUTRAL	O	AVOID	

Monkfish is an excellent fish to cut into chunks and dredge in flour for sautéeing. It can also be used for grilled kabobs on a skewer. Monkfish is often referred to as the poor man's lobster. When cooked, its taste and texture is said to resemble that of the prized crustacean.

1½ lbs. monkfish
3 tablespoons olive oil
1 teaspoon dried oregano

brown rice or spelt flour
1 to 2 eggs
salt

- Cut the monkfish into 1-inch cubes.
- Heat oil in a heavy cast-iron skillet over medium heat.
- Combine oregano and flour. Beat the eggs well.
- Dip the monkfish pieces in the egg, a few pieces at a time, then roll them in the seasoned flour.
- Slide floured fish into skillet, but do not overcrowd the pan.
- Sauté gently, several minutes on each side, until batter is crisp and fish is done. Season with salt.   *Serves 4.*

TUNA STEAK MARINATED
IN LEMON AND GARLIC

HIGHLY BENEFICIAL	AB	NEUTRAL	O, A, B	AVOID	

Tuna is certainly a popular fish, though most people are more familiar with canned tuna than with any other kind. Maybe this simple but elegant recipe will help to change that.

Serve this tuna with basmati rice, using the cooked marinade as a light sauce over the rice.

1-lb. tuna steak
2 to 3 tablespoons olive oil
juice of 1 lemon
3-inch piece lemon peel
4 cloves garlic, crushed and
   peeled
2 tablespoons fresh cilantro,
   chopped

1-inch piece fresh ginger,
   grated
1 to 2 tablespoons tamari
   sauce
water

■ Place tuna in glass or ceramic bowl. Combine oil, lemon juice, lemon peel, garlic, cilantro, ginger, and tamari, and pour over fish.

■ Allow to marinate 2 hours, turning a couple of times.

■ Heat a heavy cast-iron skillet over medium heat.

■ Put tuna in the skillet. Add marinade and a tablespoon or two of water and bring to a simmer.

■ Cover and steam 8 to 10 minutes. Watch carefully; cooking time will vary according to the thickness of the fish and your preference. Add additional water, 1 tablespoon at time, if necessary. *Serves 4.*

STEAMED WHOLE RED SNAPPER

HIGHLY BENEFICIAL	O, AB	NEUTRAL	A, B	AVOID	

Any small, whole, white-fleshed fish can be steamed by this method. Varying the sauce permits you a wide range of possibilities! (See "Dressings and Sauces.") Steam fish on a heavy, restaurant-style platter that fits inside the top of a steaming utensil. A large wok, bamboo steamer, or a traditional fish poacher with removable colander tray modified to lift fish above the boiling water are all suitable alternatives. It is worth working out some kind of system for this recipe because not only is it easy, it provides a meal for all blood types, using their personalized sauces.

1½- to 2-lb. red snapper, head and tail on, washed, cleaned, scaled, and trimmed
3 tablespoons olive oil
3 cloves garlic
5 scallions, thinly sliced

1-inch piece fresh ginger, slivered
2 tablespoons tamari sauce
1 scallion, slivered lengthwise
½ cup chopped fresh cilantro

- Steam fish 10 to 15 minutes.
- Meanwhile, prepare sauce: Heat oil in heavy cast-iron skillet over low to medium heat. Add garlic, scallions, and ginger, and gently sauté until softened but not browned. Remove pan from heat and add tamari.
- When fish is done, drain off accumulated juices and pour sauce over fish. Garnish with slivered scallion and cilantro. *Serves 3 to 4.*

Tofu and Tempeh

Soy Good!

OFU IS THE JAPANESE NAME FOR THE CURD PRODUCED FROM THE milklike liquid extracted from the soybean. It originated in China, where it was known as *doufu*. The soybean is one of the five sacred grains of China, and tofu is a staple throughout Asia. It is the primary source of protein for millions of people. Tofu's texture ranges from soft to firm to extra firm. The silken tofu, however, is soft, delicate, and custardy. Tofu is eaten in countless ways, its bland taste making it perfect for flavorful sauces, spices, and seasonings and its texture lending itself to almost any cooking method.

In particular, Blood Types A and AB should experiment with tofu. Try using it in soups and stews, in place of meat or chicken. It is very inexpensive, easy to find, lasts for several days in the refrigerator, and can be served at any meal.

Tempeh has been a food staple in Indonesia for over two thousand years. It can be found today in many supermarkets and health-food stores in the refrigerated section. Tempeh is a fermented and pressed rectangular cake composed of soybeans and a fermenting culture called *Rhizopus oligosporus*. This is a filamentous fungus that produces a white mold that spreads throughout the tempeh cake. The tempeh texture alters, and the mold forms a sort of cheeselike rind around its outside. The tempeh becomes extremely nutty and chewy, with a dense, almost meatlike consistency. Some people compare it to a nutty veal. Tempeh can also be made with rice, quinoa, peanuts, kidney beans, wheat, oats, barley, or coconut. It is very popular in vegetarian cuisine worldwide.

Tempeh is substantial, satisfying, and versatile. Great on the grill, fried, baked, or sautéd, tempeh is a perfect protein. It can last unopened in the refrigerator for a couple of weeks, but once opened it should be cooked within a few days. Tempeh should be steamed whole before additional cooking, but if it's left to marinate long enough, the steam step can be eliminated. Black spots on the surface are normal, but if tempeh turns color or smells sour, it should be discarded.

TOFU AND CURRIED VEGETABLE STEW

HIGHLY BENEFICIAL	A, AB	NEUTRAL	O	AVOID	B

Curried vegetables are easy to prepare, and when combined with tofu and brown rice, they form the base for a high protein meal. Choose the most suitable vegetables for your stew, and adjust proportions to balance flavors. The stew may seem a bit thin, but if you include white potato or okra, they will thicken the broth.

2 tablespoons olive oil
4 cloves garlic, chopped
1 medium onion, diced
1 to 2 tablespoons curry
   powder
2 cups water
2 small turnips, halved and
   thinly sliced
1 small sugar pumpkin, cut
   into 1-inch cubes
1 small winter squash, cut
   into 1-inch pieces
1 carrot, thinly sliced

1 parsnip, thinly sliced
1 white potato, diced
   (Type AB)
1 sweet potato, diced
   (Types O, AB)
½ head cauliflower, cut into
   "flowers" (Types A, AB)
½ head broccoli, cut into
   "flowers"
12 okra, stemmed and left
   whole
1 large cake tofu, cubed
½ cup cilantro, chopped

- Heat oil in a large, heavy skillet over medium heat. Add garlic and onion and cook, stirring, until just colored.
- Sprinkle curry powder to taste over vegetables in pan, and continue to gently sauté everything about 5 minutes, being careful not to scorch the garlic and curry.

- Add water and bring to a boil.
- Begin adding ingredients, starting with those that require the longest cooking times.
- When the water has returned to a boil, cover, lower heat, and simmer about 15 minutes, or until all the vegetables are nearly tender. The cauliflower, broccoli, and okra should be put in at this time, and the stew simmered another 10 to 15 minutes or so.
- Add the tofu for the final 5 minutes, just to heat it through.
- Ladle over bowls of brown rice and top with a little cilantro. *Serves 6 to 8.*

TOFU-VEGETABLE STIR-FRY

HIGHLY BENEFICIAL	A, AB	NEUTRAL	O	AVOID	B

Stir-fry meals always seem quick, with surprisingly little clean-up. By the time the brown rice is cooked, which takes about forty-five minutes, you'll have had plenty of time to prepare and cut up the rest of the ingredients. Once you begin to stir-fry, the meal will be ready and on the table in a little over 10 minutes.

2 tablespoons olive oil
1 medium onion, diced
1 head broccoli, cut into "flowers," stems sliced
1 small bunch bok choy, cut into 1-inch pieces
6 cloves garlic, crushed and peeled

½ cup vegetable stock or water
½ lb. snow peas
1 cake tofu, cut into ½-inch cubes
1 tablespoon tamari sauce
arrowroot flour (optional)

- In a wok or a large, heavy skillet, heat oil over fairly high heat. Add onion, stirring constantly, until the onions are soft.
- Add broccoli, stirring a moment or two. Add bok choy, stirring again. Add garlic.
- Add about ½ cup vegetable stock or water and let come to a boil.
- Cover pan and reduce heat and steam vegetables several minutes, until broccoli is tender but still crisp.

- Add snow peas, then tofu. Reduce heat and let the mixture steam a few minutes.
- Add tamari, toss gently, and serve.
- If you prefer a thick sauce, push the vegetables to one side, add a teaspoon or so of arrowroot flour to the liquid, and stir until thickened. Gently toss with the vegetables before serving.
Serves 4 to 6.

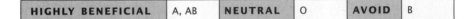

TOFU-SESAME FRY

HIGHLY BENEFICIAL	A, AB	NEUTRAL	O	AVOID	B

Tofu can make a satisfying breakfast when served with some brown rice and miso, a deeply complex and salty paste made from fermented soybeans.

2 tablespoons olive oil
1 cake tofu
1 to 2 tablespoons white
   sesame seeds
   (Type A and O)
1 to 2 tablespoons black
   sesame seeds
   (Type A and O)
2 to 4 tablespoons peanuts,
   coarsely chopped (Type AB)

salt
lemon juice
3 to 4 tablespoons tahini
   (Types A and O)
juice of ½ lemon (optional)
1 teaspoon tamari sauce
   (optional)

- Heat oil in a heavy skillet over medium to high heat.
- Slice tofu about ½ inch thick. Coat half the slices with the white seeds, the other half with the black, or coat slices with chopped peanuts.
- Carefully sauté tofu in the oil, a few minutes on each side.
- Serve with a dash of salt and a squeeze of lemon. Or drizzle a little tahini, thinned with a little lemon juice and 1 teaspoon tamari, over the tofu. Allow 2 slices per serving.
Serves 3 to 4.

QUINOA TEMPEH WITH RICE NOODLES

HIGHLY BENEFICIAL	A, AB	NEUTRAL	O	AVOID	B

1 package tempeh (any
  variety)
2 tablespoons olive oil
1 onion, thinly sliced
2 cloves garlic, crushed and
  peeled
3 tablespoons chopped fresh
  cilantro

2 Portobello mushrooms
¼ cup dry cooking sherry
1 package fresh spinach,
  cleaned and chopped
1 tablespoon tamari sauce
1 lb. rice noodles

- Bring a large pot of water to a boil. Boil tempeh 5 to 10 minutes.
- With a large slotted spoon or strainer, lift tempeh out of boiling water, reserving the water for the noodles; set tempeh aside.
- In a large skillet, heat oil over medium to high heat. Add onion, garlic, cilantro, and mushrooms and sauté.
- Slice the tempeh and add the onion and mushroom mixture.
- Add the sherry, the spinach, and the tamari. Cover and simmer 15 minutes.
- Meanwhile, cook noodles according to directions and drain.
- Divide noodles among 4 plates and serve each with 2 slices of tempeh and vegetables.   *Serves 4.*

RICE STICKS AND TOFU WITH VEGETABLES

HIGHLY BENEFICIAL	A, AB	NEUTRAL	O	AVOID	B

These rice sticks are not the same as the rice spaghetti you find in the stores. They are, instead, similar in texture to bean threads. Of course, many vegetables are wonderful to use in this dish, so feel free to experiment with what is available in the market or your refrigerator.

MARINADE

½ cup tamari sauce

⅓ cup rice wine

1 tablespoon turbinado sugar

5 cloves garlic, crushed and
  peeled or put through a
  press

5 scallions, thinly sliced

1-inch piece fresh ginger,
  grated

2 tablespoons canola oil

2 containers firm tofu,
  drained

- Combine marinade ingredients in medium bowl. Add tofu and marinate at least 1 hour.
- Preheat grill or broiler.
- Cook tofu for 5 minutes on each side; set aside.

1 package rice sticks

1 package fresh spinach,
  washed and stems removed

1 lb. green beans or sugar
  snap peas, washed and
  stems removed

¼ cup chopped fresh cilantro

- Cook noodles according to directions, until tender.
- Drain and rinse in warm water; drain well. Transfer to a platter.
- Arrange the steamed vegetables around the noodles.
- Slice the tofu and place on top of noodles. Pour marinade over the tofu and top with chopped cilantro. *Serves 4.*

TEMPEH KABOBS

HIGHLY BENEFICIAL	A, AB	NEUTRAL	O	AVOID	B

These kabobs are great cooked on the barbecue and served over steamed rice or Wild and Basmati Rice Pilaf (see page 287).

1 package tempeh (any variety)

BARBECUE SAUCE

6 oz. plum jam

2 oz. pineapple juice (from
the pineapple)

3 tablespoons tamari sauce

2 cloves garlic, put through a
press

2 scallions, thinly sliced

2-inch piece fresh ginger,
grated

FOR THE SKEWERS

1 large onion, quartered and
separated into layers,
2 layers per piece

2 Portobello mushrooms, cut
into 1 × 1-inch pieces

2 medium zucchini, cut into
1-inch-thick slices

2 cups 1 × 1-inch pineapple
chunks

- Prepare grill.
- Steam tempeh 10 to 15 minutes.
- Meanwhile, combine barbecue sauce ingredients and prepare vegetables.
- When the tempeh is cool enough to handle, slice into pieces the same size as the vegetables.
- Assemble the skewers, alternating vegetables with the tempeh and pineapple. When skewering the zucchini, do so through the green rind. The flesh becomes pulpy when cooked, and won't hold on well.
- Brush with sauce and grill over medium heat until nicely browned.
- Serve on a bed of rice. *Serves 4.*

TOFU AND BLACK BEAN CHILI

HIGHLY BENEFICIAL	A	NEUTRAL	O	AVOID	B, AB

A truly fragrant and spicy main course that isn't peppery, but full of freshly ground flavor. The paleness of the tofu contrasts nicely with the black beans.

¼ cup canola or olive oil
2 onions, diced
1 red pepper, diced (Type O only)
½ tablespoon ground chili (Type O only)
½ tablespoon ground cayenne (Type A omit)
1 tablespoon ground coriander
1 tablespoon fresh thyme
1 teaspoon ground cloves
2 tablespoons spelt flour

1 tablespoon sherry
1 container firm tofu, drained and cubed
2 cans black beans, drained and rinsed, or 1 cup dried black beans, soaked overnight and cooked al dente
1 to 1½ cups chicken stock
1 bay leaf
6 cloves garlic, peeled and chopped

- In a large pot, heat oil over medium heat. Add onions and ground chili and cook 2 minutes, until onions are wilted.
- Add the remaining spices, stirring and toasting well to release the flavors.
- Add the flour and cook 2 more minutes. Be careful not to burn the spice paste.
- Deglaze with sherry, then add the black beans, stirring well to coat with the spices.
- Add 1 cup of chicken stock, then the bay leaf and garlic, stirring until incorporated.
- Simmer 30 minutes, adding more chicken stock as needed.
- For the last 10 minutes of cooking, add the tofu. Since tofu can be rather fragile, handle it gently, using a wooden spoon. Be sure to remove the bay leaf before serving.
- Serve with rice or homemade tortillas. *Serves 4 to 6.*

SILKEN TOFU SCRAMBLE

HIGHLY BENEFICIAL	A, AB	NEUTRAL	O	AVOID	B

Silken is the smoothest, most custardy type of tofu available, and it makes a wonderful substitute for eggs, ricotta cheese, and even yogurt.

1 tablespoon olive oil
1 teaspoon Garlic-Shallot
   Mixture (see page 375)
1 small carrot, grated
1 small zucchini, grated

5 oz. silken tofu
salt
1 tablespoon chopped fresh
   parsley or basil

- In a small skillet, heat the oil over low heat. Add the shallot-garlic mix and sauté 2 minutes.
- Add the grated carrot and cook another 3 to 4 minutes.
- Add the zucchini and silken tofu. With the side of a spoon, chop the tofu as it warms, and stir until cooked. Season with salt and freshly chopped herbs. *Serves 2.*

GRILLED WILD-RICE TEMPEH

HIGHLY BENEFICIAL	A, AB	NEUTRAL	O	AVOID	B

1 package wild-rice tempeh

SIMPLE MARINADE

3 tablespoons olive oil
2 tablespoons tamari sauce
2 tablespoons Garlic-Shallot
   Mixture (see page 375)

2 tablespoons chopped fresh
   cilantro
2 tablespoons lemon juice

- Remove tempeh from wrapper and place in shallow bowl.
- In a small bowl, mix together the remaining ingredients and pour over the tempeh, turning once.
- Refrigerate for several hours. For a quicker marinade, first steam tempeh for 20 minutes, then marinate 1 hour.
- Prepare grill.
- Cook tempeh over medium heat, turning and basting with the marinade about 15 minutes, until nicely browned. Let sit for a few minutes before slicing.
- Serve with brown rice pilaf and a crisp romaine salad. *Serves 4.*

FRUIT-SILKEN TOFU SCRAMBLE

HIGHLY BENEFICIAL	A, AB	NEUTRAL	O	AVOID	B

This alternative breakfast is so delicious, in fact, that it can also be served as a nutritious dessert. Quick and easy to prepare.

TYPE O

2 tablespoons unsalted butter
1 banana, sliced
¼ cup blueberries

8 oz. silken tofu, drained
salt to taste

TYPE A AND TYPE AB

2 tablespoons canola
  margarine
1 peach, pitted and sliced

¼ cup blueberries
8 oz. silken tofu, drained
salt to taste

- In a medium skillet, melt butter or margarine over low heat.
- Add fruit and gently cook 2 to 3 minutes. Let the bananas or peaches caramelize a bit, then add the berries and sauté 2 to 3 minutes.
- Push the fruit aside and add the silken tofu, chopping and warming it 2 to 3 minutes. The fruit and silken tofu are kept separate so that the tofu doesn't pick up all of the berries' color.
- At the final minute of cooking, toss them together and add the salt. Serve in a fruit bowl. *Serves 2.*

BAKED TOFU "FRIES"

HIGHLY BENEFICIAL	A, AB	NEUTRAL	O	AVOID	B

⅓ cup rye cracker crumbs
2 tablespoons quinoa flour
2 tablespoons spices (ground
　　cumin or cayenne,
　　or oregano and garlic)

1 teaspoon salt
1 cake firm tofu, drained,
　　pressed, and cut into
　　finger-size sticks

- Preheat oven to 350 degrees F.
- Combine first four ingredients and roll the tofu sticks in the crumb mixture to cover evenly.
- Brush a cookie sheet with a light coating of oil.
- Arrange the sticks in a single layer and bake for 35 minutes. Check for crispness, turn over, and bake 10 minutes longer, if necessary. *Serves 2.*

Pasta

Try Something New

S INCE MOST PASTA IS MADE OF DURUM SEMOLINA WHEAT
flour, many people aren't aware of the wonderful nonwheat varieties. Try rice, buckwheat, Jerusalem artichoke, spelt, quinoa, and
spinach pastas. The tastes and textures of these pastas differ considerably from those of the ubiquitous pasta, but they are quite delicious. Sauces also do wonderful things for any pasta. A good sauce
can be made from just about anything—the simpler, the better.

Spelt flour produces a taste and texture closest to those of traditional pasta. There are two kinds of spelt spaghetti, just as there are
two kinds of spelt flour. Like wheat flour, spelt is available in whole
grain or white. For the most part, it's always nutritionally beneficial
to choose the whole grain. However, the white spelt pasta most
resembles the pasta we're all familiar with. If you want a more
robust pasta, then the whole-spelt noodles or *soba* buckwheat noodles certainly provide that.

The recipe for pizza dough works with both whole-grain or white
spelt flour. Be aware that the whole-grain spelt flour doesn't rise so
much as the white spelt flour, which doesn't rise so much as white
wheat flour.

Some of these recipes mention adding a dusting of pecorino
romano or Parmesan, which is the way many people like to eat their
pasta. This is optional, although a dusting won't do any harm.

STUFFED SHELLS WITH PESTO

HIGHLY BENEFICIAL	B, AB	NEUTRAL	A	AVOID	O

This pasta, made without tomatoes, is Highly Beneficial to Type B and Type AB, particularly if it's made with rice flour. Semolina or spinach shells are all right; it's the dairy that counts here. Children love these shells, so make plenty of them.

1 lb. shell pasta, either spelt, semolina, or rice flour
1 lb. ricotta cheese

½ lb. mozzarella cheese, grated
½ cup vegetable stock
Basil Pesto (see page 369)

- Boil the pasta until done, undercooking by a minute or two, because this dish will cook further once it's assembled.
- Drain the cooked pasta; set aside.
- Preheat oven to 375 degrees F.
- In a bowl, combine the ricotta and grated mozzarella.
- Spoon about 1 tablespoon of this mixture into each shell, then place the shells in an oiled glass baking dish, lining them up in neat little rows.
- When all the shells are filled, pour in the vegetable stock, cover the baking dish with aluminum foil, and bake about 20 minutes.
- Remove from oven and serve hot, accompanied by a bowl of pesto to spoon over the shells.   *Serves 4 to 6.*

GREEN VEGETABLE PASTA

HIGHLY BENEFICIAL		NEUTRAL	O, A	AVOID	B, AB

This beautiful dish is as its name describes—all green. It's a delicious way to incorporate a variety of beneficial vegetables.

¼ cup extra-virgin olive oil
plus extra for tossing pasta

2 scallions, sliced

1 lb. asparagus, trimmed and
cut on the diagonal
into 1-inch pieces

2 green zucchini, sliced on
diagonal

4 artichoke hearts, quartered

1 lb. Jerusalem artichoke
pasta

salt

¼ cup chopped fresh basil

grated romano cheese

- Bring a large pot of water to a boil.
- In a large skillet, heat oil over medium heat. Add scallions and cook gently until wilted, about 3 minutes.
- Add asparagus, zucchini, and artichoke hearts. Cook 3 more minutes. Meanwhile, cook and drain pasta. Rinse well with warm water and drain again.
- Toss pasta with a little olive oil and season with salt. Cover and keep warm.
- The vegetables should be tender but still a little crisp. Toss with pasta, sprinkle on the basil, and serve with grated cheese. *Serves 4.*

SOBA NOODLES OR SPELT PASTA WITH PUMPKIN AND TOFU

HIGHLY BENEFICIAL	A	NEUTRAL	O, AB	AVOID	B

Soba noodles, pumpkin, and tofu are all Highly Beneficial for Type A. Type O and Type AB can substitute rice or spelt pasta. This is a simple dish. Steamed broccoli or a mesclun salad makes a satisfying complement.

olive oil

6 cloves garlic, crushed and
peeled

1 medium leek, thinly sliced

water

1 small fresh sugar pumpkin

1 lb. soba noodles or 1 lb.
rice or spelt pasta

1 lb. tofu

- Bring a large pot of water to a boil.
- In a large, heavy skillet, heat 2 tablespoons oil over medium heat. Add garlic and leek, stirring for a few moments.

- Add ½ cup water, cover, and steam over low heat until leeks are tender, 10 to 15 minutes, adding more water if necessary.
- Meanwhile, cut pumpkin in half, remove seeds (save for toasting later), and carefully peel. Cut into 1-inch pieces and add to the skillet with the garlic and leeks.
- Add an additional ½ cup water and steam pumpkin until tender, 10 to 15 minutes.
- The water for the noodles or pasta should be boiling. Add the noodles or pasta and cook according to package directions.
- When all the vegetables are done, cut the tofu into ½-inch pieces. Add tofu to the skillet and heat thoroughly.
- Spoon the mixture over the drained hot noodles.   *Serves 4 to 6.*

FETTUCCINE WITH GRILLED LAMB SAUSAGES AND VEGETABLES

HIGHLY BENEFICIAL	B	NEUTRAL	O, AB	AVOID	A

Once the fettuccine is cooked, serve with a simple salad of mixed greens.

2 red peppers (Type AB omit)
2 yellow peppers (Type AB omit)
2 Portobello mushrooms
2 cloves garlic, crushed and peeled
¼ cup olive oil

1 to 1½ lbs. lamb sausages
1 lb. rice fettuccine
salt
¼ cup chopped fresh basil and parsley
romano cheese

- Prepare grill.
- Prepare vegetables: Slice peppers in half lengthwise and remove seeds and stems. Remove stems from mushrooms so they lie flat on the grill. Slice eggplants ½-inch thick. Slice zucchini ½-inch thick on diagonal.
- Rub all of the vegetables with garlic, reserving a small amount, then brush with oil.

- Grill the lamb sausages over medium-hot coals until nicely browned and juices run clear, about 20 to 25 minutes.
- Move the sausages to the side of the grill to keep them warm while the vegetables are cooking.
- In the meantime, cook the fettuccine in plenty of boiling water. Drain cooked pasta, rinse with warm water, and drain again.
- Pour remaining olive oil over pasta, and season with salt and pepper.
- When all the vegetables are nicely grilled, soft but not burned, slice into long strips and toss with garlic.
- Serve over the fettuccine with a couple of sausages. Sprinkle with fresh herbs and grated romano cheese. *Serves 4.*

GREEN LEAFY PASTA

HIGHLY BENEFICIAL	A	NEUTRAL	O, B, AB	AVOID	

Nutritious leafy greens braised in olive oil and a bit of their own water make a nutritious sauce. Except for the Jerusalem artichoke pasta, this is another all-green meal!

1 lb. spinach pasta (Type B and Type AB) or 1 lb. Jerusalem artichoke pasta (Type O and Type A)
¼ cup olive oil
2 leeks, washed and sliced
2 cloves garlic, chopped

1 bunch spinach, washed and rinsed
1 bunch Swiss chard, washed and trimmed
salt
romano cheese

- Bring a large pot of water to a boil.
- Cook the vegetables as you cook the pasta, drain, and dress with a little oil. Keep covered; the vegetables will be ready soon.
- In a large skillet, heat oil over medium heat. Add leeks, turning to coat with the oil, and cook them gently several minutes, until they begin to soften and wilt.

- Add the garlic and stir. A few moments later, add the spinach and Swiss chard, tossing to coat with oil and garlic. The greens will begin to wilt.
- Steam uncovered several more minutes, or until the greens are fully cooked. Season to taste and grate on some romano. *Serves 4.*

CELLOPHANE NOODLES WITH GRILLED SIRLOIN AND GREEN VEGETABLES

HIGHLY BENEFICIAL	O	NEUTRAL	B	AVOID	A, AB

This is a great dish for company. The Asian-inspired flavors of this dish are refreshing. The bean noodles are light and slippery, absorbing the pungent flavors of the fresh ginger, scallion, and cilantro. Best served at room temperature.

MARINADE

½ cup tamari sauce
⅓ cup rice wine
5 cloves garlic, minced or put through a press
1 tablespoon turbinado sugar

2 scallions, thinly sliced
2 tablespoons olive or canola oil

2 lbs. lean sirloin steak

- Combine marinade ingredients.
- Put steak on large platter. Pour marinade over steak, turning at least once.
- Marinate for 1 hour, but the longer the better.

cellophane noodles (made from beans)
2 cloves garlic, crushed and peeled
1 lb. sugar snap peas or haricot verte, or delicate string beans, stems removed

1 bunch fresh spinach
Dipping Sauce (see page 376)
¼ cup chopped fresh cilantro
1-inch piece fresh ginger, peeled and grated

- While steak is marinating, prepare grill.
- Drain steak and grill until medium-rare, about 8 minutes each side; set aside.
- Bring a pot of water to a boil for the noodles, and a smaller pot of water to steam the vegetables.
- Soften the noodles in hot water, and then cook according to directions, or until tender.
- Rinse in warm water and drain thoroughly. Pile high on platter.
- Steam garlic and peas for 1 minute or so, then add spinach and steam 2 more minutes.
- Arrange the vegetables around the noodles.
- Slice the steak, place on top of the noodles, and drizzle with dipping sauce. Top with fresh cilantro and grated ginger. *Serves 4.*

PENNE WITH SAUSAGE AND PEPPERS

HIGHLY BENEFICIAL		NEUTRAL	O, B	AVOID	A, AB

This is an updated version of a classic southern Italian dish. Type B needs to eliminate the tomato sauce. But the dish is just as satisfying "dry." The pasta, of course, is spelt or rice noodles.

8 turkey sausages
¼ cup olive oil
1 large onion, thinly sliced
1 tablespoon Garlic-Shallot
   Mixture (page 375)
   or 4 cloves garlic, minced
2 peppers, thinly sliced

¼ cup chopped parsley
2 tablespoons sherry
2 cups tomato sauce
   (Type B omit)
salt
1 lb. penne (rice or spelt)

- In a heavy skillet, brown sausages. When nicely browned, transfer them to a plate.
- In the same skillet, heat oil over medium heat. Add onion and Garlic-Shallot Mixture and cook until wilted.
- Add peppers and parsley and cook a few more minutes, then add sherry. Add tomato sauce and salt to taste.

- Return sausages to pan and simmer 20 minutes.
- While sausages are simmering, cook pasta; drain well.
- Transfer pasta to large platter. Spoon sausages and peppers over the pasta. *Serves 4.*

SAUTÉED VEGETABLES
WITH QUINOA PASTA

HIGHLY BENEFICIAL	A, AB	NEUTRAL	O	AVOID	B

Although this pasta appears to be neutral for all blood types, it's not always. It cannot be stressed enough how important it is to read the labels on all packaged items. Quinoa pasta found in the stores usually lists corn flour as the first ingredient, then quinoa flour. It's wonderfully tasty and quite yellow—a dead giveaway to its origins—but it's suitable only for Type A. All other blood types should use a beneficial pasta, such as spelt, buckwheat, or rice.

¼ cup olive oil
4 cloves garlic, crushed and peeled
¼ cup chopped fresh parsley
2 Portobello mushrooms, thinly sliced
¼ cup sherry
1 container firm tofu (optional)
1 small head radicchio, washed and sliced
1 bunch dandelion greens, broccoli rabe, or spinach, washed well and tough stems removed
salt
1 lb. rice pasta
olive oil (for pasta)
romano cheese (optional, according to blood type)

- Boil water for the pasta.
- In a very large skillet, heat the oil over low heat and gently cook the garlic, being sure not to darken the cloves, which will make them bitter.
- Add parsley and cook 2 minutes.
- Add mushrooms and cook until soft, about 5 minutes.

- Add sherry, and cook 1 minute to burn off the alcohol.
- Add tofu, if using, radicchio, and greens. The volume will seem unmanageable at first, but it will quickly reduce. Turn the greens over as they cook, so that the somewhat wilted bottoms are on top.
- Cover and cook 10 minutes. Season with salt to taste.
- Meanwhile, add the pasta to the water and cook according to directions.
- Drain and rinse with warm water. Toss with a little olive oil to keep it from sticking.
- Place the pasta on the plate first, then smother with the vegetables. Top with grated romano cheese. *Serves 4.*

COLD SOBA NOODLES WITH
THAI PEANUT SAUCE

HIGHLY BENEFICIAL	A	NEUTRAL		AVOID	O, B, AB

1 package buckwheat (soba) noodles
1 cup Peanut Butter Sauce (see page 374)
2 cups shredded romaine, washed and dried

1 cup grated carrots
2 scallions, thinly sliced
chopped fresh cilantro

- Cook noodles in plenty of water according to package directions.
- Drain, then rinse in tepid water and drain again. Toss with sauce.
- On a platter or 2 serving plates, spread the lettuce, then the shredded carrots.
- Roll noodles on top. Sprinkle with sliced scallion and fresh cilantro and serve. *Serves 2.*

FIFTEEN

Beans and Grains

Protein Plus

Legumes *aka* Beans

Legumes are plants that produce edible seeds within a pod. Legumes constitute an enormous family with more than six hundred genuses and thirteen thousand species. Beans, broad beans, soybeans, peas, lentils, and peanuts are all legumes. They provide a sizable amount of protein and some complex carbohydrates. Unlike animal proteins, legumes are incomplete proteins, lacking some of the essential amino acids. However, many cultures rely heavily on legumes as their primary source of protein, instinctively combining them with grains and some dairy products to gain all of the essential amino acids necessary to form complete proteins.

For many people, beans cause considerable difficulty during digestion, leading to flatulence and intestinal discomfort. Some beans cause worse distress than others. If you don't regularly consume beans, start slowly and cautiously. Preparation is the key to success. When soaking beans, drain them every few hours and add fresh water to continue soaking off the enzymes that are the source of the bean's digestive aftereffects. Use fresh water when you cook the beans. Drain and rinse canned beans well. And be sure to cook dried beans thoroughly! They must be tender. Cook them longer than you might otherwise, even if you are following directions. Many things can affect the cooking time of beans, such as the age of the beans, type of water, altitude, and where the beans were grown. Eat a small amount. Start with a tablespoon or two with a grain dish such as rice.

LIMA BEANS WITH GOAT CHEESE AND SCALLIONS

HIGHLY BENEFICIAL	B	NEUTRAL	O	AVOID	A, AB

Lima beans are neutral benefit for Type O and are highly beneficial for Type B. They're very creamy with a mild flavor. They're so creamy, in fact, that they're often referred to as butter beans. Don't overcook lima beans; they turn mushy very quickly once they've softened. Also, be aware that cooking lima beans produces a lot of foam, so they're not necessarily the best bet for a pressure cooker. They can make a delicious main-course salad, with a lemon vinaigrette dressing—Types B and AB can have oil and vinegar—and sprinkled with goat cheese and scallions.

1 package frozen baby limas
   or 1 cup dried lima beans
   or 2 cups fresh lima beans
1 tablespoon olive oil
2 scallions, thinly sliced
2 cloves garlic, crushed and
   peeled

dressing of choice
4 oz. goat cheese
3 tablespoons fresh parsley,
   minced

- Prepare lima beans and put them in a serving bowl.
- In a skillet, heat oil over medium to high heat. Add the scallions and sauté a minute or two until fragrant. Add garlic, turning briefly until it just begins to color.
- Add scallions and garlic to the lima beans.
- Pour 2 to 3 tablespoons of dressing over the beans and toss gently.
- Crumble goat cheese over the top and garnish with parsley. Serve at room temperature. *Serves 4.*

BLACK-EYED PEAS WITH LEEKS

HIGHLY BENEFICIAL	O, A	NEUTRAL		AVOID	B, AB

If you use canned beans, or if you plan ahead and soak some the night before, this is an easy, delicious dish, served either hot or cold. Serve it hot with rice for dinner or cold (or room temperature) with a dressing of olive oil and lemon juice for a quick lunch.

2 cups cooked black-eyed peas
1 tablespoon olive oil
1 small leek, thinly sliced
1 clove garlic, crushed and
    peeled

¼ cup water
pinch of salt
¼ cup fresh cilantro, chopped

- Put the beans in a pot to heat.
- In a cast-iron skillet, heat oil over low heat. Add leek and garlic, turning well to coat with oil.
- Add water, cover, and braise leek until soft. Add more water as needed, 1 tablespoon at a time.
- When leek is tender, add it to the beans and heat thoroughly. Toss gently with cilantro and salt. *Serves 4.*

LENTIL SALAD

HIGHLY BENEFICIAL	A, AB	NEUTRAL		AVOID	O, B

This lentil salad tastes great, and is an excellent accompaniment to other, interesting ingredients. This is a slightly "sweet" salad that is perfect for lunch and dinner.

2 cup lentils
8 cups water
½ cup dried cherries
½ cup raisins
½ cup walnuts, broken into
    pieces

2 tablespoons olive oil
juice of ½ lemon
pinch of salt

- Cook the lentils in the water, gently simmering, until done, 30 to 40 minutes. Start checking at 30 minutes because lentils can overcook very quickly.
- Drain and let cool.
- Add cherries, raisins, and walnuts.
- Whisk together oil, lemon, and salt. Pour dressing over salad, mixing gently and thoroughly. *Serves 4 to 6.*

PURÉED PINTO BEANS WITH GARLIC

HIGHLY BENEFICIAL	O, A, AB	NEUTRAL		AVOID	B

With brown rice and braised kale, these beans make a very filling and quick dinner. Also try this as a different and delicious dip for raw vegetables.

2 tablespoons olive oil
1 medium onion, diced
6 cloves garlic, crushed
1 can pinto beans, drained
    and rinsed, or 1 cup
    dry pinto beans, soaked
    and cooked

1 teaspoon ground cumin (or
    to taste)
generous pinch of salt
3 tablespoons chopped fresh
    cilantro

- In a cast-iron skillet, heat 2 tablespoons oil over very low heat. Add diced onion and cook about 10 minutes, stirring frequently, until onion is golden brown.
- Add garlic and sauté a few minutes more. Add beans and spices, then cook another few minutes.
- Transfer mixture to blender and purée until very smooth. You might have to scrape down the blender once or twice to get it all.
- Serve sprinkled with the cilantro. *Serves 4.*

Grains

There is a very wide variety of life-sustaining grains. Today, long forgotten or ignored grains such as spelt and quinoa have been rediscovered and are being cultivated. For people with wheat intolerance, alternative grains are a real boon, whether these grains are used as flours in breads, pastas, and cereals or as whole grains cooked like buckwheat or rice. Many of these rediscovered grains have unfamiliar tastes and textures, which make them exciting and different. There's a world of grains to discover.

Rice

HIGHLY BENEFICIAL	AB	NEUTRAL	O, A, B	AVOID	

The second largest food crop in the world behind wheat, rice has almost eight thousand varieties. Wild rice belongs to a different species altogether. Rice is an extraordinarily compatible grain that can be enjoyed by all blood types. There are many kinds of rice sold under various trademarks: basmati, Texmati™, wild pecan, Lundberg Royal™, Wehani™, Black Japonica™, Jasmati™, arborio, white and brown sushi, short- and long-grain white and brown, sweet brown, and many others.

Mixed-blood type families as well as guests always appreciate a main course with rice. The rule of thumb is 2 cups of water to 1 cup rice. Allow about 20 to 25 minutes of cooking time for white rice, and 35 to 40 minutes for brown rice.

Wild Rice

HIGHLY BENEFICIAL	AB	NEUTRAL	O, A	AVOID	B

Not a rice at all but an aquatic grass, wild rice is truly a native American crop, the uncultivated varieties of which grow in the wetlands around many northern lakes and rivers. Wild rice has a more complex taste and aroma than those of most grains, and its beautiful, dark color and crunchy texture set it apart from domesticated grains. Wild rice is now grown commercially in California, but there are those who still prefer the hand-harvested wild rice.

Because of its variations, it is hard to gauge the amount of water needed to cook wild rice. For 1 cup wild rice, begin with 2 to 2½ cups water and keep an eye on it. Bring to a boil, then reduce heat to low. The rice is done when it's tender and some of the individual grains have burst open. Add more water, a tablespoon at a time, or cook the rice a little longer to absorb the last of the water.

Amaranth

HIGHLY BENEFICIAL	A	NEUTRAL	O, AB	AVOID	B

A tiny grain from a majestic, maroon-headed plant, amaranth was a staple food of the Aztecs. It is high in protein, calcium, phosphorus, iron, and fiber as well as the amino acids lysine and methionine. Toast these seeds lightly before cooking by tossing the seeds in a preheated cast-iron pan over a medium-low heat. Allow 1 cup of amaranth to 1 cup water.

Buckwheat

HIGHLY BENEFICIAL	A	NEUTRAL	O	AVOID	B, AB

Buckwheat originated in Asia, and it is actually a seed rather than a true grain. Buckwheat is high in protein, B vitamins, vitamin E, iron, and calcium. It is best known as kasha, a hearty porridge, and it also makes an excellent pancake. Buckwheat can also substitute for corn and makes a wonderfully rich and different polenta.

Kamut

HIGHLY BENEFICIAL		NEUTRAL	O, A	AVOID	B, AB

An ancient Egyptian grain, kamut is a distant relative of modern hybrid wheat. It contains far more protein than wheat while being far less allergen-producing. The kernels are larger than wheat berries and have a nutty taste and smooth texture. Kamut resembles rice in shape and is a good choice for salads and pilafs.

Millet

HIGHLY BENEFICIAL	B, AB	NEUTRAL	O, A	AVOID	

One of the most ancient of grains, common millet is grown in China, India, Russia, southern Europe, and parts of North America. Foxtail millet is among China's five most sacred crops. There is no one millet—the name is given to a number of cereal grains that don't even belong in the same genus. Pearl millet is cultivated in India; sorghum in India, Africa, and China. Another strain of millet is cultivated in the Philippines as well as in Ethiopia, where it's called *teff* and is the essential ingredient of *injera*, the Ethiopian flatbread. In its various forms it has been eaten as a porridge for millennia. Millet has been grown as a grain to stave off famine, because it is so hardy and grows in such inhospitable environments. Rich in phosphorus, iron, calcium, riboflavin, and niacin, it also contains the amino acid lysine, something that cornmeal doesn't. Eaten in combination with tofu or beans, millet forms a complete protein.

Quinoa

HIGHLY BENEFICIAL		NEUTRAL	O, A, B, AB	AVOID	

The tiny quinoa seed contains a germ with far more protein than any other grain, and of higher quality. Its amino acids are more balanced than those of other grains, with high levels of lysine, methionine, and cystine. Not really a grain at all, quinoa's genus can be found in the herb family. It was a sacred food of the Incas for centuries. It ideally complements beans for a complete protein meal. Among its many recommendations, quinoa is a source of iron, magnesium, zinc, copper, potassium, riboflavin, thiamin, niacin, and phosphorus. Quinoa has reemerged from obscurity and is finding its way into more people's diets every day. Quinoa's high protein and low gluten contents, nutty flavor, and crunchy texture make it a worthwhile addition to anyone's diet, particularly since it can readily substitute for most other grains, and its reaction is neutral for all blood types.

Spelt

HIGHLY BENEFICIAL		NEUTRAL	O, A, B, AB	AVOID	

A nonhybridized wheat that was a staple in biblical times, spelt will soon become a modern-day staple, not only for its nonallergenic properties, but for its great nutritive value. Spelt contains more protein, amino acids, B vitamins, and minerals than does its distant cousin, hybridized wheat. Spelt is available in many different forms. Whole-spelt and white-spelt flours can be substituted pretty closely for any wheat recipe, and pastas made from spelt are good replacements for durum and semolina, although the current cost is three times higher than that of wheat products. Whole-spelt flour makes for a denser dough than white-spelt flour, which is still slightly denser than that made from commercial white flour. Spelt berries are large, moist, slightly chewy, and flavorful, similar in texture to barley. The spelt berries make excellent grain salads.

FARO PILAF

HIGHLY BENEFICIAL		NEUTRAL	O, A, B, AB	AVOID	

Faro *is the Italian word for "spelt," and it makes a different, nuttier alternative to rice in this recipe for pilaf.*

1 cup faro
2 cups water
olive oil
3 cloves garlic, crushed and
   peeled

2 small zucchini, diced small
2 tablespoons fresh parsley,
   chopped
salt
pecorino romano cheese

- Combine faro and water in a saucepan and bring to a boil. Reduce heat, cover, and steam until all water is absorbed, about 20 minutes.
- Meanwhile, heat about 2 tablespoons oil in a heavy cast-iron skillet over medim-low heat. Add garlic and sauté a few moments.
- Add zucchini and stir until coated with oil. Cover and steam until soft, about 5 to 8 minutes.
- Add parsley, cover pan, and allow to steam another minute.
- Remove from heat and place in bowl with faro; mix together. Add salt to taste. Grate a little pecorino romano over the dish. *Serves 3 to 4.*

WILD AND BASMATI RICE PILAF

HIGHLY BENEFICIAL	AB	NEUTRAL	O, A	AVOID	B

The following recipe is easy to prepare, as it calls for the most basic of ingredients and a modest cooking time.

1 cup wild rice, cooked in 2 to 3 cups water
1 cup basmati rice, cooked in 2 cups water
3 green scallions, sliced
¼ cup olive oil
2 teaspoons salt

- Cook the rices in separate pans.
- When the rices are cooked, combine them, toss with the scallions and olive oil, and salt to taste.   *Serves 4 to 6.*

MILLET TABBOULEH

HIGHLY BENEFICIAL	B, AB	NEUTRAL	O, A	AVOID	

Millet's versatility makes it a perfect choice for recipes calling for bulghur wheat. Traditionally, tabbouleh is a parsley and mint salad with the occasional sprinkling of grain. Here we have replaced the traditional cracked bulghur with millet. Feel free to increase the fresh herbs as desired.

2½ cups water (vegetable stock makes for more flavor)
1 cup millet, lighly toasted without oil
3 scallions, thinly sliced
1 cucumber, peeled, seeded, and diced small

3 plum tomatoes, chopped (optional)
¼ cup chopped fresh parsley
¼ cup chopped fresh mint
2 tablespoons olive oil
juice of 1 lemon
salt

- Bring water to a boil. Add millet, stir, and return to boil.
- Reduce heat and simmer 15 to 20 minutes, or until all water is absorbed. Let sit off heat 10 minutes.
- Transfer cooked millet to a bowl and let cool slightly.
- Add scallions, cucumber, tomatoes, if using, parsley, and mint; mix well.
- Dress with oil and lemon. Add salt to taste.   *Serves 3 to 4.*

MILLET COUSCOUS

HIGHLY BENEFICIAL	B, AB	NEUTRAL	O, A	AVOID	

Couscous is not just a grain, but the name of the national dish of North African countries such as Algeria, Morocco, and Tunisia. It is produced from semolina, the flour that results from the milling of the endosperm of hard durum wheat. Couscous is produced by mixing the resulting semolina with flour and sprinkling the two with cold salted water. It is then rolled and pressed (usually by hand) to produce the tiny beads of couscous. This variation of the traditional couscous is made from the ubiquitous millet, and is quite good eaten on its own, though it marries easily with vegetables, meats, soups, stews, or salads. This recipe uses the millet couscous as part of a deliciously textured salad.

1 cup millet, lightly toasted without oil

2½ cups water or vegetable stock

2 carrots, diced small

1 small red onion, diced small

¼ cup raisins, plumped (by soaking in hot water)

3 tablespoons sunflower seeds (Types O, A) or 3 tablespoons chopped walnuts (Types O, B, and AB)

2 tablespoons olive oil

juice of 1 lemon

salt

- Cook millet and transfer to a bowl.
- Add carrots, red onions, raisins, and sunflower seeds or walnuts.
- Whisk together the olive oil and lemon juice and pour over the millet. Add salt to taste. Also quite good when topped with silken tofu. *Serves 3 to 4.*

SPELT BERRY AND BASMATI RICE PILAF

HIGHLY BENEFICIAL		NEUTRAL	O, A, B, AB	AVOID	

The chewy spelt berries give this pilaf additional body and flavor.

1 cup cooked spelt berries

1 cup cooked basmati rice (increase amount of rice if desired)

2 scallions, diced

2 tablespoons olive oil

salt

- Combine all ingredients and let sit for at least 15 minutes. Serve at room temperature. *Serves 4.*

SPELT BERRY AND RICE SALAD

HIGHLY BENEFICIAL	AB	NEUTRAL	O, B	AVOID	A

This is a slighly different version of the pilaf recipe offered previously. The colors alone make for an appealing dish, but the taste and textures add their own interesting note.

1 cup cooked spelt berries
1 to 2 cups cooked rice (any variety)
1 yellow pepper, diced small (Type AB substitute 1 cup sautéed maitake mushrooms)

3 tablespoons chopped fresh parsley
1 tablespoon diced jalapeño peppers (Type AB omit)
3 tablespoons olive oil
salt

- Combine all ingredients and serve at room temperature. Feel free to add scallions, garlic, and complementary spices such as coriander and a dusting of cumin. The dish can hold in the refrigerator up to 4 days. *Serves 4 to 5.*

QUINOA RISOTTO

HIGHLY BENEFICIAL		NEUTRAL	O, A, B, AB	AVOID	

Traditional Italian risotto is cooked with the classic round rice known as arborio. The rice is first cooked in oil or butter for a few minutes while being constantly stirred. Liquid is added, and then the mixture is simmered until the liquid is absorbed. Cooked in this manner, the rice remains separate and firm. Using quinoa in place of the rice doesn't change the essential texture of the dish and adds a tremendous protein boost to the meal, as quinoa contains far more protein than do most other grains.

2 tablespoons olive oil
1 onion, diced
2 cloves garlic, minced
1 red pepper, minced (Types O and B only)
3 tablespoons chopped fresh flat-leaf parlsey

2 cups quinoa, rinsed and drained
3¼ cups vegetable broth
salt

- Heat oil in a medium saucepan over medim heat. Add the onion and garlic and cook a few minutes, being careful not to burn the garlic. Add the red pepper and parsley and continue cooking another minute.
- Add the quinoa and cook a few moments, thoroughly coating the quinoa with the oil and vegetables, then add the stock. Water may be used, although vegetable broth adds flavor to the dish.
- Bring to a boil, then reduce to a simmer, cover, and cook 15 minutes. Season with salt to taste. Serve immediately. This dish is also good served cold.   *Serves 4.*

BROWN RICE PILAF

HIGHLY BENEFICIAL	AB	NEUTRAL	O, A, B	AVOID	

Any brown rice will do for this pilaf, but brown basmati rice has a slightly nutty flavor that is quite pleasing. Some of the colored rices added in any proportion to the brown rice also provide variations in texture and are quite decorative.

1 cup brown rice
2 cups water
2 tablespoons olive oil
4 cloves garlic, crushed and peeled

1 large carrot, diced
½ cup water
¼ cup fresh cilantro, chopped
salt

- Combine rice and 2 cups water in a saucepan and bring to a boil. Reduce heat, cover, and steam 40 minutes, or until all water has been absorbed. Always check your rice toward the end of the cooking time. Rice cooking times are specific to the variety and will vary.

- While the rice cooks, heat 2 tablespoons oil in a heavy skillet over medium heat. Add garlic and sauté gently a few moments. Add carrot, stir to coat with oil, and add remaining ½ cup water.
- Reduce heat, cover pan, and simmer until carrot is tender but not soft. Check carefully to be sure there is sufficient water to braise the carrot, adding water in small quantities if necessary.
- Add coriander in the last few minutes, letting it steam.
- When rice is cooked, place carrot and rice in bowl, mixing gently. Add salt to taste.   *Serves 4.*

WILD RICE SALAD

HIGHLY BENEFICIAL	AB	NEUTRAL	O, A	AVOID	B

Here's a chance to use wild rice in a festive and interesting way. This is a very pretty dish that makes an admirable accompaniment to squab, Cornish game hens, lamb, and venison.

1 cup hand-harvested wild rice
1 cup dried apricots, diced
1 cup walnuts, chopped
1 cup dried cherries

¼ cup olive oil
juice of 1 lemon
1 tablespoon maple syrup
salt

- Bring 3 cups water to a boil. Add wild rice. Cover, reduce heat, and simmer about 45 minutes, or until tender.
- Drain any remaining water and reserve for stock. Toss rice lightly with fork.
- Plump dried apricots by pouring boiling water over them; let sit until soft.
- When rice has cooled for a while, add walnuts, cherries, and apricots, mixing well.
- Whisk together olive oil, lemon juice, maple syrup, and pinch of salt. Pour over salad, turning well. Adjust seasoning to taste. The wild rice salad tastes best when served at room temperature. *Serves 3 to 4.*

SPELT BERRY SALAD

HIGHLY BENEFICIAL		NEUTRAL	O, A, B, AB	AVOID	

Spelt berries suit all of the blood types. Make this salad for lunch, or serve it with fish or tofu for dinner.

1 cup spelt berries
1 cucumber, peeled and diced
2 scallions, finely sliced
¼ cup red onion, finely chopped
¼ cup fresh cilantro, chopped

2 tablespoons olive oil
juice of 1 lemon
salt
2 tablespoons crumbled goat cheese

- Cook spelt in 4 cups water about 45 minutes, until tender and chewy.
- Add cucumber, scallions, red onion, and cilantro, and mix gently.
- Dress with olive oil, lemon juice, and salt to taste.
- Sprinkle with goat cheese.   *Serves 4.*

Vegetables

The Simpler, the Better

*T*HE FLAVORS AND TEXTURES OF MOST VEGETABLES ARE best expressed through simple treatment. Eaten raw, steamed, baked, or sautéed, vegetables should accompany every meal; the more, the better.

The recipes that follow provide creative ways to prepare vegetables when you're looking for something different and interesting. Just remember: the simpler the preparation, the better.

GLAZED TURNIPS AND ONIONS

HIGHLY BENEFICIAL	O, A	NEUTRAL	B, AB	AVOID	

Turnips are an often overlooked vegetable choice. Cook them as you would carrots. Small turnips don't need to be peeled if they're fresh and unwaxed. Otherwise, peel the turnip and put in hot water 10 minutes. This makes them easier to digest and reduces their rather sharp, pungent odor. Highly Beneficial for Type O and Type A, they are of Neutral value to Type B and Type AB. Turnips are a terrific source of vitamin C, potassium, and folic acid. Turnip greens are rich in vitamins A, B, and C as well as potassium and magnesium. The greens can be cooked as you would spinach.

2 tablespoons butter (Type A use olive oil)

2 tablespoons olive oil

1 yellow onion, quartered

4 turnips, cut into wedges

4 cloves garlic, crushed and peeled

¾ to 1 cup chicken stock (Type A and Type AB use water)

salt

3 to 4 tablespoons fresh parsley, chopped

■ In a heavy skillet, melt the butter in the oil over low heat. Add onion, turning to coat with butter and oil, and cook over very low heat until soft and deep golden in color, about 20 minutes.

■ Add turnips and garlic, turning well.

■ Add chicken stock or water and a little salt and bring to boil.

■ Reduce heat, cover, and simmer until done, about 20 minutes. Check to be sure there is always liquid in the skillet. Add a few tablespoons at a time as needed. There should be very little liquid left.

■ Remove lid and allow the last of the liquid to evaporate. Continue to turn vegetables. Serve at once, spooning sauce over them and sprinkling with parsley. *Serves 4.*

CARROTS AND PARSNIPS WITH GARLIC, GINGER, AND CILANTRO

HIGHLY BENEFICIAL	O, A, B, AB	NEUTRAL		AVOID	

Carrots and parsnips, humble root vegetables that they are, reach new heights of gustatory delight when paired with garlic, ginger, and cilantro. The depth and sweetness of the carrot and the savory richness of the parsnip provide a wonderful complement to the sharp zing of the fresh ginger.

olive oil

2 carrots, sliced on the diagonal

2 parsnips, sliced on the diagonal

6 cloves garlic, crushed and peeled

½- to 1-inch piece of fresh ginger, minced

water

4 tablespoons fresh cilantro, chopped

salt

- Heat 1 to 2 tablespoons oil in a heavy skillet over medium heat. Add vegetables, and turn in the oil a few moments until coated. Add garlic and ginger, stirring another moment.
- Add ½ cup water and bring to a boil.
- Reduce heat, cover, and braise 15 to 20 minutes, or until carrots and parsnips are tender. Be sure that there is always a little water in the skillet, adding a tablespoon or two as needed. As the dish nears completion, water should be absorbed.
- At the last moment of cooking, add the chopped cilantro and salt to taste. *Serves 3 to 4.*

SWEET POTATO PANCAKES

HIGHLY BENEFICIAL	O, B, AB	NEUTRAL		AVOID	A

Sweet potatoes are a vitamin A-packed treat. They are lovely when baked, and are great in casseroles and stews. These pancakes are a perfect accompaniment to grilled meats and roasts, and are equally delicious with poultry and fish.

1 large sweet potato, or
  4 cups grated
¼ red onion, grated
2 tablespoons chopped fresh
  cilantro

1 large egg
¼ cup spelt flour
¼ teaspoon salt
¼ cup olive or canola oil for
  cooking

- Wash and rinse sweet potato; do not peel. Grate over a large plate.
- Add onion and cilantro.
- Mix in egg and flour until well incorporated, then add salt. The mixture will be loose, but will form patties.
- In a large skillet, heat oil and carefully pan-fry each cake 4 to 5 minutes on each side. Once cooked, the pancakes can be kept warm in a 250-degree F oven for an hour or so. *Makes 6 large dinner-size pancakes, or 15 appetizer-size pancakes.*

CAULIFLOWER WITH GARLIC AND PARSLEY

HIGHLY BENEFICIAL	B, AB	NEUTRAL	AB	AVOID	O

Cauliflower is a densely packed flowering vegetable with a potent nutritional wallop. Its mild flavor is an excellent foil for many different flavors, in particular garlic, curry, and nutmeg. This is a Highly Beneficial vegetable for Type B and Type AB. While of Neutral value for Type A, its benefits make it a valuable addition to the diet. And don't forget the hybrid of broccoli and cauliflower, broccoflower, a pale green cruciferous vegetable loaded with nutritional goodness.

1 head cauliflower
2 tablespoons olive oil
4 to 6 cloves garlic, crushed
   and peeled
water
3 to 4 tablespoons chopped
   fresh parsley
salt

- Cut cauliflower into fairly uniform sections.
- In a large, heavy skillet, heat 2 tablespoons oil. Add garlic, sautéeing until fragrant.
- Add cauliflower pieces and turn in the oil. Then add about a cup of water and bring to a low boil.
- Cover pan and let the cauliflower steam. When cauliflower is soft but firm, the water should be almost absorbed. If not, remove the lid and let most of the excess liquid boil away, leaving a rich oil and garlic sauce.
- With the back of a wooden spoon, coarsely mash cauliflower. Add parsley and salt to taste.
- Served with pan-roasted chicken or fish, this is also a satisfying pasta sauce. *Serves 4.*

BRAISED FENNEL AND GARLIC

HIGHLY BENEFICIAL		NEUTRAL	O, A, B, AB	AVOID	

Fennel has a sweet, earthy flavor lightly tinged with anise that goes well with fish. This simple preparation seems well suited to this often over-looked but glorious vegetable.

1 bulb fennel
2 tablespoons olive oil
3 cloves garlic, crushed and
   peeled

water
½ teaspoon salt
3 to 4 tablespoons fresh
   parsley, chopped

- Cut fennel into ¼-inch-thick slices, using as much of the fennel as possible. The stalks are a little fibrous, but can be saved for stock or used here.
- Heat oil in a heavy skillet over low to medium heat. Add sliced fennel and stir to coat with oil.
- Add garlic, ½ cup water, and salt, and bring to a gentle simmer.
- Cover and cook until tender, 15 to 20 minutes. Be sure to keep a little water in the skillet, adding extra by the tablespoon as needed.
- During the last few minutes of cooking, add parsley.
  Serves 3 to 4.

STEWED STRING BEANS WITH TOMATOES AND GARLIC

HIGHLY BENEFICIAL		NEUTRAL	O, AB	AVOID	A, B

This is a traditional Greek method of preparing string beans. The long, slow cooking in the acidic tomato and pungent garlic makes the beans tender. String beans are a Neutral value for all the blood types, and tomatoes are Neutral for Type O, so slide this dish to your side of the table and enjoy.

2 tablespoons olive oil

4 cloves garlic, chopped

1 to 1½ lbs. string beans, washed and stems removed

28-oz. can whole plum tomatoes

1 teaspoon dried oregano

salt

- Heat oil in a casserole dish over medium heat. Add garlic and sauté briefly. Add beans and stir to coat with oil.
- Add the plum tomatoes, crushing them before they go into the pot. You can use a knife to coarsely chop them, or break them up by hand.
- Bring to a boil, and then reduce heat to a low simmer.
- Stir in oregano and a generous pinch of salt, cover, and cook mixture 45 minutes to 1 hour. The beans should be very tender and the tomato liquid almost absorbed.
- For the last several minutes of cooking, slide the lid aside so that most of the steam escapes, leaving a rich, thick sauce.

Serves 4 to 6.

MASHED PLANTAINS

HIGHLY BENEFICIAL		NEUTRAL	B, AB	AVOID	O, A

Plantains look a lot like bananas and are easy to find, usually in the tropical foods section of the produce aisle. They're of Neutral value to Type B and Type AB, but can be a welcome change from potatoes.

2 ripe plantains

1 tablespoon butter

1 tablespoon olive oil

salt

- Peel plantains. Though similar in appearance to bananas, plantains don't peel like bananas. You'll probably have to cut them into smaller pieces first.
- After peeling, cut them into 1-inch-thick slices and place in a pot. Cover them completely with water and bring to a boil.

- Cook until they are fully tender, 20 to 30 minutes. Keep an eye on them, because riper plantains will cook more quickly. Don't overcook.
- Drain, reserving a little of the broth. Mash well, adding butter and olive oil. Season with salt to taste. You may want to use the cooking water, a spoonful at a time, in the mashing process. *Serves 3 to 4.*

BRAISED GREENS WITH GARLIC

HIGHLY BENEFICIAL	O, A, B, AB NEUTRAL		AVOID	

There is a rich, nutritious world of mildly bitter to sharply bitter greens waiting to be discovered and cooked. Greens are easy to prepare, available year-round, and complement anything from grains to tofu, fish, meats, and poultry. And greens are compatible for all blood types. What better recommendation could they possibly have? The following recipe is a general guide for braising these great greens. Braising them slowly makes them easier to digest, and their nutrients are better assimilated in our bodies. The flavors vary tremendously, from mildly piquant to bitter, with a number of the greens having a hot, peppery bite. Recommended are chard, mustard greens, collards, kale, escarole, chicory, dandelion greens, broccoli rabe (sometimes sold as rappini), beet greens, and turnip greens.

1 bunch greens	water
2 tablespoons olive oil	salt
4 to 6 cloves garlic, crushed and peeled	

- Wash the greens very well, because some of them are exceptionally gritty, and carelessness at this stage of preparation can result in a less than pleasant dining experience.
- Some greens have leaves that are very wide. Cut them against the grain of the stems at 1-inch intervals into long strips, and don't discard the stems. Eat them, too.

- Heat oil in a heavy skillet with a lid over medium heat. Add garlic and sauté until it softens.
- Add cut green leaves, turning them in the oil. The leaves will be voluminous, but they will reduce in size substantially by the time they're ready to be eaten.
- Reduce heat and cook for several minutes. The moisture retained during washing should be all the water the greens initially need.
- After several minutes, add ½ cup water and cover skillet.
- Check frequently to be sure there is still water, adding a few tablespoons at a time as necessary. Doneness varies from green to green. They should be soft and limp, and most of the water should have evaporated. Add salt to taste.   *Serves 2 to 3.*

PURÉED CAULIFLOWER WITH PESTO

HIGHLY BENEFICIAL	B, AB	NEUTRAL	A	AVOID	O

The swirl of green pesto in this pure white purée is very pretty, and the taste is unusual.

1 head cauliflower	salt
2 cloves garlic, crushed and peeled	Basil Pesto (see page 369)

- Quarter cauliflower, place in top of double boiler, and sprinkle with garlic.
- Pour boiling water over cauliflower and garlic, and steam until cauliflower is soft enough to pierce with a straw, 15 to 20 minutes.
- Transfer to blender or food processor and purée until smooth. Add salt to taste.
- At the table, spoon a dollop of pesto onto each serving.   *Serves 4.*

VEGETABLE FRITTERS

HIGHLY BENEFICIAL	O, A, B, AB	NEUTRAL		AVOID	

Fritters can be a light supper on their own or an excellent accompaniment to chicken or fish. Depending on your blood type, squash, sweet potatoes, yams, carrots, and turnips are all good choices for this fritter recipe. Grate the vegetables finely. If there's any excess liquid, drain and reserve before adding the rest of the ingredients.

3 cups grated vegetables
1 tablespoon finely minced
  onion

2 eggs
olive oil
salt

- Mix grated vegetables with onion and eggs. The batter will be quite wet.
- In a large, heavy skillet, heat 3 tablespoons oil over medium heat.
- Lightly shape a handful of the batter for each fritter and gently drop into the oil, taking care not to splatter yourself. Flatten the fritters with a spatula.
- Let them brown over medium heat until the bottoms begin to color. Turn the fritters over and fry for several more minutes.
- Drain on paper towels, sprinkle with salt, and serve. You can also keep them warm in a preheated 250-degree F oven while you cook the rest of the batter.   *Serves 4 to 6.*

STEAMED ARTICHOKE

HIGHLY BENEFICIAL	O, A	NEUTRAL		AVOID	B, AB

Everyone has developed his or her own approach to artichokes, and if it works for you, carry on. Remember: Although the meat at the bottom of the leaves contains small amounts of the very potent sugar produced in the artichoke heart, the prized and succulent heart itself is a treasure trove of potassium, magnesium, and folic acid. While arti-chokes are Highly Beneficial for Type O and Type A, they are on the Avoid list for Type B and Type AB. It pays to know your blood type!

1 stalk lemongrass, peeled and cut into pieces (large is okay)	1 teaspoon olive oil
	4 cloves garlic, crushed and peeled
1-inch piece fresh ginger, peeled and julienned	1 artichoke per person

■ Place all ingredients in the steamer. With or without trimming, the stem left long or cut short, the bottom up or tips down, an arti-choke usually takes between 45 and 55 minutes to thoroughly cook. Keep plenty of water in the bottom of the pan, and the pot mostly covered.

■ Serve with a squeeze of lemon juice or a dipping sauce. Allow 1 artichoke per person.

SWISS CHARD WITH SARDINES

HIGHLY BENEFICIAL	O, A, B, AB	NEUTRAL		AVOID	

This recipe is suited to all of the blood types if the tomato is eliminated for Types A and B. Swiss chard is Highly Beneficial for Types O and A, and is a Neutral value to Types B and AB, offset by the tremendous nutritional boost of the sardines, which are loaded with calcium.

2 lbs. Swiss chard	1 tomato, chopped (Types O and AB)
2 tablespoons olive oil	
3 cloves garlic, minced	salt
1 small onion, thinly sliced	
6 sardines, packed in water, drained and chopped	

■ Wash chard well, slice into 1-inch strips, and steam quickly. Remove from pan and set aside.

- In a large skillet, heat oil over medium heat. Add garlic and onions and cook until slightly browned and soft.
- Add sardines and tomato. Add greens and toss lightly, cooking all ingredients together for a few more minutes. Season with salt to taste. *Serves 4.*

GARDEN RATATOUILLE

HIGHLY BENEFICIAL		NEUTRAL	O, A, B, AB	AVOID	

If you are lucky enough to have your own garden, or a generous neighbor who does, this recipe will come in handy at the end of the summer, when there is always an overabundance of green and yellow squash, plum and cherry tomatoes, and basil. There are no hard and fast rules here. If your vegetable bin yields a mushroom or two, so much the better. Of course, choose only the best vegetables for your blood type. The basic recipe is as simple and elegant as the result is nutritious and delicious!

3 tablespoons olive oil
1 medium onion, diced
5 cloves garlic, chopped
3 green zucchini (medium),
    sliced lengthwise,
    then cut into chunks
3 yellow squash (medium),
    prepared as above

1 or 2 cups tomatoes,
    chopped, or cherry
    tomatoes, halved (Types A
    and B omit)
salt
½ cup fresh basil, chopped
grated pecorino romano
    cheese (optional)

- In a large, heavy skillet, heat oil, add onion, and cook 3 minutes, then add garlic and cook another 3 minutes.
- Add squash and cook, turning every 5 minutes, for 15 minutes.
- Types O and AB add tomatoes, reduce heat, and continue to cook another 10 minutes.
- Season with salt, toss with fresh basil, and top with grated cheese, if desired.
- Serve with rice or pasta as a main course, or with grilled meats, chicken, or fish. *Serves 6.*

BRAISED COLLARDS

HIGHLY BENEFICIAL	O, A, B, AB	NEUTRAL		AVOID	

Collard greens were traditionally cooked for hours with a piece of fatback bacon. For our purposes, however, a little olive oil replaces the bacon fat. Collard greens are not only delicious and nutritious, but Highly Beneficial for all of the blood types. Collards also are great as cold leftovers. You can use them as a filling for a frittata or an omelette. For Type O, Type B, or Type AB, there is no better way to fuel the body for a day's excursions than an omelet or frittata with leftover collards.

3 tablespoons olive oil
1 large onion, thinly sliced
1 large bunch fresh collard
   greens, washed well, tips
   of stems removed (the
   stems are quite delicious)

2 tablespoons soy sauce or
   tamari sauce (optional)
small amount of water, as
   needed

- Heat oil in a very large skillet or saucepan. Add onion and cook 5 minutes.
- Meanwhile, slice collards by rolling them into 1 large bunch, then cutting across the leaves in 1-inch intervals. Wash them, and with water on their leaves add all the collards to the pot at once, cover, and reduce heat.
- After 5 minutes, turn the collards so the wilted greens are on top. Add soy sauce or tamari, if using, and replace cover.
- Cook another 40 minutes, turning collards occasionally to make sure they cook evenly. Add a tablespoon or two of water at a time, as needed. Unlike other greens, collards are tastier if allowed to cook longer.   *Serves 4.*

GRILLED PORTOBELLO MUSHROOMS

HIGHLY BENEFICIAL		NEUTRAL	O, A, B, AB	AVOID	

These dense, meaty mushrooms are a great vegetarian substitute for hamburgers. Try them with garlic over pasta, or serve them as a satisfying and tasty side dish. Be sure to brush liberally with garlic and olive oil.

4 large Portobello mushrooms, stems removed (reserve for soups or stews)
4 teaspoons Garlic-Shallot Mixture (see page 375)

4 slices soy cheese (optional)
1 tablespoon olive oil
salt
chopped fresh parsley or basil
4 homemade spelt buns

- Prepare grill.
- Brush mushrooms liberally with Garlic-Shallot Mixture, olive oil, and herbs. Grill over medium heat 5 to 8 minutes. Turn over.
- If using soy cheese to make cheeseburger substitutes, place cheese on top.
- Whether you use cheese or not, grill another 5 to 8 minutes.
- Season with salt, sprinkle with fresh herbs, and serve on homemade spelt buns. Or, serve with grilled meat, poultry, fish, tempeh, and a nutty brown rice. *Serves 4.*

BRAISED LEEKS

HIGHLY BENEFICIAL	O, A	NEUTRAL	B, AB	AVOID	

Leeks are Highly Beneficial for Type O and Type A, while of Neutral value to Type B and Type AB. Try braising them with other vegetables, or use them in soups, stews, and casseroles.

1 large leek
2 cloves garlic, sliced
2 tablespoons olive oil

salt
½ cup water or vegetable stock

- Wash leeks thoroughly, removing green tops and root ends; slice thinly.
- Heat oil in a heavy cast-iron skillet over medium heat. Add sliced garlic and sauté a few moments.
- Add leeks and stir to coat with oil and garlic.
- Cover pan and gently cook leeks, adding a tablespoon of water at a time, until they are soft and thoroughly cooked. Season with salt.   *Serves 3 to 4.*

Soups and Stews

Old-Fashioned Comfort

OUPS AND STEWS HAVE SUSTAINED NATIONS. THE APOCRYPHAL story of rock soup isn't that far from the truth. Somehow, the concept of a communal pot into which any ingredient could be added became the metaphor for cultures and civilizations. Soups and stews are much the same, varying only in the proportion of broth to solid ingredients. They are filling and nutritious, providing a simple, one-pot, cook-ahead meal that often tastes even better on the second or third day. Soups and stews are avenues to dietary inspiration. The majority of refrigerators, pantries, and gardens contain ample ingredients for a soup. Frozen meat, fish, chicken, or vegetable stock; vegetables; beans; pasta; leftover meats, chicken, fish—the list of potential ingredients is endless. Soups and stews provide a terrific opportunity to use up leftovers and can be prepared in sufficient quantity to supply more than one meal.

The first two recipes that follow are for basic homemade stocks. These stocks are vastly superior to canned broths and bouillon cubes.

BASIC TURKEY STOCK

HIGHLY BENEFICIAL	AB	NEUTRAL	O, A, B	AVOID	

Homemade stocks frozen in individual batches provide a great head start for preparing any number of sumptuous dishes. A good stock is basic to any sauce, soup, or stew. Creating a stock really takes very little effort. There are a number of ways to approach it. For instance, you can roast a turkey and set aside the carcass, neck, and giblets for a stock. Or purchase necks and backs from the butcher, and use these as the basis for a hearty stock. Either of these methods will provide a tasty stock. Turkey is Neutral for Type O, Type A, and Type B, and Highly Beneficial for Type AB—a perfect stock for all blood types! Turkey, once considered only a holiday bird, is now available year-round. The ingredients should always be fresh. A turkey stock can also be enhanced by mushroom stems, herbs, onion peels, leek stalks, or celery leaves. Don't add vegetables such as broccoli, cauliflower, or Brussels sprouts; they are cruciferous vegetables which will add an unpleasantly sulphurous taste and odor to the stock.

1 medium turkey carcass, picked fairly clean (reserve any leftover meat for soup)

2 onions, roots removed, skins on, and cut into quarters

3 large carrots, cut into chunks

3 stalks celery, washed and cut into large pieces

¼ bunch fresh parsley, including stems, washed

fresh herbs, such as thyme, rosemary, oregano, basil, to taste

bay leaf or sage

- Fill a very large (5- to 6-quart) stock pot three-quarters full with water. Add all of the ingredients and bring to a boil.
- Reduce heat and simmer at least 2½ hours. The stock should reduce by a third.
- Let cool to room temperature, and skim any scum or fat from the surface.

- Refrigerate. Once cold, the fat will harden on top of the stock. At the same time, the scum will sink to the bottom. Stock made with bones will gel when cold.
- The stock can be frozen in convenient pint and quart containers. *Makes approximately 4 quarts.*

BASIC VEGETABLE STOCK

HIGHLY BENEFICIAL	O, A, B, AB NEUTRAL		AVOID	

Vegetable stock is simmered only 40 minutes, unlike turkey stock which needs to cook slowly over many hours to develop its rich flavors. This vegetable stock is "sweet" and clean-tasting, and full of nutrients. Again, don't use the cruciferous vegetables broccoli, Brussels sprouts, or cauliflower; they will dominate the taste of the broth.

1 large yellow onion, cut into quarters	parsley stems
	garlic skins
2 carrots, washed, trimmed, and cut into large pieces	apple skins and cores
	mushroom stems
2 stalks celery, washed and cut	parsnips
	leeks

- Fill a very large (5- to 6-quart) stockpot three-quarters full with water and bring to a boil.
- Add all the vegetables and herbs and simmer 40 minutes.
- Cool and strain out the vegetables. Refrigerate or freeze. *Serves 4 to 6.*

INDIAN LAMB STEW WITH SPINACH

HIGHLY BENEFICIAL	B, AB	NEUTRAL		AVOID	O, A

Buy a leg of lamb, cut it in half, and use part for this stew and the other half for shish kabobs. The meat for the stew should be cut into cubes smaller than those for the skewers. This is a good way to prepare two dinners at the same time.

3 tablespoons olive oil
1 large onion, chopped
2 tablespoons ground
　mustard
2 tablespoons ground cumin
2 tablespoons ground
　coriander
4-lb. leg of lamb, cut in half
　and cubed small
　(reserve other half for
　kabobs)

1 cup plain yogurt (low-fat is
　good)
water
4 to 5 cloves garlic, peeled
　and diced
2-inch piece fresh ginger,
　peeled and diced
2 lbs. fresh spinach, cleaned
　and chopped
salt

- In a large stew pot or saucepan, heat oil over medium heat. Add onion and cook several minutes, until translucent.
- Add all the spices and cook 2 to 3 minutes to release the flavors. Add lamb, mixing to coat well with the spices.
- Bit by bit, stir in yogurt and add enough water to cover.
- Stir in garlic and ginger and simmer meat, covered, until tender, about 1 hour and 15 minutes. Remove cover and simmer another 15 minutes, if necessary, to reduce liquid.
- Add spinach in batches, stirring it down to incorporate it into the stew. It will cook in just a few minutes.
- Season with salt to taste, and serve with saffron rice and mango chutney (Type B only.)
- Like all other stews, this one can be made ahead and even frozen. It really does improve the second day.　*Serves 4.*

BEEF STEW WITH GREEN BEANS AND CARROTS

HIGHLY BENEFICIAL	O	NEUTRAL	B	AVOID	A, AB

The great thing about stews is that there are no hard and fast rules on the seasonings and various ingredients. If you have some mushrooms, throw them in at the last minute. (If they are dried, put them in with the carrots.) If you prefer thyme, oregano, and rosemary, use those herbs instead of the ground spices. Follow the parameters of the recipe and create your own version according to blood type. Replacing the beef with cubed lamb would make this a Highly Beneficial dish for Type O, Type B, and Type AB, if you omit the chili powder. The beef stew is only Highly Beneficial for Type O and is of Neutral benefit for Type B.

2 lbs. stew beef, cut into
 1-inch cubes
¼ cup spelt flour (or less, for
 dredging meat)
3 tablespoons olive oil
1 tablespoon ground cumin
½ tablespoon ground kelp
1 tablespoon chili powder
1 teaspoon salt
⅓ cup red wine

2 to 3 cups stock (chicken,
 vegetable, or meat)
1 tablespoon Garlic-Shallot
 Mixture (see page 375)
 or 1 medium onion plus
 2 cloves garlic, chopped
4 skinny carrots, peeled and
 sliced on the diagonal
1 lb. green beans

- Cut away any fat from the meat. Dredge lightly in flour and shake off any excess.
- Heat oil in a large pot over moderate heat and brown beef in 2 batches. After the second batch is nearly done, return first batch of meat to the pot, then add all the spices and salt.
- Cook 5 minutes on low heat, then add wine to deglaze. Add 2 cups stock, then stir in shallot mixture. If using onions and garlic, add them.
- Cover pot and simmer 1 hour, checking periodically to see if more liquid is needed. Add if necessary.
- Add carrots, cover, and simmer another 30 minutes. Check for tenderness.

- Add green beans and cook another 10 to 15 minutes.
- Serve with buttered rice noodles or with rice and homemade bread. A terrific leftover.   *Serves 6.*

CUCUMBER YOGURT SOUP

HIGHLY BENEFICIAL	B, AB	NEUTRAL	A	AVOID	O

This light, refreshing soup makes a simple, healthy lunch on a hot summer's day. Allow one cup of yogurt and one cucumber for every two servings.

1 cucumber	pinch of salt
1 cup yogurt	½ cup fresh dill for garnish
squeeze of lemon	

- If the cucumber skin isn't too tough or covered with a preserving wax, leave it on.
- Dice cucumber and put it in the blender with the yogurt, dill, lemon, and salt. Blend until almost smooth.
- Pour into a serving bowl and garnish with some fresh dill. If it's too thick, thin with water to desired consistency.   *Serves 2.*

ADZUKI BEAN & PUMPKIN SOUP OR NAVY BEAN SOUP

HIGHLY BENEFICIAL	O, A, B, AB	NEUTRAL		AVOID	

This delicious soup is Highly Beneficial for Type O and Type A if you use pumpkin, and the same for B and AB if you replace adzuki beans with navy beans.

2 tablespoons olive oil

2 medium leeks, washed well and thinly sliced

6 large cloves garlic, chopped

6 cups water

1 small (6 to 8 inches across) sugar pumpkin or 1 acorn

or butternut squash, peeled and cut into ½-inch pieces

1 can adzuki beans, drained and rinsed well

generous handful chopped parsley

salt

- In a heavy pot, heat oil over medium heat. Add leeks and garlic and turn to coat with oil. Cook a few minutes, until they begin to color.
- Add enough water to cover them and bring to a boil. Reduce heat and simmer 10 minutes.
- Meanwhile, prepare squash. Add squash to pot, cover with water, and bring to a boil.
- Reduce heat and simmer 15 to 20 minutes, depending on variety of squash, or until tender.
- Stir in drained beans and heat through. Add parsley for the last minute or two of cooking. Add salt to taste.   *Serves 4 to 6.*

HEARTY FISH SOUP

HIGHLY BENEFICIAL	O, A, B, AB	NEUTRAL		AVOID	

Fish soup can make an elegant and special meal. Each of the blood types should choose a fish that is Highly Beneficial. Monkfish proves fine for everyone, so it can be used for a mixed-blood type family. Combinations of various fish also make for a hardy soup. Cod, snapper, grouper, and hake are just a few examples of excellent soup fish.

2 tablespoons olive oil

1 small leek, finely sliced

6 to 8 cloves garlic, crushed and peeled

7 to 8 cups water

½ large parsnip, diced small

1 medium yellow pepper, diced small (Types O and B only)

1 to 1½ lbs. fish, cut into ½-inch pieces

1 to 2 cups tender, young leaves from celery, or any greens, finely slivered

1 yellow tomato, chopped (Type O and Type AB only)

½ cup chopped parsley

salt

- In a large soup pot, heat oil over medium heat. Add leek and sauté a few minutes. Add garlic and continue to cook another moment or two, being careful not to let the garlic burn, which turns it bitter.
- Pour in water and bring to a boil. Add parsnips and simmer 5 minutes.
- Add peppers and simmer 5 to 8 minutes.
- Add fish and return soup to a boil. Reduce heat at once.
- Add greens and tomato, then simmer 5 to 8 minutes longer, or until the fish is cooked. Stir in parsley and salt to taste. Serve at once.   *Serves 4.*

WHITE BEAN AND WILTED GREENS SOUP

HIGHLY BENEFICIAL		NEUTRAL	O, A, B, AB	AVOID	

This is an easy soup to make, and it's a great mixed-blood type pleaser. The cannellini beans are Neutral for all blood types. The Swiss chard is Neutral as well. As a colorful bonus, the chard tints the white cannellini beans a light pink.

1 can cooked cannellini beans, drained and rinsed	1½ to 2 cups stock or water
1 clove garlic, peeled and end trimmed	1 cup chopped Swiss chard
	½ teaspoon salt

- In a 2-quart saucepan, bring beans, garlic, and stock to a boil. Reduce heat and simmer 10 to 15 minutes.
- With a slotted spoon, scoop out beans and transfer to a food processor or blender with ½ cup of liquid. If you have one of those handheld blenders, leave soup in the saucepan and purée until smooth.
- Return purée to saucepan and stir until blended. Add greens, season with salt, and cook another 5 minutes.   *Serves 2.*

CREAM OF WALNUT SOUP

HIGHLY BENEFICIAL	O, AB	NEUTRAL	A, B	AVOID	

2 cloves garlic, peeled and
   end trimmed
1½ cups walnuts
3 cups homemade turkey
   stock

½ cup dry white wine
½ cup soy, rice, or almond
   milk
salt and pepper
3 scallions, thinly sliced

- Purée garlic in a food processor. Add walnuts and, while adding 2 cups of turkey stock, grind the nuts.
- Pour mixture into saucepan with remaining cup of stock.
- Add wine and soy milk and heat through. Season to taste with salt and pepper.
- Sprinkle with scallions before serving. *Serves 4 to 6.*

MUSHROOM-BARLEY SOUP WITH SPINACH

HIGHLY BENEFICIAL		NEUTRAL	O, A, AB	AVOID	B

The flavor and textures of this classic soup are extremely satisfying. The slightly honeyed essence of the barley and its smooth texture contrasts nicely with the mushroom and spinach. The spinach is best when fresh and added to the soup at the last minute, so it's still green and only slightly wilted.

1 tablespoon olive oil
1 small onion, diced
½ cup barley (uncooked)
1 tablespoon sherry
1 Portobello mushroom,
   halved and sliced
8 cups liquid, either turkey or
   vegetable stock (water is
   acceptable, but the flavor
   will not be as rich)

1 teaspoon salt
2 cups fresh spinach, washed
   and stems cut or chopped

- In a large pot, heat oil over medium heat. Add onion and cook 2 minutes, or until onion is wilted.
- Add uncooked barley, stirring until it is incorporated, and cook 2 minutes. Stir in sherry and mushrooms.
- Cover, reduce heat, and simmer 2 minutes. When mushrooms have softened, add stock and bring to a boil.
- Reduce heat and simmer 45 to 50 minutes.
- Season with salt and add spinach. It will wilt very quickly. *Serves 4.*

CURRIED CARROT SOUP

HIGHLY BENEFICIAL	A, B	NEUTRAL	O, AB	AVOID	

This soup has eye-pleasing color, and the addition of the curry provides a spicy taste that contrasts wonderfully with the slightly sweet carrots.

½ stick butter (Type B) or canola-oil margarine (Type A) or 3 tablespoons olive oil
1 large onion, peeled and diced
2-inch piece fresh ginger, peeled and grated
1 tablespoon curry powder
3 cloves garlic, crushed and peeled

2 lbs. carrots, washed and trimmed
1 cup dry white wine (optional)
7 cups chicken, turkey, or vegetable stock
1 sweet potato, peeled (Types O, B, AB only)
salt and pepper

- In a large pot, melt butter or margarine or heat oil over low heat. Add onion, ginger, curry, and garlic, and cook until onions are translucent.
- Coarsely cut carrots and add with sweet potato to stockpot. Add wine and cook 1 minute, or until all the alcohol burns off.
- Add stock and simmer 45 minutes.
- Let cool slightly. Transfer mixture in batches to a food processor and purée.

- Return mixture to pot and season with salt and pepper to taste.
- If soup is too thin, reduce by simmering another 10 minutes, or until desired consistency is achieved. *Serves 10 to 12.*

WILD RICE AND MUSHROOM SOUP

HIGHLY BENEFICIAL	A	NEUTRAL	O	AVOID	B, AB

This soup combines the taste of deep, earthy, wild mushrooms with the intense flavors of the dark, nutty-textured wild rice.

2 cups wild mushrooms (abalone, Portobello, or tree oyster) or 4 oz. dried, reconstituted
6 tablespoons butter (Type O) or canola-oil margarine (Type A) or 4 tablespoons olive oil
2 leeks, washed well and finely chopped
¼ cup minced garlic
⅓ cup spelt flour
8 cups chicken stock
½ cup dry white wine (optional)
1 cup wild rice
4 cups water for cooking rice
¼ cup sherry (optional)
sprig fresh thyme
salt

- If using dried mushrooms, soak in water until soft. Drain, reserving soaking liquid, and chop mushrooms.
- In a soup pot, melt butter or canola-oil margarine, or heat olive oil. Add leeks and garlic, and sauté 1 minute.
- Add mushrooms and cook another 2 minutes. Add flour all at once and cook, stirring well, 2 minutes.
- Meanwhile, warm chicken stock and add 2 cups at a time to pot, whisking to incorporate. Add wine, if using. This is a basic gravy or roux, which is used to thicken sauces. Try to do this step slowly and in stages to avoid lumps.
- Simmer 1 hour.
- Separately boil the wild rice in plenty of water and drain while still al dente.
- Add rice to the simmering soup and cook 30 minutes longer.
- Add sherry, if using, and thyme, and cook 5 more minutes. Season with salt. *Serves 8 to 10.*

CUBAN BLACK BEAN SOUP

HIGHLY BENEFICIAL	A	NEUTRAL	O	AVOID	B, AB

This is a thick and lemony bean soup that may be served either hot or cold. It becomes slightly grayish-purple with the addition of the lemon. Garnish by placing a slice of lemon on top of each serving. It's acceptable to use canned beans, and doing so makes for a really fast soup.

¼ lb. dried black beans or
    2 cans beans, drained and
    rinsed
1 onion, peeled and chopped
4 cloves garlic, crushed and
    peeled
4 to 5 cups chicken or
    vegetable stock

juice of 2 lemons, or ¼ cup
    juice
2 teaspoons salt
lemon slices for garnish or
    plain yogurt (Type A only)

- Wash and soak dried beans in three times the amount of water needed to cover and refrigerate overnight or for at least 8 hours.
- Drain and rinse beans.
- Combine beans, onion, garlic, and stock in large pot. Cook beans slowly over low heat until very tender, about 1 hour.
- Let cool slightly, then transfer to a food processor and purée in batches, adding liquid from pot to obtain desired consistency.
- Stir in lemon juice and salt. Serve immediately with a slice of lemon on top, or chill and serve with a dollop of plain yogurt (Type A only). *Serves 6 to 8.*

WHITE GAZPACHO

HIGHLY BENEFICIAL	B, AB	NEUTRAL	A	AVOID	O

This is a wonderful variation of the classic tomato-based cold soup for those sweltering nights when one's appetite has been dimmed by the dog days of summer.

3 cucumbers, peeled and
   seeded
2 green peppers, washed and
   seeded (Types A and AB
   omit)
1 red onion, cut in quarters
2 cups plain, organic yogurt
1 cup green grapes, coarsely
   chopped

vegetable stock as needed
2 tablespoons chopped fresh
   cilantro
2 tablespoons chopped fresh
   mint
salt

- Cut cucumbers, peppers, and red onion into medium-size pieces.
- Combine them in a food processor and pulse on and off until they're not quite puréed. The texture should remain a bit chunky.
- Transfer to a large mixing bowl and whisk in yogurt. Thin as desired with vegetable stock or water with a little bit of white grape juice.
- Stir in the fresh herbs and grapes, and season with salt to taste.
Serves 6 to 8.

SIMPLE FISH SOUP

HIGHLY BENEFICIAL	A, B, AB	NEUTRAL	O	AVOID	

Exactly as its name describes it, this soup is simple. It can be served either hot or cold with a tossed green salad, crusty homemade spelt bread, and cheese—if it's permitted on your Blood Type Diet.

1 tablespoon olive oil
1 carrot, diced small
2 small stalks celery, diced
   small
½ onion, diced small
1 tablespoon sherry
   (optional)

4 cups water
¾ lb. grouper, cut into 1-inch
   pieces
2 tablespoons chopped fresh
   parsley

- Heat oil in a saucepan over medium heat. Add carrot, celery, and onion, and sauté several minutes.
- Add water. Add sherry, if using, and cook until vegetables are soft, about 10 minutes.
- Add grouper and simmer a few minutes longer, until the fish is thoroughly cooked. Sprinkle parsley over each serving. *Serves 2.*

Breads, Batters, and Muffins

Better Baked Goods

*T*HIS CHAPTER COVERS A WIDE VARIETY OF BAKED GOODS. Bread baking is both an art and a science, but it is an art that anyone can learn, and making your own bread is very rewarding. Children love to bake bread because it is a tactile, interesting experience, and they get to eat the results! The many steps to traditional bread baking are all quite simple. They just take time, attention, and patience.

There are also many delicious breads available commercially. Most natural breads can be found in a health-food store, but carefully check the listed ingredients. Increasingly, commercial bakeries are using clever packaging to make their breads seem more wholesome, but refined wheat flour is still often the main ingredient. Essene and Ezekiel are the two commercial loaves that we highly recommend, but breads made with spelt, rice, and rye flours are also becoming more widely available.

To be a successful bread baker, it is important to remember these key points: Read the directions for the recipe before you start to bake. Always have the ingredients at room temperature. Try to be as precise in measuring all of the ingredients as possible. Make sure that your oven's temperature is correct. A variation of as little as twenty-five degrees can affect the baking process. The exciting news is that your baking skills will improve with each loaf of bread you make.

Hand-Kneaded Breads

FRENCH BREAD

HIGHLY BENEFICIAL	AB	NEUTRAL	O, A, B	AVOID	

1¼ cups warm water
¼ teaspoon sugar
1½ teaspoons active dry yeast
4 to 5 cups spelt flour
   (4 cups white spelt flour,
   1 cup whole-grain spelt)

½ teaspoon salt
2 tablespoons cornmeal or
   rice flour (if necessary, for
   baking sheet only)
egg wash (1 beaten egg)

- Combine water, sugar, and yeast in a large mixing bowl. Stir until dissolved and let set 10 minutes.
- Add 4 cups white spelt flour and salt. Mix well with a dough hook attachment on a mixing machine or with a wooden spoon.
- When the dough is well mixed and still sticky, turn it onto a well-floured surface. Begin to knead by hand, adding in more flour (whole grain) as needed. Knead 10 minutes, or until dough is smooth and elastic.
- Put the dough in an oiled bowl, turn once to cover with oil, and cover with a clean dish towel. Place in a warm spot in your kitchen and let rise 2 hours. The back of the stove with a pilot light is ideal. Near a radiator or a warm stove is also good.
- When the dough has doubled in size, punch down and divide in half.
- Roll into baguettes by folding the dough into itself, then rolling it with your hands from the middle outward.
- Place in French-bread pans, or place on a baking sheet dusted with cornmeal or rice flour. Brush each loaf with egg wash, cut 3 diagonal gashes about ¼ inch deep, and let rise a second time, about 30 minutes.
- Preheat oven to 375 degrees F and bake loaves 30 to 35 minutes. Bread should sound hollow when tapped on the underside.
Yields 2 loaves.

Note: To double this recipe, you may find that it only takes 7½ to 8 cups of flour. You can also substitute half whole-grain spelt and half white spelt flour for a denser, coarser texture.

RAISIN-PUMPERNICKEL BREAD

HIGHLY BENEFICIAL	AB	NEUTRAL	O, A	AVOID	B

A dark, flavorful loaf full of moist, sweet raisins. Delicious still warm out of the oven. Also delicious toasted.

½ tablespoon (1½ teaspoons)
  dry yeast, or ½ package
  yeast
1½ cups lukewarm water
½ cup molasses
1 tablespoon strong coffee, or
  2 teaspoons instant coffee
  (Type O omit)
1 tablespoon salt

2 cups rye flour
2 cups whole-grain spelt flour
2 cups white spelt flour
2 tablespoons canola oil
1 cup raisins
¼ cup cornmeal or rye
  cracker crumbs (for pan
  only)

- Dissolve yeast in a bowl with lukewarm water. Let sit 5 minutes, then add molasses, coffee, and salt, and stir well.
- Add 5 cups flour all at once, and mix well with a heavy spoon. Turn onto a well-floured surface and knead in remaining 1 cup flour 8 to 10 minutes. Rye-flour breads tend to be a little stickier and take longer to rise than lighter doughs.
- Place in an oiled bowl, turn over once, and cover with a clean dish towel. Place in a warm area of the kitchen, allowing the dough to rise until three times its original size. It will take approximately 2 hours.
- Turn dough onto a floured surface, and fold in the raisins by kneading the dough once more.
- Return to bowl, cover, and let rise again, but only until doubled. It will take approximately 30 to 40 minutes for this second rising.
- Turn dough onto a floured surface and cut into thirds. Shape into three loaves or make small breakfast rolls.
- Dust baking sheet with cornmeal (or rye cracker crumbs) and set loaves apart from one another, leaving enough room for each loaf to rise. Cover until doubled in size.
- Preheat oven to 375 degrees F and bake 35 to 40 minutes for bread, 20 to 25 minutes for rolls.
- Let cool on a rack.   *Yields 3 loaves or 18 rolls.*

Muffins and Tea Cakes

Muffins and tea cakes take only a few moments to prepare, cook fairly quickly, freeze well, and come in dozens of variations. They can make a healthy snack for children, are a perfect breakfast, or a satisfying little meal with a cup of green tea and a piece of fruit. Muffin and tea cake batters are raised with baking powder and baking soda. Unlike yeast-raised doughs, they don't need to rise before baking. They also require much less handling, so the lighter the touch, the better. Texture is dramatically affected by overmixing these batters.

A plethora of dried and fresh fruits, as well as nuts and seeds, can make endless combinations in these sweet breads. Feel free to substitute other fruits, nuts, and seeds according to your blood type.

BANANA-WALNUT BREAD OR MUFFINS

HIGHLY BENEFICIAL		NEUTRAL	O, B	AVOID	A, AB

The bananas make this bread sweet and moist, and the walnuts create an interesting counterpoint to the banana flavor.

oil for pans
2 cups white spelt flour
1 teaspoon salt
2 teaspoons baking soda
⅔ cup canola oil (Type B use butter)

1 cup turbinado sugar
1½ cups ripe banana chunks (about 2 large bananas)
3 eggs, beaten
½ cup chopped walnuts

- Preheat oven to 350 degrees F.
- Prepare pans. If nonstick, they don't need greasing; otherwise, oil and flour the pans. If you're making muffins, you can use paper liners.
- Mix all dry ingredients in one bowl and all wet ingredients in another.

- Blend together and add walnuts for the last few turns with the spoon. *Don't overmix the batter.*
- Fill prepared pans three-quarters full, and bake 25 to 30 minutes for muffins, 30 to 35 minutes for prepared breads, or until a cake tester comes out clean.
- Let cool on rack. This is a great breakfast treat. *Makes 1 dozen muffins or 3 small loaves.*

Note: For a whole-grain banana bread, substitute 1 cup whole-spelt flour for 1 cup white spelt flour.

BLUEBERRY MUFFINS

HIGHLY BENEFICIAL	A	NEUTRAL	O, B, AB	AVOID	

These muffins are both beautiful and dramatic. If you use buckwheat, they're dark and dense. But with any flour, the muffins take on a deep purple hue from the berries. They aren't too sweet and are great with a complementary all-fruit preserve.

oil or paper liners for muffin tins
1 cup buckwheat flour (Type O and Type A)
1 cup oat flour (Type B and Type AB)
1 cup white spelt flour
2½ teaspoons baking powder
½ teaspoon salt
⅔ cup sugar
2 tablespoons honey
1 cup soy milk
¼ cup canola oil (Type B should substitute butter)
1 egg, beaten
½ cup blueberries, fresh or frozen

- Preheat oven to 350 degrees F.
- Grease muffin tins or use paper liners.
- In a large bowl, mix dry ingredients together.
- In another bowl, stir together the honey, soy milk, oil, and egg.
- Lightly combine the dry and wet ingredients. Fold in blueberries.
- Fill each muffin cup to top.
- Bake 20 minutes, or until a toothpick comes out clean.
  Makes 12 muffins.

CORN BREAD

HIGHLY BENEFICIAL		NEUTRAL	A	AVOID	O, B, AB

Corn bread is a favorite accompaniment with soups and stews, as well as meat and bean dishes.

grease for pan
¾ cup white spelt flour
¾ cup stone-ground cornmeal
½ cup buckwheat flour
2 tablespoons brown sugar
2½ teaspoons baking powder

pinch salt
2 eggs
4 tablespoons canola-oil
   margarine, melted
1 cup soy milk

- Grease a 9-inch square pan or cast-iron skillet and preheat in 425-degree F oven.
- Mix spelt flour, cornmeal, buckwheat flour, brown sugar, baking powder, and salt in one bowl.
- In another bowl, beat eggs well. Add melted margarine and soy milk, and stir until blended.
- Add liquid ingredients to dry, stirring quickly until just mixed. *Do not overmix.*
- Pour into hot pan or skillet and bake 20 to 25 minutes. Serve hot. *Makes 12 pieces.*

QUINOA-ALMOND MUFFINS

HIGHLY BENEFICIAL		NEUTRAL	O, A, B, AB	AVOID	

These are moist and full of the unique flavor of quinoa, which has a light, almost hazelnut, taste to it.

butter, oil, or paper liners for
   pan
1 cup quinoa flour
1 cup white spelt flour
⅓ cup turbinado sugar
2½ teaspoons baking powder

¼ teaspoon salt
1 egg
1 cup soy or rice milk
½ cup canola oil (Type B
   should substitute light
   olive oil or butter)

- Preheat oven to 400 degrees F.
- Prepare muffin tins using butter, oil, or paper liners.
- In one bowl, combine all dry ingredients.
- In another bowl, beat egg. Add milk and oil, and stir until blended.
- Add liquid ingredients to dry, stirring quickly until just mixed.
- Fill tins to almost full. Add water to remaining empty tins, and bake 15 to 20 minutes. *Makes 12 muffins.*

BANANA-PLUM BREAD

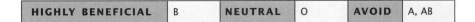

HIGHLY BENEFICIAL	B	NEUTRAL	O	AVOID	A, AB

Serve this moist, not-too-sweet loaf for breakfast. Type Bs can try spreading it with a little sweetened ricotta, while Type Os can use fresh goat cheese. Add the larger amount of nuts and lemon rind if you prefer. Type O can use all-spelt flour.

butter for pans
1 cup spelt flour
¾ cup oat flour
2½ teaspoons baking powder
½ teaspoon salt
5 tablespoons softened butter
⅔ cup turbinado sugar

1 to 2 teaspoons grated
   lemon rind
1 to 2 eggs, beaten
1 cup mashed banana
3 ripe plums, diced
½ to 1 cup walnuts, broken
   into pieces

- Preheat oven to 350 degrees F.
- Liberally butter two 8½ × 4½ × 2-inch loaf pans.
- Sift flours, baking powder, and salt into one bowl.
- In another bowl, blend butter, sugar, and lemon rind until creamy. Beat in eggs and mashed banana.
- Add dry ingredients to butter mixture in 3 parts, beating well after each addition.
- Fold in plums and walnuts. Pour into prepared loaf pans.
- Bake about 40 minutes, or until a straw comes out clean. Cool. This slices well. *Makes 2 small loaves.*

LEMON TEA CAKE

HIGHLY BENEFICIAL		NEUTRAL	O, B	AVOID	A, AB

With the addition of the lemon glaze, this cake stays moist for several days. Refrigerate to retard spoilage.

¾ cup butter, at room
   temperature
¾ cup turbinado sugar
3 eggs, beaten
1 tablespoon lemon juice

zest of same lemon
1½ cups white spelt flour
¾ teaspoon baking powder
¼ teaspoon salt

LEMON GLAZE

1 cup water
juice of 2 lemons

¼ cup honey

- Preheat oven to 350 degrees F.
- Butter and flour two 8½ × 4½ × 2-inch loaf pans.
- In a mixing bowl, blend butter and sugar until light and fluffy. Add eggs, lemon juice, and zest (the outer, colored portion of the lemon).
- Gradually add flour, baking powder, and salt, scraping down the sides of the bowl. *Do not overmix.*
- Fill prepared pans to almost three-quarters full, and bake 25 minutes.
- Meanwhile, prepare glaze: Combine all ingredients in a small saucepan and simmer about 10 minutes. The glaze should be thick but still pourable.
- While cake is still warm, pour glaze over top, allowing it to run down sides. Let cool.

PUMPKIN-ALMOND BREAD

HIGHLY BENEFICIAL		NEUTRAL	O, A, AB	AVOID	B

A moist, sweet, slightly spicy tea bread with an interesting texture, thanks to the ground almonds.

butter or oil for pan
1 cup white spelt flour
¾ cup ground almonds
½ teaspoon baking powder
1 teaspoon baking soda
½ teaspoon salt
½ teaspoon cinnamon (Types A and AB)
⅛ teaspoon cloves
⅛ teaspoon nutmeg (Type O omit)

½ teaspoon ginger
¾ cup turbinado sugar
¼ cup butter, at room temperature (Type O only; Type A and Type AB may substitute canola-oil margarine)
2 eggs
1 cup pumpkin
⅓ cup soy milk
½ cup raisins or chopped figs

- Preheat oven to 350 degrees F.
- Grease a 9 × 13-inch glass pan.
- In a large bowl, mix flour, ground almonds, baking powder, baking soda, salt, cinnamon, cloves, nutmeg, and ginger.
- In a separate bowl, beat the sugar, butter or margarine, and eggs until very light. Add pumpkin and beat again.
- Swiftly add dry ingredients alternately with soy milk in two additions. Stir in raisins or figs.
- Pour into prepared pan and bake about 30 minutes, or until a straw comes out clean.   *Yields: 1 loaf.*

Batters for Pancakes and Waffles

Pancakes and waffles don't have to be weekend luxuries. They don't even have to be eaten for breakfast. If you keep a mixture of the dry ingredients in a container, all you have to do to enjoy these filling pancakes or dessert crêpes is to heat the griddle or waffle iron, add the wet ingredients, and pour the batter.

BARLEY AND SPELT PANCAKES

HIGHLY BENEFICIAL		NEUTRAL	O, A, AB	AVOID	B

1 cup barley flour
1 cup spelt flour
2 teaspoons baking powder
pinch of salt
2 eggs

1½ cups soy milk
water as needed
butter, margarine, or oil for
   skillet

- Combine flours, baking powder, and salt in a large bowl. Stir well to combine.
- In a separate bowl, beat eggs very well and stir in soy milk.
- Pour liquid into dry ingredients and stir until blended. The addition of water here depends on whether you prefer thick or thin pancakes.
- Heat butter, margarine, or oil in a heavy skillet. When hot, ladle in batter.
- Cook on low heat until bubbles fully cover the surface of the pancakes. Turn over and cook until beautifully colored.
- Serve with maple syrup, honey, or your favorite all-fruit preserves. *Makes 15 to 20 medium-size pancakes.*

MILLET, SPELT, AND SOY PANCAKES

HIGHLY BENEFICIAL	B, A, AB	NEUTRAL	O	AVOID	

1 cup millet flour
½ cup spelt flour
½ cup soy flour
1 tablespoon baking powder
pinch of salt

2 eggs
1½ to 2 cups soy milk
water as needed
butter, margarine, or oil for
   skillet

- Combine flours, baking powder, and salt in a large bowl. Stir well to combine.
- In a separate bowl, beat eggs and add soy milk, mixing well.
- Pour liquid into dry ingredients and blend thoroughly.
- Heat butter, margarine, or oil in a heavy skillet. When hot, ladle in batter.
- Cook over low heat until bubbles fully cover surface of pancakes. Flip over and cook until lightly colored on underside.
- Serve with maple syrup, honey, or your favorite all-fruit preserves. *Makes 15 to 20 pancakes.*

AMARANTH PANCAKES

HIGHLY BENEFICIAL		NEUTRAL	A, AB	AVOID	O, B

Served with honey, maple syrup, or just fresh fruit, these pancakes are full of the exceptional protein, vitamins, and minerals that amaranth can provide. Amaranth contains twice the iron and four times the calcium of wheat—an excellent way to provide nutritious fuel for the day's labors.

1 cup amaranth flour
1 cup white spelt flour
1 teaspoon sugar
½ teaspoon salt
1 teaspoon baking powder
2 eggs, beaten

1 cup low-fat ricotta cheese
1 cup water
½ teaspoon almond extract
butter, margarine, or oil for
  skillet

- In a medium bowl, mix flours, sugar, salt, and baking powder. Stir well to combine.
- In another bowl, blend eggs, ricotta, water, and almond extract.
- Pour liquid into dry ingredients and blend without overmixing. The batter may seem a bit thin, but it thickens after sitting 5 minutes.
- Heat butter, margarine, or oil in a heavy skillet. When hot, spoon in batter.
- Cook over medium heat until bubbles form on surface. Turn over and cook until lightly colored.   *Makes 15 to 20 pancakes.*

BROWN RICE AND SPELT PANCAKES

HIGHLY BENEFICIAL	B, AB	NEUTRAL	O, A	AVOID	

These are delicious pancakes, and the combination of whole-spelt and brown rice flours gives them a lot of natural sweetness and body. They are spectacular with fresh berries. Type Bs be sure to check the label on your rice milk. Some brands use canola oil.

1 cup brown rice flour	1½ cups rice milk
1 cup whole-spelt flour	butter, margarine, or oil for
1 teaspoon baking powder	skillet
2 eggs	

- In a medium bowl, combine flours and baking powder, mixing well. Beat in eggs and rice milk.
- Heat butter, margarine, or oil in a heavy skillet. When hot, ladle in batter.
- Cook over medium low heat until bubbles appear on the surface. Flip over and cook until lightly browned.
- Serve with maple syrup, honey, or a favorite all-fruit preserve.
Makes 15 to 20 medium-size pancakes.

Salads

Beyond Rabbit Food

*E*ACH OF THE BLOOD TYPES HAS A TASTY VARIETY OF vegetables to choose from. Blood types are limited only by the vegetables that have been indicated as Avoid on their individual lists. Even though many vegetables are listed as of Neutral value for a specific type, the tastes, textures, and valuable nutrients should be enjoyed anyway for their aesthetic and food value.

COLE SLAW

HIGHLY BENEFICIAL	B	NEUTRAL	AB	AVOID	O, A

This colorful version of the American classic has more bite and crunch than its simpler predecessor.

½ head white cabbage
¼ head red cabbage
½ head Chinese cabbage
2 carrots, grated
1 red onion, chopped
¾ to 1 cup Olive-Oil
   Mayonnaise (see page 364)

2 tablespoons horseradish
½ teaspoon celery salt
1 teaspoon caraway seeds
¾ to 1 cup walnuts, broken
   into pieces

■ ■ ■ ■

- Finely sliver the leaves of all 3 cabbages to make 6 to 8 cups.
- In a large bowl, combine cabbage with grated carrots and chopped onion and toss until well mixed.
- Combine mayonnaise, horseradish, celery salt, and caraway seeds in a small bowl. Pour dressing over cabbage leaves and toss to combine.
- Let marinate in the refrigerator several hours to develop flavors.
- Add walnuts just before serving.   *Serves 6 to 8.*

MESCLUN SALAD

HIGHLY BENEFICIAL		NEUTRAL	O, A, B, AB	AVOID	

Mesclun is a salad of mixed greens that was difficult to find in any but the finest gourmet restaurants until a couple of years ago. Mesclun is readily available in the markets now. Even organic mesclun is widely available. There are varied mixtures, but certain lettuces are inevitably part of the ingredients: Swiss chard and spinach are standard greens, as are frisée, red- and oak-leaf lettuces, radicchio, arugula, and watercress. The slightly peppery arugula and watercress contrast nicely with the colorful, crunchy radicchio, and the entire salad is quite pretty. A fresh white apple sliced over the top with a drizzle of olive oil and a squeeze of lemon make a lovely presentation.

1 lb. mesclun greens
2 medium tomatoes, sliced
  (Type O and Type AB
  only)
1 cucumber, peeled and sliced

¼ cup crumbled feta or mild
  goat cheese
Olive Oil & Lemon Dressing
  (see page 370)

- Spoon 2 tablespoons of dressing into a large bowl. Add the mesclun. Toss with another tablespoon of the dressing so there's a light coating on the greens.
- Top with sliced tomato and/or cucumber and crumbled feta or goat cheese.   *Makes 4 large salads.*

SPINACH SALAD WITH EGG & BACON

HIGHLY BENEFICIAL	A	NEUTRAL	B, AB, O	AVOID	

Fresh is best, but wilted spinach with a warmed vinaigrette is also very pleasing.

1 lb. fresh spinach
Olive Oil & Lemon Dressing
   (see page 370)
1 hard-boiled egg, chopped
2 slices organic turkey bacon,
   cooked and chopped

2 tablespoons grated romano
   cheese
salt

- Wash the spinach several times to clean it of dirt and grit. Remove tough stems. Pat or spin dry. Place in a large salad bowl.
- Heat dressing and pour it over the spinach. Toss well to mix. If not wilted enough, then put spinach and dressing back into the pan for a minute.
- Top with chopped egg, turkey bacon, and grated cheese. Add salt to taste. *Serves 2.*

GREEK SALAD

HIGHLY BENEFICIAL	O, A	NEUTRAL	B, AB	AVOID	

Certain ingredients need to be toyed with and others omitted from this all-time favorite, but the basic flavors remain the same. The romaine lettuce is highly beneficial to Type O and Type A, and of Neutral value to Type B and Type AB, which makes it fine for all.

⅓ cup Olive Oil & Lemon
Dressing (see page 370)
1 tablespoon fresh mint,
chopped
2 tablespoons fresh basil,
chopped
2 tablespoons fresh parsley,
chopped
2 cucumbers, washed, peeled,
and sliced
1 green pepper, halved,
seeded, and cut into
bite-size pieces (Type A
and Type AB omit)

2 stalks celery, chopped
1 small red onion, sliced
1 clove garlic, diced
1 head crisp romaine,
washed, dried, and torn
into bite-size pieces
¼ cup crumbled Greek feta
cheese
Greek olives (Type AB only)
1 teaspoon fresh or dried
oregano

- In a large salad bowl, mix the dressing, the herbs, and all of the vegetables. Reserve the romaine, cheese, and olives.
- Cover vegetables and marinate in refrigerator 1 to 2 hours.
- Toss the romaine with the marinated vegetables. Top with the crumbled feta and the olives. Sprinkle with a dusting of oregano. Mix well.   *Serves 2 to 4.*

MIXED MUSHROOM SALAD

HIGHLY BENEFICIAL		NEUTRAL	O, A, B, AB	AVOID	

This salad is often found as an antipasto in Italian restaurants. However, it's also delightful as a side dish served on a bed of shredded romaine.

10 to 12 oz. mushrooms,
according to blood type
1 cup vinaigrette
2 tablespoons chopped fresh
parsley

2 tablespoons chopped fresh
chives
2 cups shredded lettuce

- Choose a salad dressing for your blood type. For many, the Sweet Vidalia Onion Dressing (page 371) or oil and lemon will serve nicely.

- Marinate mushrooms in 1 cup dressing for 1 or 2 hours.
- Mix in fresh herbs.
- Divide lettuce among 4 salad plates. Using a slotted spoon, drain mushrooms and serve over lettuce. *Serves 2 to 4.*

CARROT-RAISIN SALAD

HIGHLY BENEFICIAL	A, B	NEUTRAL	O, AB	AVOID	

This updated classic provides a sweet, crunchy accompaniment to almost any light summer meal.

2 lbs. carrots, washed, trimmed, and grated
½ cup raisins, plumped in hot water
3 tablespoons mayonnaise (Type A substitute olive oil and lemon dressing)

3 tablespoons chopped fresh Italian parsley or chopped fresh cilantro
1 scallion, thinly sliced, or 1 tablespoon chopped fresh chives

- Place carrots in a serving bowl. Drain the raisins and mix with the carrots.
- Add remaining ingredients and toss well. *Serves 4.*

GRILLED SWEET-POTATO SALAD

HIGHLY BENEFICIAL	O, B, AB	NEUTRAL		AVOID	A

This is a very refreshing side dish that makes great use of extra cooked sweet potatoes.

2 lbs. sweet potatoes, sliced raw and then grilled
3 tablespoons olive oil
1 scallion, sliced
2 tablespoons chopped fresh parsley

2 tablespoons chopped fresh cilantro
juice of 1 lime

- Cube the sweet potatoes after they've cooled. If you can refrigerate them for a while, they'll taste even better.
- In a large bowl, combine sweet potatoes with remaining ingredients, toss well, and serve. *Serves 4 to 6.*

ALDER-SMOKED MACKEREL SALAD

HIGHLY BENEFICIAL		NEUTRAL	O, A, B, AB	AVOID	

This works for lunch or hors d'oeuvres on rye or rice crackers. However, smoked fish should be eaten rarely and only if you have no digestive problems. Try it as a filling for scooped-out cherry tomatoes for Type O and Type AB. Put a half-spoonful on cucumber slices or at the base of small endive leaves.

4 smoked mackerel fillets, skinned and boned	⅓ to ½ cup Olive-Oil Mayonnaise (see page 364)
½ red onion, diced small	juice of 1 lemon

- Chop fillets by hand.
- Combine fillets and remaining ingredients in small bowl. Mix well and serve with crackers. *Yields approximately 2 cups.*

COLD GRILLED CHICKEN SALAD

HIGHLY BENEFICIAL		NEUTRAL	O, A	AVOID	B, AB

Grill chicken parts on hot grill, turning to cook each side, about 40 minutes. After chicken parts have finished grilling, set them aside and let them cool. Remove skin, take meat from the bone, and slice into smaller pieces until you have between one and two cups. White breast meat is the least fatty of chicken parts.

1 to 2 cups diced chicken
3 tablespoons Olive-Oil
   Mayonnaise (see page 364)
juice of 1 lime
3 tablespoons chopped fresh
   cilantro
2 scallions, thinly sliced

1 red pepper, either roasted
   or grilled, with skin
   removed, or fresh, cut
   in half, then sliced
   (Type O only)
salt

- Put the prepared chicken in a bowl. Thin mayonnaise with lime juice and add to chicken.
- Add remaining ingredients, toss well, and serve with crackers, on Ezekiel bread, or rolled in a romaine leaf. *Serves 2 to 4.*

GREEN BEANS, CHÈVRE, AND WALNUTS

HIGHLY BENEFICIAL	O, A	NEUTRAL	B, AB	AVOID	

This is simple to prepare and great for entertaining. The green beans are Highly Beneficial for Type A and the walnuts are Highly Beneficial for Type O, but all blood types can enjoy this dish. This dish is best served at room temperature, but during the warmer summer months you may want to chill it first.

2 lbs. green beans, stems
   removed
¼ cup walnut pieces and
   halves
2 tablespoons crumbled goat
   cheese

2 tablespoons extra-virgin
   olive oil
squeeze of lemon juice
salt

- Quickly blanch the green beans by throwing them into a pot of boiling water and counting to a slow 30. Then transfer them to an ice bath. Drain well and dry.
- On a serving plate, layer the beans, walnuts, and crumbled goat cheese.
- Dress with good olive oil and a squeeze of lemon juice. Add salt to taste. *Serves 4 to 6.*

Sandwiches and Eggs

Simple and Inexpensive

ERE ARE A WIDE RANGE OF SIMPLE, INEXPENSIVE recipes that provide wonderful ways to use leftovers. You can also use whatever you happen to have in your vegetable bin or pantry. A few staples can form the basis for a satisfying and quick supper, or for an elegant meal for unexpected company. It's a good idea to have the fundamentals for these recipes on hand: A loaf of fresh or frozen bread, eggs, a couple of cheeses, pasta, olive oil, a jar or two of preserves, nut butters, sardines, tuna, fresh vegetables, and a pot or two of fresh herbs gracing your window. Dried herbs are just fine, though.

Leftovers are the key to many of the recipes offered in this chapter, and there's no better way to plan ahead than when the grill or oven is already heated up for some other meal. Pull whatever you have out of the vegetable bin—carrots, onions, sweet potatoes, mushrooms, leeks, tempeh, tofu, apples—cut into pieces, brush with olive oil, sprinkle with salt, and grill or broil, five minutes on each side. Let cool, refrigerate, and in the next day or two, incorporate the mélange of grilled vegetable leftovers into your meals.

Sandwiches

For many people sandwiches are a way of life—or at least a way of *lunch*. However, sandwiches work better in your diet if you eat them only occasionally. At those times, you can enjoy a variety. Here are some blood type–friendly combinations that you can try. They all contain Highly Beneficial or Neutral ingredients.

Place the sandwich fillings either on the commercially made Ezekiel or Essene breads, or on slices of those loaves you make yourself. The sandwiches based on vegetables and cheese are especially good on spelt baguettes. For roll-up sandwiches, or "wraps" as they're popularly called, you can make your own flour tortillas or crêpes. There is also a wide variety of pitas and flat breads available. Don't hesitate to serve these elegant and filling sandwiches to company or to your family when you're pressed for time. With a bowl of soup and a simple salad, these sandwiches can be a sumptuous treat for dinner.

Grilled Peppers (all varieties) and Goat Cheese	Blood Types O, B
Grilled Eggplant and Feta Cheese	Blood Types A, AB
Sliced Tomatoes, Fresh Mozzarella, and Basil	Blood Types O, AB
Braised Red Peppers and Onions with Feta	Blood Types O, B
Roasted Red Peppers and Goat Cheese	Blood Types O
Grilled Eggplant, Braised Shiitake Mushrooms, and Goat Cheese	Blood Type B
Almond Butter and Sliced Banana	Blood Types O, B
Peanut Butter, Raisins, and Honey	Blood Types A, AB
Tofu, Avocado, Alfalfa Sprouts, and Lemon Vinaigrette	Blood Type A
Tofu, Tomato, Chopped Olives, and Lemon Vinaigrette	Blood Type AB
Sunflower Butter and Plum Preserves	Blood Types O, A
Persimmons, Tahini, and Sprouts	Blood Types O, A
Grilled Chicken Breast	Blood Types O, A
Sliced Lamb with Mango or Peach Chutney	Blood Types O, B

These are acceptable for all blood types:

Fresh Mozzarella, Sautéed Zucchini, and Garlic
Ricotta, Chopped Walnuts, Raisins, and Honey
Soft Goat Cheese and Preserves
Mashed Sardines and Minced Garlic
Quick Tuna Salad (see page 344)
Curried Egg Salad (see page 344)
Turkey Burgers on Spelt Buns

Quick Common-Sense Suggestions

GRILLED OR ROASTED PEPPER
ON RYE CRACKERS WITH CHÈVRE

HIGHLY BENEFICIAL		NEUTRAL	O, B	AVOID	A, AB

2 red or yellow peppers,
   grilled or roasted with
   some olive oil

4 rye crisp crackers (Type O)
   or rice crackers (Type B)
2 oz. crumbled goat cheese

- Slice peppers to size of cracker. Crumble goat cheese on top.
Serves 2.

GRILLED GOAT CHEDDAR
ON EZEKIEL OR SPELT BREAD

HIGHLY BENEFICIAL	B, AB	NEUTRAL	O, A	AVOID	

2 slices Ezekiel bread
3 to 4 slices goat Cheddar

2 tablespoons butter or soft
   canola-oil margarine

- Spread butter or margarine on one slice of bread, and add goat
cheese. Slice sandwich on the diagonal.   *Serves 1.*

CURRIED EGG SALAD

HIGHLY BENEFICIAL	O	NEUTRAL	A, B, AB	AVOID	

4 hard-boiled eggs, peeled
and mashed
2 tablespoons Olive-Oil
Mayonnaise (see page 364)

1 teaspoon salt or to taste
1 teaspoon good-quality
curry powder

- Mix all ingredients together and serve with Ezekiel bread or rice crackers. *Serves 3.*

QUICK TUNA SALAD

HIGHLY BENEFICIAL	AB	NEUTRAL	O, A, B	AVOID	

1 can chunk light tuna,
packed in water
1 can solid white tuna,
packed in water

2 tablespoons Olive-Oil
Mayonnaise (see page 364)
1 scallion, thinly sliced or
¼ red onion, diced

- Drain tuna, but leave some liquid. Mix all ingredients well and serve on spelt toast.
- For a tuna melt, add any acceptable cheese. Soy cheese slices are also quite good. *Serves 2.*

Eggs

Eggs have received a lot of bad press over the last few years. Many people have banished them from their diets. All of that cholesterol! Well, further research has proven that it's not the cholesterol in the egg; it's how the body produces cholesterol that accounts for harmful or healthy levels of dietary cholesterol in an individual. As a result of this new information, a lot of nutritionists are backpedaling, and eggs have been returned to the list of good foods we should eat, albeit on a limited basis.

Fried, poached, scrambled, soft-boiled, hard-boiled, or in omelettes and frittatas, eggs are little powerhouses of protein. Enjoy them according to the frequency recommended for your blood type and your particular health needs.

SINGLE-EGG OMELET

HIGHLY BENEFICIAL		NEUTRAL	O, A, B, AB	AVOID	

1 tablespoon olive oil
1 small green zucchini,
    washed and grated
1 large organic egg

2 fresh basil leaves
2 tablespoons grated romano
salt

- In a medium frying pan, heat oil over medium heat and quickly cook zucchini 2 to 3 minutes, then set aside on a plate.
- Briskly beat egg, add 1 tablespoon water, and beat again. The idea is to get the egg as fluffy as possible.
- Add another bit of olive oil to grease the pan and reheat. Pour in egg, letting egg run around the whole bottom of the pan. Since there's only 1 egg, it's bound to be thin.
- Quickly add the zucchini, basil, and romano cheese.
- With a spatula, lift the edges of the omelet and carefully fold over the filling to make a half moon. Roll the omelet out of the pan and onto the plate. Season with salt to taste. *Serves 1.*

Alternative Fillings for Omelets and Frittatas

With just a little forethought, any vegetables left over from yesterday's meal can become the filling for a breakfast or lunch egg dish.

If you've run out of ideas for fillings, remember that almost anything will do. Here's a short list of ideas that may inspire you!

Asparagus

Braised collards

Broccoli

Steamed carrots

Freshly grated carrot with crumbled goat cheese
    and fresh dill

Sautéed onions

Tomato and basil

Tofu, scallion, and cilantro

Wild rice tempeh with basmati rice

Be sure to warm any of your leftovers before using them to fill an omelet.

Frittatas

Frittatas are a very nice change from omelets. Though comprised of many of the same ingredients, frittatas are really quite different. They are generally more substantial, and their cooking methods can vary. Frittatas can be baked, or cooked on top of the stove and browned under the broiler. Whichever way frittatas are made, they all contain a singular element: satisfaction. They're fast and pleasing to the eye. Most important, they appease the palate.

FRITTATA WITH PASTA
AND CARAMELIZED ONION

HIGHLY BENEFICIAL		NEUTRAL	O, A, B, AB	AVOID	

This is a perfect way to use up any cooked spaghetti. It's also worth making just for this purpose.

¼ cup olive oil

1 fist-sized onion, finely
    chopped

2 to 3 cups cooked spaghetti
    (buckwheat, spelt, or rice)

4 eggs

salt

2 tablespoons butter, canola-
    oil margarine, or olive oil

handful chopped fresh parsley

- Heat oil in a heavy, cast-iron skillet over low heat. Add onions, turning to coat with oil. Over low heat, cook onions until they become a beautiful golden brown. This will take quite some time, and they'll need to be stirred frequently.
- Transfer onions to a large bowl, add spaghetti, and mix well.
- In a small bowl, beat eggs until light, add a pinch of salt, then pour eggs over the spaghetti and onions. Mix them well.
- Wipe away any traces of onions or oil left in the skillet, turn heat to medium, and add butter or margarine. When hot, pour in egg mixture and spread it evenly over bottom of skillet.
- Cook about 5 minutes. Check bottom of frittata once or twice to be sure eggs are cooking thoroughly and frittata is turning a golden, crispy brown.
- When you are satisfied that the bottom is cooked through, you can either flip the frittata over, much as you would a pancake, or put it under the broiler for a moment, and cook until there is no more uncooked egg. Watch that it doesn't burn.
- Serve hot or let cool for a few minutes. Cut into wedges and sprinkle with parsley. *Serves 4 to 6.*

ZUCCHINI AND MUSHROOM FRITTATA

HIGHLY BENEFICIAL		NEUTRAL	O, A, B, AB	AVOID	

3 tablespoons olive oil
2 shallots or ½ small onion, chopped
2 medium zucchini, cut lengthwise, then crosswise on the diagonal

1 Portobello mushroom, sliced
5 eggs
¼ cup grated romano cheese
salt

- Preheat oven 350 degrees F.
- In a large heavy skillet, heat 1 tablespoon oil over medium heat and gently cook shallots. Add zucchini and sliced mushroom, and cook until soft.
- Meanwhile beat eggs with a tablespoon of water. Add cheese and vegetables to the egg mixture. Mix well.

- Add remaining 2 tablespoons oil to skillet. When oil is hot, add egg mixture.
- Cook on low heat until half done, then finish cooking in the oven. The frittata will puff up nicely. Salt to taste. *Serves 4 to 6.*

SPINACH FRITTATA

HIGHLY BENEFICIAL	O, A	NEUTRAL	B, AB	AVOID	

For a decidedly Greek flavor in this delicious frittata, use some good-quality feta cheese. Or use ¼ cup grated romano.

5 eggs
1 tablespoon water
1 bunch spinach, washed, dried, and finely chopped
2 tablespoons olive oil
1 tablespoon Garlic-Shallot Mixture (see page 375)

¼ cup crumbled feta or grated romano cheese
squeeze of lemon juice (optional)
salt

- Preheat broiler.
- Beat eggs with water. Add the spinach.
- In a large skillet, heat oil over medium heat and cook shallot mixture until softened.
- Add spinach-egg mixture all at once and cook over medium heat until almost done.
- While the top is still a bit runny, top with cheese and run under the broiler until done, about 2 or 3 minutes. Season with a squeeze of lemon, salt, and serve. *Serves 4 to 6.*

Desserts

The Perfect Ending

*D*ESSERTS ARE OFTEN AT THE CENTER OF CHILDHOOD memories, family celebrations, and holidays. Cakes, cookies, pies, tarts, and ice creams are *de rigueur* for many people. It is a universal truth that many people refuse to go a day without a sweet of some kind. But cakes and cookies aren't the only things people love to eat for dessert. Combinations of fruits and cheeses make light desserts. A ripe Anjou pear, a rich baked apple, a runny cheese—these are simple and satisfying conclusions.

Encourage children to view dessert as a real treat, and be sure to make it one. Purchase only the best ice creams, preferably organic. Make your own cookies, cakes, and pies. In this way, you are able to control the ingredients. Most families have favorite desserts. If yours doesn't yet, then establish a traditional family favorite.

Try to avoid buying commercially made baked goods. Read the nutrition label and list of ingredients. You'll see that all commercial goods are made with wheat flour, many are made with tropical oils, and most contain chemical ingredients that the majority of people can't even pronounce. That will usually stop most health-minded people right there. At least it should!

A homemade dessert can be a terrific treat. The only real problem is overindulgence. If three or four dozen cookies are lurking in the kitchen, many people feel a responsibility to eat them before they get stale or go bad. Freezing extra cookies sometimes helps, although frozen cookies don't take very long to defrost. In the world of desserts, the best advice is a gentle word or two: *A little goes a long way.*

WALNUT COOKIES

HIGHLY BENEFICIAL		NEUTRAL	O, B	AVOID	A, AB

These rich, not too sweet cookies are delicious served with a piece of ripe fruit. They make a wonderful light dessert. There are only five ingredients, so they're easy to put together.

1 stick butter
¼ cup sugar
1 cup walnuts, finely
   chopped

1 cup spelt flour
confectioners' sugar

- Preheat oven to 350 degrees F.
- Butter cookie sheets.
- In a mixing bowl, cream butter and sugar. Add nuts and flour and stir to combine.
- Drop by teaspoonfuls about 2 inches apart onto prepared cookie sheets.
- Bake approximately 25 minutes. Keep a careful watch after the first 20 minutes to make sure that the cookies don't get darker than golden. You want them to be golden brown.
- With spatula immediately remove from pans and cool on wire rack.
- Sprinkle lightly with sugar. *Makes 20 to 30 cookies.*

CARROT-GINGER RAISIN CAKE

HIGHLY BENEFICIAL		NEUTRAL	O, A, AB	AVOID	B

This spicy cake has both a great taste and texture. It is ideal for a birthday cake, especially with the Goat-Cheese Frosting.

butter, margarine, or oil for
   pans
2 cups whole-spelt flour
2 teaspoons baking soda
2 teaspoons baking powder
1 teaspoon salt
1⅓ cups canola oil

1½ cups light brown sugar
4 eggs, slightly beaten
3 cups grated carrots
2-inch piece fresh ginger,
   peeled and grated
½ cup raisins
1 cup chopped walnuts

- Preheat oven to 325 degrees F.
- Grease and flour two 8-inch round cake pans.
- In a large mixing bowl, mix dry ingredients together. In another bowl, combine oil, sugar, eggs, carrots, and ginger.
- Add carrot mixture to dry ingredients and with a minimum of folding, combine them. Stir in raisins and walnuts. *Do not overmix.*
- Fill prepared pans almost to the top. Bake 55 minutes, or until a cake tester comes out clean.
- Let cool and remove cakes from pan.
- This cake can be served plain, dusted with confectioners' sugar, or frosted with Goat-Cheese Frosting. *Makes two 8-inch rounds.*

GOAT-CHEESE FROSTING

HIGHLY BENEFICIAL		NEUTRAL	O, A, B, AB	AVOID	

4 oz. goat cheese, softened to
  room temperature
2 oz. butter or canola-oil
  margarine, softened to
  room temperature
⅔ cup confectioners' sugar

2 tablespoons honey
1 tablespoon rice milk
1 teaspoon vanilla extract
  (Types A, B, AB)
  or almond extract (Type O)
½ teaspoon lemon zest

- In a small bowl, blend goat cheese and butter using a fork. Add confectioners' sugar and blend in, but don't whip.
- Fold in honey, rice milk, vanilla or almond extract, and lemon zest.
- Spread on cooled cake. Refrigerate if not served immediately. *Makes about 1½ cups.*

WALNUT SHORTBREAD

HIGHLY BENEFICIAL		NEUTRAL	O, B	AVOID	A, AB

This is another simple but rich dessert that complements fruit salad, poached fruit, or a bunch of grapes.

1 cup butter, at room temperature

1½ cups spelt flour (Type B can substitute ½ cup oat flour for ½ cup spelt)

½ cup walnuts, ground in blender

½ cup confectioners' sugar

pinch of salt

■ Preheat oven to 350 degrees F.

■ In large mixing bowl, cream butter. Add flour, walnuts, sugar, and salt, and stir until blended. The dough will be very stiff.

■ Press dough firmly with your fingers into ungreased 9 × 9-inch pan. Prick entire surface at ½-inch intervals with a fork to let out steam.

■ Bake 25 minutes, or until just golden.

■ Remove from oven, allow to cool a few minutes, then cut into squares or narrow rectangles.

■ If you make this in a pie dish of approximately the same square-inch measurement, cut into triangles. *Makes 12 to 16 pieces.*

LEMON SQUARES

HIGHLY BENEFICIAL		NEUTRAL	O, B	AVOID	A, AB

Lemon squares are both tart and sweet—and rich. Cut the squares into fairly small pieces.

⅔ cup spelt flour

¼ cup walnuts, ground in blender

¼ cup confectioners' sugar

½ cup melted butter, cooled

⅔ cup granulated sugar

½ teaspoon baking powder

2 eggs, beaten

3 tablespoons lemon juice

3 teaspoons grated lemon peel

pinch of salt

- Preheat oven to 350 degrees F.
- In a small bowl, stir flour, walnuts, and confectioners' sugar until blended. Add butter and combine well.
- Press dough firmly with your fingers into 8 × 8-inch buttered pan. Bake until lightly colored, about 20 minutes.
- While pastry is baking, combine granulated sugar, baking powder, eggs, lemon juice, lemon peel, and salt in a mixing bowl. Beat well for just a moment.
- Pour over warm, not hot, pastry and return to oven for another 20 minutes, or until lemon topping is slightly puffed, firm, and a lovely gold.
- Cut into 2-inch squares when cool.   *Makes 12 to 16 pieces.*

SPELT BREAD PUDDING

HIGHLY BENEFICIAL		NEUTRAL	A, B, AB	AVOID	O

Spelt bread pudding began as an inedible loaf of whole-spelt French bread. As was mentioned in the "Breads" section, many attempts have to be made in the bread-baking process before a good loaf of bread is achieved. What to do with hard and heavy loaves? Milk and eggs solved the problem. Stale bread can be used for puddings, bread crumbs, croutons, and chapons, which are small rectangular pieces of stale bread, rubbed with garlic, that accompany mesclun and Niçoise salads. Hearty slices of stale bread also make good thickeners for soups. Place a slice or two at the bottom of the bowl, ladle in some soup, and let soak. Also, this pudding doubles as an excellent quick breakfast.

about 5 cups stale spelt bread
  cubes
5 cups milk or soy milk
butter for pan
4 eggs or egg substitute
1½ cups sugar

3 tablespoons vanilla extract
juice and grated rind of
  1 lemon
pinch of salt
1 cup dried cherries

- Place bread in bowl, cover with milk, and let sit 45 minutes.
- Preheat oven to 325 degrees F. Butter a 9 × 13 × 2-inch glass baking pan.

- Beat eggs until light. Add sugar, vanilla, lemon juice, lemon rind, and salt, and beat well.
- Pour into bread and milk mixture. Stir in cherries.
- Pour into prepared pan and bake 1 hour, or until set. Can be eaten warm or cold. *Serves 12.*

CRANBERRY BISCOTTI

HIGHLY BENEFICIAL		NEUTRAL	O, A., B, AB	AVOID	

Cranberry biscotti *make a wonderful tasty Christmas cookie as well as a good teething biscuit for babies.*

Dip the biscotti in your tea or coffee. Cranberries add a chewy, tart sweetness.

butter or oil for cookie sheet
3 eggs
¼ cup sugar
3 tablespoons butter or margarine, melted and cooled
1 teaspoon vanilla (Types A, B, and AB)
1 teaspoon almond extract (Type O)
zest of 1 lemon or orange

1 tablespoon pineapple juice
1⅔ cups spelt flour
1 teaspoon baking powder
¼ teaspoon salt
¼ teaspoon nutmeg (Type O omit)
½ cup chopped fresh cranberries
egg wash for glaze (made from 1 beaten egg)

- Preheat oven to 350 degrees F.
- Grease cookie sheet.
- Beat eggs until foamy, then slowly add sugar, beating until light. Add shortening, vanilla, lemon zest, and pineapple juice.
- In a separate bowl, mix all dry ingredients. Add dry ingredients to egg mixture and blend well.
- Stir in cranberries. The dough will be soft.
- Divide dough in half. On a prepared cookie sheet, mold each half into a long thin loaf, about 8 by 3 inches.

- Bake 25 minutes.
- Remove from oven and reduce heat to 325 degrees F.
- Let loaves cool 10 minutes. Place loaves on a cutting board and slice on the diagonal, into 1½-inch-thick pieces.
- Return cookies to cookie sheet and toast on one side, 5 minutes, then turn each cookie and toast on the other side another 10 minutes. Remove from oven when golden brown.
- Store for a week in a cookie jar. *Makes 32 pieces.*

RICE-CRISPY CAKES

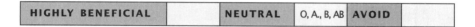

HIGHLY BENEFICIAL		NEUTRAL	O, A., B, AB	AVOID	

This crispy, chewy rice treat is an all-time favorite of children everywhere. Crispy cakes are palate pleasers, and these are every bit as sweet and delectable as the commercial versions.

2 tablespoons butter or
canola-oil margarine
(depending on Type)
¼ cup honey, maple syrup, or
brown rice syrup

2 tablespoons brown sugar
¼ tablespoon salt
3 cups crispy rice cereal
(brown rice is the nuttiest)

- In a 3-quart saucepan, melt butter or margarine, honey or other liquid sweetener, sugar, and salt.
- Add rice cereal all at once and stir to incorporate thoroughly.
- Immediately press mixture into a flat, rectangular plastic or glass container. A 5 × 8-inch dish works well. The cakes should be about 1 inch high by 2 inches square.
- Unlike those made with marshmallows, these must be refrigerated to hold together. *Makes 16 bars.*

PEANUT BUTTER COOKIES

HIGHLY BENEFICIAL		NEUTRAL	A, AB	AVOID	O, B

The fact that peanuts are listed as Highly Beneficial is always a good reason to mix up a batch of these rich and flavorful cookies. They're not too sweet, so if you'd like them sweeter, add an extra ¼ cup sugar.

grease or parchment paper
  for cookie sheets
½ cup margarine
½ cup brown sugar
¼ cup white sugar
2 eggs
1¼ cups chunky, unsalted
  peanut butter

generous pinch of salt
½ teaspoon baking soda
1 teaspoon vanilla extract
1 cup spelt flour
½ cup oat flour

- Preheat oven to 350 degrees F.
- Grease cookie sheets.
- Beat margarine until soft, then add sugars and beat until creamy. Beat in eggs, peanut butter, salt, baking soda, and vanilla, fully incorporating all the peanut butter.
- Stir in both flours, mixing well.
- Roll dough between your palms into 1-inch balls and place on greased cookie sheet, or unbuttered parchment paper. Flatten to about ¼-inch with the tines of a fork.
- Bake 7 to 10 minutes, or until cookies begin to color.
- Cool on wire racks. *Makes about 40 cookies.*

APPLE CAKE

HIGHLY BENEFICIAL		NEUTRAL	O, A, B, AB	AVOID	

This is a rich but not overly sweet cake. If you'd prefer a slightly sweeter cake, add a little more sugar. Type A and Type AB can substitute canola-oil margarine.

2 to 2½ cups peeled and
   thinly sliced apples
⅔ cup sugar
juice and grated rind of
   1 lemon
1 tablespoon spelt flour
5 tablespoons melted butter
   or margarine

½ cup white spelt flour
½ cup whole-spelt flour
1 teaspoon baking powder
pinch of salt
2 eggs or egg substitute
¼ cup soy milk

- Preheat oven to 350 degrees F.
- Butter bottom of an 8- or 9-inch pie pan deep enough to hold all the batter.
- Arrange apple slices in an attractive pattern in the pie pan. When cake has finished cooking, it will be inverted on a plate.
- Sprinkle apples with ½ cup sugar, lemon juice, and grated lemon rind.
- Type A and Type AB can sprinkle the fruit with cinnamon.
- Type B can sprinkle nutmeg.
- Dust with a tablespoon of flour, then pour melted butter or margarine over apples.
- In a bowl, combine both flours, remaining ¼ cup sugar, baking powder, and salt.
- In another bowl, beat eggs until light, then quickly stir in remaining tablespoon melted butter and soy milk.
- Add liquid ingredients to flour mixture and blend with as few strokes as possible.
- Pour batter over apples into pie pan. Bake 30 to 40 minutes, until golden brown and a straw comes out clean.
- Cover with a serving platter and reverse. *Serves 8 to 10.*

BASMATI RICE PUDDING

HIGHLY BENEFICIAL		NEUTRAL	O, A, B, AB	AVOID	

This rice pudding is a pleasant alternative to the usual milk-based ones. It's a good way to use up any leftover rice in your refrigerator. Try this substantial pudding for lunch with a fruit salad. It's also a healthy cold breakfast pudding. Quick, too!

butter for baking dish
2 cups basmati rice, cooked
4 eggs
2 cups soy milk
½ cup sugar

2 tablespoons melted butter
  or canola-oil margarine
grated rind of 1 lemon
juice of ½ lemon
½ cup raisins

- Preheat oven to 350 degrees F.
- Grease baking dish and add rice.
- In large mixing bowl, beat eggs with a whisk until frothy. Add remaining ingredients and mix thoroughly.
- Pour mixture over rice, combining well with a fork.
- Bake pudding until set, approximately 40 to 50 minutes.
  Serves 6 to 8.

PINEAPPLE UPSIDE-DOWN CAKE

HIGHLY BENEFICIAL		NEUTRAL	O, A, B, AB	AVOID	

This is an old favorite. You'll swear that this version is just like the kind mother used to make.

¼ cup butter or canola-oil
  margarine
½ cup brown sugar
6 to 9 slices canned, drained
  unsweetened pineapple
enough small pieces of fruit
  to fit into the pineapple
  "holes"; try halved pitted

cherries or halved pitted
  apricots
1 cup white spelt flour
1 teaspoon baking powder
4 eggs
2 tablespoons melted butter
  or margarine
¾ cup sugar

- Preheat oven to 350 degrees F.
- In a 9-inch round, cast-iron skillet, melt butter or margarine. Add sugar, stirring well. Distribute this mixture evenly over bottom of skillet.
- Turn off heat and add pineapple slices, fitting them neatly around perimeter of skillet, and placing 1 slice in middle. Fill the "holes" with fruit of your choice.
- In a medium bowl, mix spelt flour and baking powder well.
- In a smaller bowl, beat eggs until light. Add melted butter or margarine, then sugar, and beat until well blended.
- Add liquid to dry ingredients and stir until well blended. Pour batter over pineapple.
- Bake approximately 25 to 30 minutes, until cake is golden.
- Remove cake from oven. Place a large plate over skillet, and turn cake upside down.
- Leave on counter a few minutes, with skillet still upside down over plate, to let cake settle. Carefully remove skillet to reveal pineapple and fruit topping. *Serves 6 to 9.*

TOFU-BANANA PUDDING

HIGHLY BENEFICIAL		NEUTRAL	O	AVOID	A, B, AB

This fat-free pudding is easy to make and is a satisfying light dessert. Children love it, too. Try it for breakfast!

1 cake tofu
2 ripe bananas

- Combine ingredients in a blender and purée a few moments. Pour into individual little bowls and chill. *Serves 2 to 4.*

TOFU-PUMPKIN PUDDING

HIGHLY BENEFICIAL	O, A, AB	NEUTRAL		AVOID	B

The variations for this simple tofu treat are endless. It's a terrific way to get your soy and some healthy fruit all at the same time. So smooth and satisfying, too.

1 cake tofu
1 cup canned pumpkin

honey as needed (start with 1
to 2 tablespoons)

■ Purée all of the ingredients in a blender, pour into bowls, and chill.   *Serves 3 to 4.*

SAUTÉED PEARS OR APPLES

HIGHLY BENEFICIAL		NEUTRAL	O, A, B, AB	AVOID	

Sautéeing ripe pears and apples is a good way to use fruit that you might otherwise not eat out of hand. This is a simple fall dessert or a sublime topping for crêpes or pancakes. It is also wonderful served with cottage or ricotta cheese. Allow at least one pear or apple per person. A pinch of curry powder cooked in the butter or margarine adds a piquant flavor.

2 pears or apples
2 tablespoons butter (Type A and Type AB can use soy
   or canola-oil margarine)
cinnamon or nutmeg

■ Peel and thinly slice pears or apples.
■ Melt butter in a heavy skillet over low heat. Add fruit, turning gently to coat with butter or margarine.
■ Turn heat very low and cover pan, stewing fruit in butter or margarine and whatever juice the fruit throws off. If there doesn't seem to be enough liquid, add a tablespoon of water at a time.

- Cook 7 to 10 minutes, or until fruit is soft. There should be a little syrup.
- Type A and Type AB can sprinkle with cinnamon or nutmeg.
- Type B can sprinkle the fruit with nutmeg. *Serves 2.*

SAUTÉED BANANAS

HIGHLY BENEFICIAL	B	NEUTRAL	O	AVOID	A, AB

Ripe bananas aren't appealing to some people. Rather than tossing them out, try turning them in a little butter. Surprising and wonderful with curried dishes, they're also good for breakfast with a little ricotta or fresh goat cheese. Serve with organic vanilla ice cream. A triumph of tastes and textures, cold and hot. Allow one banana per person.

2 ripe bananas
2 tablespoons butter

1 tablespoon lemon juice
   (optional)
grated lemon rind

- Cut bananas in half crosswise, then cut in half lengthwise. The bananas should be quartered.
- Melt butter in a heavy skillet. Reduce heat to low and add bananas, turning carefully in the butter. They will brown and get softer. Don't let them burn.
- Cook 4 to 6 minutes. Sprinkle with lemon juice, if using, and lemon rind. Serve at once. *Serves 2.*

FRESH FIG SALAD

HIGHLY BENEFICIAL	O, A, AB	NEUTRAL	B	AVOID	

Fresh figs are in season for a very short time. The Black Mission and Calmyrna figs are the most widely available, but there are over 150 varieties. Eat ripe figs out of hand, or serve them as presented here, with a creamy fresh goat cheese. Allow three to four figs and a slice or two of cheese per serving.

3 to 4 figs per person
goat cheese

■ Slice figs lengthwise, exposing the complex and lovely flesh. Fan
the figs out on a plate, and top with bits of broken crumbled goat
cheese.

TROPICAL SALAD

HIGHLY BENEFICIAL		O, A, B, AB	NEUTRAL		AVOID	

*Combine these succulent and fragrant fruits according to your taste and
blood type. A generous squeeze of lemon or lime juice will keep the
colors intact, and the intense tartness is dressing enough for many
people. If you prefer, swirl Ricotta Dressing (page 365) over the top of
each portion for a richer version.*

papaya (Types O, A, B, and
  AB)
mango (Types O, B)
kiwi (Types O, A, B, and AB)
pineapple (Types O, A, B,
  and AB)

carambola (star fruit) (Types
  O, A)
banana (Types O, B)
guava (Types O, A, B)
lemon or lime juice

■ Prepare all the fruit: Peel, seed, and cut the papaya and mango.
Peel the kiwi and cut into slices or wedges. Cut pineapple into
small chunks. Slice carambola so that each piece is a little star.
Slice banana. Peel and slice guava.
■ This salad can be layered in a glass bowl, each individual fruit in
a single layer, or it can be very gently turned to mix the fruits.
■ Sprinkle each layer with lemon or lime juice, or pour juice over
salad before turning. *Allow about 1 cup prepared fruit per
person.*

FRUIT COMPOTE

HIGHLY BENEFICIAL	O, A, B, AB NEUTRAL	AVOID

Poaching fruit is an excellent way to use very ripe fruit. Don't be afraid to add some dried prunes and apricots to the mix, either. Combinations are endless, so be creative! Poached fruit over yogurt or ricotta makes a lovely breakfast or a light lunch.

1 cup water
⅔ cup sugar
juice and grated rind of
   1 lemon
3 cloves
1 cup apples, pears, peaches,
   or plums

1 cup apricots, grapes,
   nectarines, or cherries
½ cup torn fresh mint leaves
   (optional)

- A poaching syrup should be prepared first. In a large nonreactive saucepan, bring water to a boil, add sugar, lemon juice, lemon rind, and cloves.
- You don't have to peel the fruit if you don't want to. Remove all seeds and pits, slice larger fruit, and halve smaller ones, like apricots and plums. If you have a cherry pitter, leave cherries whole; if not, halve them as you remove the pits. Leave grapes whole.
- Add any combination of fruits to the boiling syrup, allowing 1 large and several smaller fruits per person.
- Poach, uncovered, about 10 to 15 minutes. Lift fruit carefully from syrup with a slotted spoon and place in a serving bowl.
- Continue to cook and reduce syrup another 8 to 10 minutes. Remove cloves and pour thickened syrup over fruits.
- Cool in refrigerator. Sprinkle with mint leaves, if desired. *Serves 2.*

Dressings and Sauces

Enticing Condiments

*D*RESSING SEEMS AN IDEAL NAME FOR ALL THOSE SIDE dishes that really do dress up other foods. We generally think of this rather extensive group as table condiments, but anyone who has ever had the taste of a dish brought alive with the introduction of a sauce or relish knows otherwise. These recipes will enable you to take something quick and easy, such as baked chicken, and transform it into something far more enticing, perhaps a Chicken with Mango-Ginger Chutney. A simple salad dressing can add a pleasant change and a nutritional boost to a fruit or mixed greens salad. Most of these recipes can be prepared very quickly. If you make them in advance and in quantity, it will be all the easier to serve a nutritious meal, even when you're pressed for time.

OLIVE-OIL MAYONNAISE

HIGHLY BENEFICIAL		NEUTRAL	O, A, B, AB	AVOID	

This is a basic mayonnaise that uses olive or canola oil and lemon or lime juice instead of vinegar. It is best to use a lighter olive oil as opposed to an extra-virgin. In this way, you achieve a flavor similar to that of canola. This mayonnaise should be used in all recipes calling for mayonnaise. CAUTION: Although many mayonnaise recipes call for the use of raw egg yolk, we suggest instead starting the recipe with a tablespoon or two of the canola-oil mayonnaise that can be found in most health-food markets. Since lemon juice is acidic, the theory of adding raw egg is that the juice cooks the egg, just as lemon or lime is used to cook the raw fish in seviche. However, the USDA no longer allows restaurants to use this method for two reasons: First, a lack of control in preparation, and second, the very real potential for food poisoning. Avoid eating raw egg at any of your meals.

1 or 2 tablespoons canola-oil mayonnaise	2 tablespoons lime or lemon juice
¼ teaspoon salt	1 cup light olive or canola oil

■ In a blender or food processor, make a basic mayonnaise by whipping the canola-oil mayonnaise and lemon juice together, and drizzling in the oil until it thickens. Keep chilled.   *Makes about 1½ cups.*

RICOTTA DRESSING

HIGHLY BENEFICIAL	B, AB	NEUTRAL	A	AVOID	O

Thinned ricotta makes a creamy dressing for those fruit salads that are served as a complete meal rather than as a dessert.

1 cup ricotta cheese
2 tablespoons honey
1 tablespoon lemon juice
2 tablespoons pineapple juice (optional), for further thinning
grated rind of ½ lemon

■ In a small bowl, combine all ingredients and stir until thoroughly mixed.   *Makes 1½ cups.*

ALMOND DRESSING

HIGHLY BENEFICIAL		NEUTRAL	O, A, B, AB	AVOID	

Like tahini, almond butter can be thinned to make a delicious dressing for fruit salads.

½ cup almond butter   ¼ cup water
1 tablespoon honey

- In a small bowl, combine all ingredients and mix until well blended.
- Drizzle over fruit. Use more water if you want a thinner, lighter dressing.   *Makes ¾ cup.*

PEANUT DRESSING

HIGHLY BENEFICIAL	A, AB	NEUTRAL		AVOID	O, B

½ cup crunchy peanut butter   pinch of salt (if using
1 tablespoon honey   unsalted peanut butter)
¼ cup water

- Combine all ingredients in a saucepan over low heat, and stir to mix well. A little more water can be added to thin the sauce if you choose.
- Serve warm over noodles or on chicken.   *Makes ¾ cup.*

TAHINI DRESSING

HIGHLY BENEFICIAL		NEUTRAL	O, A	AVOID	B, AB

Thick and creamy, sesame butter is used in a number of Middle Eastern dishes such as hummus. Try it on fruit salads.

½ cup tahini
1 tablespoon honey

1 to 2 tablespoons water (or more as needed)

■ Combine all ingredients in a small bowl and stir until blended. Drizzle over fruit.   *Makes ¾ cup.*

TOFU-MISO DRESSING

HIGHLY BENEFICIAL	A, AB	NEUTRAL	O	AVOID	B

A savory dressing for rice or vegetables.

½ cake tofu
1 tablespoon miso
2 to 3 tablespoons vegetable
  stock

2 tablespoons sesame seeds
  (Type AB omit)

■ Combine all ingredients in a blender and purée until smooth. *Makes 1½ cups.*

TOFU-PARSLEY DRESSING

HIGHLY BENEFICIAL	A, AB	NEUTRAL	O	AVOID	B

This dressing is delicious over brown rice, with a simple vegetable stir-fry. Try it instead of mayonnaise on a sandwich.

½ cake tofu
2 to 3 tablespoons fresh
  parsley

2 tablespoons lemon juice
2 teaspoons miso

■ Combine all ingredients in a blender and purée a few seconds until smooth. This dressing will stay fresh for a few days and will get thicker if allowed to sit. *Makes 1½ cups.*

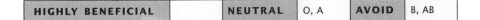

SESAME-SEED DRESSING

HIGHLY BENEFICIAL		NEUTRAL	O, A	AVOID	B, AB

This light, creamy dressing is coarser than tahini. Although the sesame seeds are ground with a mortar and pestle, they should not be ground too finely.

4 tablespoons sesame seeds
2 teaspoons soy sauce

3 tablespoons vegetable stock
1 to 2 teaspoons sugar

■ Toast the sesame seeds briefly, then grind them by hand until crushed but not too pasty. Add soy sauce, stock, and sugar.
■ Continue to grind until a little smoother. *Makes 1½ cups.*

BASIL PESTO

HIGHLY BENEFICIAL	O, AB	NEUTRAL	A, B	AVOID	

This pesto has no Parmesan cheese and substitutes walnuts for the traditional pignoli nuts. Make it with a mortar and pestle so that the pesto doesn't become too homogenized. A little coarser is better with this pesto. The proportions for the ingredients are approximate, allowing for personal taste.

1 teaspoon coarse salt
½ cup fresh basil
½ cup fresh parsley
2 to 3 cloves garlic, crushed
   and peeled

½ cup broken walnuts
olive oil

- Place salt in mortar and begin adding basil and parsley leaves. Add some garlic, continuing to work in each new addition.
- Add broken nuts, more leaves, then garlic, until mixture is well ground but not too smooth.
- Add olive oil slowly, stirring until desired consistency is reached. *Makes 2 cups.*

CILANTRO PESTO

HIGHLY BENEFICIAL	O, AB	NEUTRAL	A, B	AVOID	

Like basil pesto, this is best made with mortar and pestle. Try it on pasta, rice, or sandwiches. Stir a tablespoon into soup just before serving.

1 teaspoon coarse salt
1 cup fresh cilantro
¼ cup fresh parsley
3 cloves garlic, crushed and
   peeled

½ cup broken walnuts
olive oil

- Place salt in mortar and alternately add cilantro, parsley, garlic, and nuts, incorporating each new addition thoroughly.
- When you have a coarse paste, slowly add olive oil until you reach the desired consistency. *Makes about 2 cups.*

LEMON-HONEY DRESSING

HIGHLY BENEFICIAL	A, AB	NEUTRAL	O, B	AVOID	

This is a good marinade for fish, and a sweet and tart dressing for salads.

juice of 2 lemons
¼ cup olive oil

1 to 2 tablespoons honey
1 to 2 teaspoons tamari

- Combine all ingredients in a jar, seal tightly, and shake well. Season to taste. *Makes 1 cup.*

OLIVE OIL & LEMON DRESSING

HIGHLY BENEFICIAL	O, A, B, AB	NEUTRAL		AVOID	

A basic dressing that should be a staple in every household.

½ cup extra-virgin olive oil
juice of 2 lemons
½ teaspoon dry mustard

½ teaspoon salt
¼ teaspoon honey

- Combine all ingredients in a small bowl and whisk until blended. Serve on any salad. *Makes about ¾ cup.*

SWEET VIDALIA ONION DRESSING

HIGHLY BENEFICIAL	O, A, B, AB	NEUTRAL		AVOID	

The Vidalia onion is wonderfully sweet and mild. Joined with the tart lemon juice and green parsley, it makes a great accompaniment to mesclun or other mixed green salads.

½ small Vidalia onion
juice of 2 lemons
1 tablespoon chopped fresh
    parsley

1 teaspoon salt
½ teaspoon sugar
1½ cups olive oil

- Grate or finely chop onion. Combine onion and remaining ingredients except oil in a small bowl and allow to marinate 1 hour.
- After an hour, drizzle oil into onion and lemon mixture and whisk. If dressing separates, shake or whisk again.
Makes about 2 cups.

BALSAMIC MUSTARD VINAIGRETTE

HIGHLY BENEFICIAL		NEUTRAL	B, AB	AVOID	A, O

A slightly sweet and very satisfying salad dressing.

2 tablespoons honey
2 tablespoons Dijon mustard

½ cup balsamic vinegar
1 cup olive oil

- In a food processor, combine honey, mustard, and vinegar.
- With machine running, slowly drizzle in oil so that it is completely incorporated. This can last in the refrigerator indefinitely.
Makes about 2 cups.

CUCUMBER-YOGURT SAUCE

HIGHLY BENEFICIAL	B, AB	NEUTRAL	A	AVOID	O

This sauce is ideal with curries; with cold, sliced lamb; and with fresh vegetables for dipping.

2 cups plain yogurt
½ red onion, diced small
1 tablespoon chopped fresh mint
1 tablespoon chopped cilantro

1 small cucumber, peeled, seeded, and diced
2 teaspoons ground cumin
squeeze of lemon juice

- Combine all ingredients in a blender and purée until smooth.
  Makes about 3 cups.

PINEAPPLE CHUTNEY

HIGHLY BENEFICIAL	A, B, AB	NEUTRAL	O	AVOID	

1 small onion, diced small
2 tablespoons olive or canola oil
1 ripe pineapple, peeled, cored, and chopped small
1-inch piece fresh ginger, peeled and grated

juice of 2 lemons
1 cup brown sugar
¼ cup pineapple juice
½ cup raisins

- In a saucepan, cook onion in oil over medium heat until translucent.
- Add pineapple and ginger and cook a few minutes. Add remaining ingredients and cook down until thick, about 5 minutes.
- Cool and serve with grilled tempeh or curried tofu.
  Makes about 1 to 1½ quarts.

PINEAPPLE CHUTNEY–YOGURT SAUCE

HIGHLY BENEFICIAL	A, B, AB	NEUTRAL		AVOID	O

1 cup Pineapple Chutney (see
   page 372)
2 tablespoons plain yogurt

2 tablespoons canola or
   commercial mayonnaise

- Combine all ingredients in a blender or food processor and purée until smooth. *Makes about 1½ cups.*

FRESH MANGO AND MINT SAUCE

HIGHLY BENEFICIAL		NEUTRAL	O, B	AVOID	A, AB

Serve this sauce over fish, topped with sliced or small whole mint leaves.

1 ripe mango, peeled and
   pitted
½-inch piece fresh ginger,
   peeled
juice of 1 lime
2 tablespoons extra-virgin
   olive oil

1 teaspoon salt
zest of 1 lime
2 tablespoons fresh mint,
   rolled together, then sliced
   finely

- In a food processor or blender, combine mango, ginger, and lime juice, and purée until smooth.
- While still blending, drizzle in oil. Transfer to bowl. Stir in salt, zest, and mint. *Makes about 1⅓ cups.*

PEANUT BUTTER SAUCE (GADO-GADO)

HIGHLY BENEFICIAL	A, B, AB	NEUTRAL		AVOID	O

This sauce is a staple for those who love and can eat peanuts. It's versatile enough to use as a dip for vegetables and crackers, as a sauce for fish destined for the broiler, but, above all, as a perfect accompaniment to tempeh and tofu. Double the recipe and keep it in the refrigerator. It lasts a good ten days, if not longer.

1 clove garlic, crushed and peeled
2 scallions
¼ cup coarsely chopped fresh cilantro
½ cup peanut butter

¼ cup tamari sauce
2 tablespoons lemon juice
½ cup water
1 teaspoon peeled and chopped fresh ginger

- In a food processor, chop garlic, scallion, and cilantro.
- Add peanut butter, tamari, and lemon juice, and pulse until blended, scraping down bowl as necessary. The mixture will be very thick.
- With machine running, slowly add some water until desired consistency is reached.   *Makes about 2 cups.*

LIME DRESSING

HIGHLY BENEFICIAL		NEUTRAL	O, A, B, AB	AVOID	

A very tasty dressing for mixed greens that is also delicious on fish. The canola oil can be replaced entirely with olive oil in this recipe.

½ teaspoon Garlic-Shallot Mixture (see page 375), or 2 shallots, finely chopped

2 teaspoons dry mustard
juice and zest from 2 limes
½ teaspoon salt
1 cup canola oil or olive oil

- Combine Garlic-Shallot Mixture or 2 shallots, mustard, lime juice, zest, and salt in a small bowl.
- While whisking briskly, drizzle the oil in a steady stream until it has all been incorporated. For a smoother dressing, use a blender. *Makes about 1½ to 2 cups.*

GARLIC-SHALLOT MIXTURE

HIGHLY BENEFICIAL	O, A, AB	NEUTRAL	B	AVOID	

This recipe cuts down on both preparation and cooking time! There are so many recipes that call for chopped garlic, or onions, or both. This is a terrific substitute. Spoon a teaspoon or so into any dish that you're making.

10 cloves garlic, peeled
10 shallots, peeled
olive oil to cover

- In a food processor or blender, combine garlic and shallots and pulse on and off, scraping down sides of bowl as necessary, until finely chopped.
- When desired consistency is reached, transfer to an airtight container and cover with oil. This will be good, refrigerated, for about 10 days or longer.

DIPPING SAUCE

HIGHLY BENEFICIAL		NEUTRAL	O, A, B, AB	AVOID	

Use as a dip or marinade for tempeh, fish, or meats.

¼ cup tamari sauce
juice of 1 lime
1 tablespoon sesame oil
(Type O only) or olive oil
2 tablespoons chopped fresh
cilantro

1 tablespoon sugar
2 tablespoons brown rice
vinegar, or 2 tablespoons
lemon juice
1 clove garlic, crushed and
peeled

- Combine all ingredients in a small bowl.
- For a great marinade, just add an additional ½ cup olive oil.
Makes about 1 cup.

TWENTY-THREE

Snacks and Munchies

Healthy Treats

$\mathcal{S}$NACKS ARE BY NO MEANS ESSENTIAL TO GOOD EATING. But let's face the facts: They're here to stay, especially if you have kids. Why not give them a healthy boost? Rather than letting children fill up on the highly processed junk foods that are heavily advertised to appeal to kids, making a little extra effort can provide some delightful alternatives.

Snacks for kids should be quick, easy, and on hand. Whatever you choose not only has to satisfy between-meal hunger, but also has to provide a good, nutritious boost to their systems. Snacks should be something older kids can serve themselves. Healthy snacks can be on the kitchen table, ready to eat, a few minutes after the kids walk in the door from school or play.

Trail Mix

Originally a high-calorie energy sustainer for extended hiking, trail mix started becoming very popular in the late 1960s. Affectionately nicknamed Gorp, the basic recipe has been modified to suit the different blood types. Ingredients for trail mix can be adjusted according to your taste. It is made primarily of nuts, seeds, and dried fruits, which are concentrated energy sources, so a little trail mix goes a long way. For school, in the car, or on a hike, trail mix may be one of the most satisfying treats ever invented. The crunch of the nuts and seeds and the intense sweetness of the dried fruits combine to provide a filling, satisfying combination. Trail mix is very simple to prepare. The following recipes provide three variations of the basic mix for each of the four blood types. Merely combine all ingredients and store in a tightly covered glass container.

Type O Trail Mixes

TYPE O TRAIL MIX #1

1 cup walnuts, broken into pieces
½ cup filberts, halved
½ cup dried apricots, quartered
½ cup dried cherries
½ cup dairy-free semisweet chocolate or carob chips

TYPE O TRAIL MIX #2

1 cup pumpkin seeds
½ cup sunflower seeds
½ cup dried pears, chopped
½ cup dried pineapple, chopped

TYPE O TRAIL MIX #3

1 cup dried cranberries
1 cup sunflower seeds
½ cup walnuts, broken into pieces
½ cup dairy-free chocolate chips

Type A Trail Mixes

TYPE A TRAIL MIX #1

1 cup peanuts
½ cup dried apricots,
    quartered

½ cup raisins

TYPE A TRAIL MIX #2

1 cup pumpkin seeds
½ cup sunflower seeds
½ cup walnuts, broken into
    pieces

1 cup dried pineapple,
    chopped

TYPE A TRAIL MIX #3

1 cup almonds, chopped
1 cup dried cherries

½ cup dairy-free semisweet
    chocolate or carob chips

Type B Trail Mixes

TYPE B TRAIL MIX #1

1 cup Brazil nuts, chopped
½ cup dried bananas, sliced

½ cup dried apricots,
    quartered

TYPE B TRAIL MIX #2

1 cup macadamia nuts,
  halved
1 cup dried pineapple,
  chopped

1 cup dried cranberries

TYPE B TRAIL MIX #3

½ cup pecans, broken into
  pieces
½ cup almonds, chopped
½ cup raisins

½ cup dried cherries
1 cup semisweet chocolate or
  carob chips

Type AB Trail Mixes

TYPE AB TRAIL MIX #1

1½ cups peanuts
1 cup walnuts, broken into
  pieces

½ cup raisins
½ cup dried apricots,
  quartered

TYPE AB TRAIL MIX #2

½ cup cashews
½ cup toasted pignoli

½ cup dried cranberries

TYPE AB TRAIL MIX #3

½ cup pistachios
1 cup dried cherries
½ cup dried pineapple,
  chopped

1 cup dairy-free semisweet
  chocolate or carob chips

All of the trail-mix combinations can be endlessly adjusted and altered, so you need never get bored. Consult your Blood Type lists and take it from there. A final note of caution: Sitting around and watching TV while eating trail mix can be hazardous to your waistline. Remember, nuts, seeds, and dried fruits are not only high in vitamins, minerals, and fiber, they're also high in fat and calories. These mixes are best eaten to sustain energy during performance-oriented activities such as hiking, cycling, or other high calorie-burning sports.

Candies, Toasted Seeds, & Dips

ALMOND-BUTTER CANDY

HIGHLY BENEFICIAL		NEUTRAL	O, A	AVOID	B, AB

1 cup plus 2 tablespoons
  ground sesame or
  sunflower seeds
¼ cup dried figs, finely sliced

¼ cup dried apricots, finely
  sliced
½ cup almond butter
1 to 2 tablespoons honey

- Reserve 2 tablespoons sesame or sunflower seeds.
- Grind the rest of the seeds in a blender until powdery.
- Sprinkle several tablespoons over dried fruit, and toss to coat and separate the sticky little pieces of fruit.
- Add remainder of ground seeds to almond butter and stir until blended. Add honey, then dried fruit, blending well with a fork or your hands.
- Form mixture into balls and roll each one in sesame seeds.
  Makes 20 to 24 candies.

PEANUT-BUTTER CANDY

HIGHLY BENEFICIAL	A, AB	NEUTRAL		AVOID	O, B

Without honey this is a delicious but not very sweet candy. Add a tablespoon or more of honey to the recipe as you prepare it, adjusting the sweetness to taste.

1 cup chunky peanut butter	honey
6 tablespoons powdered goat's milk	½ cup walnuts, chopped
½ cup dried cherries, halved	
½ cup dried apricots, quartered	

- Combine peanut butter and 5 tablespoons of the powdered goat's milk in a small bowl and stir until blended.
- Sprinkle remaining tablespoon of powdered goat's milk over the dried fruit to separate it somewhat.
- Mix fruit with peanut butter and honey to taste, adding additional powdered milk if necessary for desired consistency.
- Shape into balls, and roll in the chopped walnuts.
  Makes 20 to 24 candies.

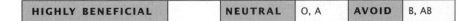

TAMARI-TOASTED SUNFLOWER SEEDS

HIGHLY BENEFICIAL		NEUTRAL	O, A	AVOID	B, AB

4 oz. raw shelled sunflower seeds	1 tablespoon tamari sauce
	½ cup of raisins

- In a large skillet, heat sunflower seeds over medium heat until almost popping. Flip around to toast evenly, turn off heat, then add tamari.
- Toss seeds only a few more seconds. The seeds should be well coated, but don't let the tamari burn. Mix with raisins for a sweet and savory snack.   *Serves 2.*

TAMARI-TOASTED PUMPKIN SEEDS

HIGHLY BENEFICIAL	O, A	NEUTRAL		AVOID	B, AB

4 oz. raw pumpkin seeds
1 tablespoon tamari sauce

- In a large skillet, heat pumpkin seeds over medium heat until almost popping. Pumpkin seeds behave a lot like popcorn. Shake pan so bottoms of seeds don't burn.
- Toss a few times, turn off heat, then add tamari.
- Toss again and cook a few more seconds. Remove seeds from pan and cool.   *Serves 1 to 2.*

Note: This same treatment can be applied to a wide range of nuts as well. Raw cashews, almonds, filberts, peanuts, and Brazil nuts can all be quickly toasted and coated with the salty tamari sauce, according to your blood type.

CURRY DIP

HIGHLY BENEFICIAL		NEUTRAL	O, A, B, AB	AVOID	

Use this spicy dip for fresh vegetables and apples. It also makes an unusual substitute for plain mayonnaise in salads and on sandwiches.

1 cup Olive-Oil Mayonnaise
   (see page 364) (Type B
   should substitute
   commercial mayonnaise)
1 tablespoon lemon juice
1 tablespoon good-quality
   ground curry powder

1 tablespoon ground cumin
1 tablespoon ground
   coriander powder
1 tablespoon ground mustard
   seed

- Mix all ingredients together until well blended and serve. Store in a tightly covered glass container.   *Makes about 1½ cups.*

BLACK BEAN DIP

HIGHLY BENEFICIAL	A	NEUTRAL	O	AVOID	B, AB

This dip is very easy to put together and tastes great. If a spicy black bean dip is desired, Type O can add chopped jalapeño peppers or a hot pepper sauce to the basic recipe.

2 cups cooked black beans,
   or 1 can black beans,
   rinsed well and drained
juice of ½ lemon
1 teaspoon salt
½ to 1 cup vegetable stock or
   water

1 small red onion, diced
   small
1 tablespoon chopped
   cilantro

- In a food processor or blender, purée beans. Add lemon juice, salt, and a little of the liquid, and blend until desired consistency is achieved.
- Transfer to mixing bowl. Stir in red onion and cilantro.
- Adjust seasonings and serve chilled with homemade quinoa tortilla chips.   *Makes 4 cups.*

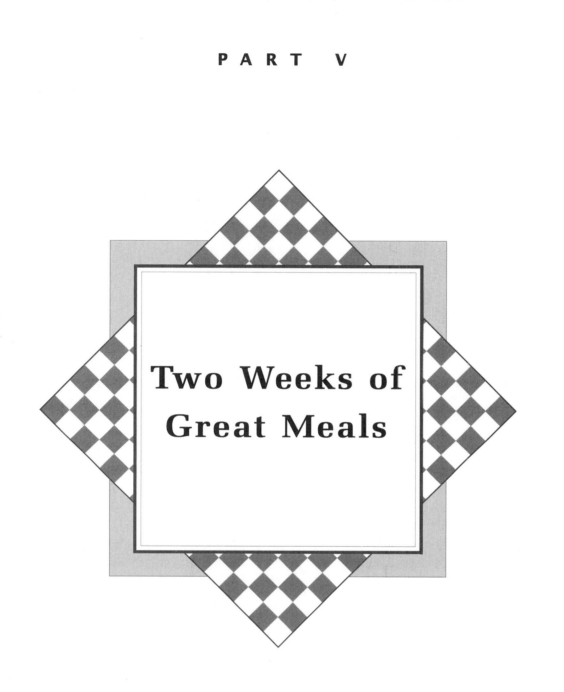

PART V

Two Weeks of Great Meals

*W*HEN YOU DECIDED TO FOLLOW THE BLOOD TYPE DIET, you made a very big commitment to change the way you eat and live. But you may still feel some uncertainty about exactly what your meals will look like. These menus offer a road map for your blood type. They show you how to take the food lists and the recipes and organize them into a daily diet that will set you on the path to staying healthy, living longer, and achieving your ideal weight.

Included here is a two-week menu plan for each blood type. As you grow accustomed to eating right for your type, you'll eventually develop a menu plan of your own. The goal is to reach a stage where it becomes natural for you to eat the foods that are going to do you the most good. Note that beverages are listed with most meals, but I suggest you drink them one half hour before or after eating, rather than with the meal. Be sure to determine the specific requirements of your personal situation—for example, if you need to lose weight, suffer from a medical condition, or have a special susceptibility to disease because of your blood type. Eating well and living well are on the same path.

Everyday Menus for Type O

Meals for Meat-Eaters

DAY 1	
BREAKFAST	**SNACK**
Single-egg omelet with grated carrot and zucchini	Carrot–ginger juice
Glass of pineapple juice	**DINNER**
Rose hips tea	Fettuccine with lamb sausages
	Green salad with honey–lemon dressing
SNACK	Spelt baguette
2 plums	Glass of wine
Glass of soy milk	Fresh figs
LUNCH	
Tuna salad on rye crisps	
Iced fenugreek tea	

DAY 2

BREAKFAST
1 slice of Ezekiel toast with
   black cherry preserves
Ginger tea

SNACK
Fresh pineapple
Grape juice and seltzer

LUNCH
Hamburger with melted
   goat Cheddar and slice of
   tomato
Iced seltzer water
Handful of grapes

SNACK
Tamari pumpkin seeds

DINNER
Roast turkey with sage and
   rosemary
Brown-rice pilaf with
   carrots and onions
Steamed broccoli
Seltzer

DAY 3

BREAKFAST
Single-egg omelet with
   broccoli and rice pilaf
Slippery elm tea

SNACK
½ grapefruit
Glass of soy-rice milk

LUNCH
Sliced turkey on spelt bread
   with mayonnaise, lettuce,
   and tomato
Cranberry juice and seltzer

SNACK
Handful of walnuts and
   raisins

DINNER
Grilled whole salmon with
   basil pesto
Grilled sweet potatoes
Romaine salad with Caesar
   dressing
Glass of white wine

DAY 4

BREAKFAST
Silken tofu scramble with
banana and blueberries
Rose hips tea

SNACK
Rice cake with soy butter
and jam
Green tea

LUNCH
Salmon salad with mayon-
naise and chopped fresh
dill on a bed of greens
Rye crisps
Iced fenugreek tea

SNACK
Pear
Glass of soy milk

DINNER
Rice spaghetti with meat
sauce
Steamed artichoke
French baguette
Chamomile tea

DAY 5

BREAKFAST
Poached egg on toasted
Ezekiel bread
½ grapefruit
Slippery elm tea

SNACK
Banana–silken tofu shake
with peach juice

LUNCH
Turkey vegetable soup
French bread
Glass of seltzer

SNACK
Figs with goat cheese and
walnuts

DINNER
Grilled swordfish with lime
wedge
Sweet potato salad (from
leftover grilled sweet
potatoes)
Grilled red peppers
Glass of white wine

DAY 6

BREAKFAST
Wild rice–flour pancakes
    with maple syrup
Fresh berries
Mulberry tea

SNACK
Banana–silken tofu shake

LUNCH
Quinoa tortilla filled with
    leftover rice, red peppers,
    and romaine, served with
    a tahini dressing
Seltzer
2 apricots

SNACK
Carrot–ginger juice

DINNER
Curried leg of lamb
Basmati rice
Fresh mango chutney
Spinach salad with grated
    hard-boiled egg
Glass of red wine

DAY 7

BREAKFAST
Single-egg omelet with fresh
    spinach and feta cheese
Fenugreek tea

SNACK
Mixed plums
Ginger tea

LUNCH
Sliced cold lamb on a bed
    of romaine with mint
    sauce
Iced rose hips tea

SNACK
Carrot sticks and pan-fried
    onion dip

DINNER
Country vegetable stew
    with pinto beans
Wild rice salad
Fresh sliced peaches,
    nectarines, figs, and
    plums
Shortbread

DAY 8

BREAKFAST
Rice crackers with almond
    and prune butters
Sarsaparilla tea

SNACK
Apple with walnuts and
    raisins

LUNCH
Grilled turkey burger with
    melted goat Cheddar
Sliced tomato and
    cucumbers
Glass of seltzer and
    pineapple juice

SNACK
Banana–soy milk smoothie

DINNER
Stir-fried shrimp with bok
    choy, red pepper,
    broccoli, garlic, onion,
    and tamari sauce
Sushi rice
Iced ginger tea
Fig cookies

DAY 9

BREAKFAST
Frittata with leftover
    vegetables and rice
Peppermint tea

SNACK
Plums and apricots
Prune juice and seltzer

LUNCH
Grilled goat Cheddar on
    Ezekiel bread
Iced ginseng tea

SNACK
Apple–carrot juice

DINNER
Turkey burritos with
    quinoa tortilla
Rice and black beans
Jicama sticks with
    pineapple salsa
Beer

DAY 10

BREAKFAST
French toast with sautéed
blueberries
Rose hips tea

SNACK
Banana–soy milk smoothie

LUNCH
Cuban black bean soup
Glass of seltzer and cherry
juice

SNACK
Apple and goat Cheddar
slices with rye crisp

DINNER
Grilled liver with Vidalia
onions
Steamed broccoli with
dipping sauce
Brown rice pilaf

DAY 11

BREAKFAST
Fried egg on brown rice
pilaf
Fenugreek tea

SNACK
Banana spelt muffin
Peppermint tea

LUNCH
Grilled chicken breast on
toasted spelt bread with let-
tuce and tomato
Mixed plums
Mineral water

SNACK
Tamari pumpkin seeds
Carrot–ginger juice

DINNER
Grilled filet of beef with
Portobello mushroom
sauce
Braised leeks
Spinach salad with lemon
vinaigrette
Glass of red wine
Shortbread

DAY 12

BREAKFAST
Spinach frittata
Fenugreek tea

SNACK
Fresh or dried figs
   or apricots
Glass of seltzer with lemon

LUNCH
Curried carrot and ginger
   soup
Lettuce and tomato salad
Prune juice and seltzer

SNACK
Walnut cookies
Ginseng tea

DINNER
Pasta with green
   vegetables
Caesar salad
Plum tart
Rose hips tea

DAY 13

BREAKFAST
Banana–nut muffin
Peppermint tea

SNACK
Fresh carrot juice

LUNCH
Slices of roast beef with
   pan-fried onion dip rolled
   in a romaine leaf
Pears and walnuts
Mineral water

SNACK
Rye crisps with soy–nut
   butter

DINNER
Braised veal shanks
Onion and fennel confit
Rice
Stir-fried sugar snap peas
Glass of wine

DAY 14

BREAKFAST
1 poached egg on Ezekiel
  bread
½ grapefruit and sliced
  banana
Mint tea

SNACK
Walnuts, raisins, and
  chocolate chips
Mineral water

LUNCH
Turkey burger
Lettuce and tomato
Glass of seltzer

SNACK
Red pepper strips with
  curry dip
Ginseng tea

DINNER
Indian lamb stew with
  spinach
Basmati rice
Mango chutney
Fenugreek tea

Everyday Menus for Type A

Feast on Vegetables and Grains

DAY 1

BREAKFAST
Silken tofu scramble with
  Vidalia onion and
  broccoli
Bowl of blueberries
Coffee
Glass of water with lemon

SNACK
Yogurt with raisins,
  sunflower seeds, and
  honey

LUNCH
Quinoa-flour tortillas filled
  with adzuki beans, goat
  Cheddar, diced onion,
  and sprouts
Pineapple salsa
Iced ginseng tea

SNACK
Iced vanilla nut coffee
  with rice milk

DINNER
Rice spaghetti with stir-
  fried spinach, carrots,
  Portobello mushrooms,
  onion, and garlic
1 slice spelt French bread
Glass of wine

DAY 2

BREAKFAST
Rice cakes with almond
   butter and cherry
   preserves
Rose hips tea

SNACK
2 plums
Apricot juice

LUNCH
Black bean soup
1 piece of corn bread
Iced burdock tea

SNACK
Carrot juice

DINNER
Tofu with peanuts and
   apricots
Brown rice
Steamed spinach

DAY 3

BREAKFAST
Buckwheat pancakes with
   blueberry syrup
Toasted almond coffee with
   almond milk

SNACK
Fresh pineapple–soy
   milk shake

LUNCH
Salad of romaine, grated
   carrot, onion, and flaked
   salmon with lime
   vinaigrette
Carrot cucumber juice

SNACK
Handful of raisins and
   peanuts

DINNER
Quinoa tortillas with
   black beans
Brown rice
Braised escarole
Glass of red wine
Fresh pineapple

DAY 4

BREAKFAST
Quinoa muffins with
  raspberry preserves
Coffee with soy milk

SNACK
Handful of cherries

LUNCH
Soba noodles in miso soup
Green tea

SNACK
Carrot-ginger juice

DINNER
Grilled red snapper
Basmati rice
Steamed artichoke
Chamomile tea
Frozen yogurt

DAY 5

BREAKFAST
Kasha with brown sugar
  and soy milk
Stewed prunes
Saint John's wort tea

SNACK
Bowl of ricotta with raisins
  and cinnamon

LUNCH
Peanut butter and blueberry
  jam on soy-flour bread
Glass of goat's milk
2 apricots

SNACK
Fresh vegetables with
  tahini dip
Water with lemon

DINNER
Lasagna with rice noodles,
  spinach, ricotta, and basil
  pesto
Portobello mushrooms with
  white sauce
Romaine salad with
  mustard vinaigrette
Glass of wine
Oatmeal cookies

DAY 6

BREAKFAST
Silken tofu scramble with
   peaches and blueberries
½ grapefruit
Hazelnut coffee

SNACK
Fresh figs
Glass of goat's milk

LUNCH
Salad pizza with whole-spelt
   crust, fresh greens,
   and slivers of melted
   mozzarella
Fenugreek tea

SNACK
Carrot–celery juice

DINNER
Broiled grouper with
   peanut sauce, served on a
   bed of red lentils and rice
Steamed pumpkin
Valerian tea

DAY 7

BREAKFAST
Blueberry–oat bran muffin
Fresh pineapple
Cinnamon coffee

SNACK
Peanuts and raisins
Glass of soy milk

LUNCH
Grilled soy cheese on
   Ezekiel bread
Sliced apples and walnuts
Lemonade

SNACK
Broccoli–carrot juice

DINNER
Sesame chicken
Spelt noodles with grated
   pecorino romano cheese
Braised collard greens
Glass of red wine
Sliced mixed plums

DAY 8

BREAKFAST
Silken tofu scramble with
  brown rice and leftover
  collards
Ginger tea

SNACK
Fruit smoothie with soy
  milk, peaches, and
  pineapple

LUNCH
White bean soup with
  wilted greens and garlic

1 slice of pumpernickel
  and raisin toast
Iced fenugreek tea

SNACK
Goat cheese on rye crackers
Pineapple juice

DINNER
Broiled salmon, marinated
  in tamari dipping sauce
Kasha
Stewed okra and onion
Glass of red wine

DAY 9

BREAKFAST
Single-egg omelet filled with
  okra and kasha, topped
  with goat cheese
Grapefruit juice
Cinnamon coffee

SNACK
2 plums
Green tea

LUNCH
Millet tabbouleh with
  squares of silken tofu
Iced ginger tea

SNACK
Sliced apples and goat
  Cheddar

DINNER
Artichoke pasta with garlic,
  fresh spinach, walnuts,
  feta cheese, and black
  olives
Braised carrots, garlic, and
  ginger
Spelt baguette
Glass of red wine

DAY 10

BREAKFAST
Blueberry buckwheat
  muffin
Apricot juice
Vanilla-nut coffee

SNACK
Silken tofu shake with
  pineapple juice

LUNCH
Lentil soup with leeks and
  carrots
Fenugreek tea

SNACK
Rice cakes with soy butter
  and cherry preserves

DINNER
Cornish game hen roasted
  with onions and parsnips
Wild and basmati rice pilaf
Tossed green salad with
  mustard vinaigrette
Fresh figs
Rose hips tea

DAY 11

BREAKFAST
Millet porridge with raisins,
  dates, sunflower seeds,
  and soy milk
Black coffee

SNACK
Carrot sticks with peanut
  butter
Saint John's wort tea

LUNCH
Avocado, goat cheese,
  cucumber, and sprouts on
  sprouted-wheat bread
Pineapple juice

SNACK
2 apricots
Glass of soy milk

DINNER
Grilled, marinated tempeh
Quinoa risotto
Broccoli sautéed with
  walnuts and walnut
  oil–lemon dressing
Glass of red wine
Gingerbread

DAY 12

BREAKFAST
1 slice of sprouted-wheat
  toast with blackberry
  preserves
Coffee with soy milk

SNACK
Yogurt shake with apricot
  juice and peaches

LUNCH
Black bean, barley, and
  corn salad
Guacamole and chips
Lemonade

SNACK
Carrot juice with fresh
  ginger

DINNER
Portobello mushroom
  burgers, topped with
  mozzarella and onions,
  on spelt buns
Tofu fries
Carrot–raisin salad
Glass of red wine
Watermelon slices

DAY 13

BREAKFAST
Oat-flour waffles with
  maple syrup
Cinnamon coffee
Fresh pineapple

SNACK
Walnuts and raisins
Ginseng tea

LUNCH
Escarole soup with grated
  pecorino romano
1 slice of whole-spelt bread
  with melted soy cheese
Glass of water with lemon

SNACK
Carrot–cucumber juice

DINNER
Grilled tuna steak
Grilled zucchini, onions,
  and Portobello
  mushrooms
Brown rice pilaf
Dandelion and watercress
  salad with mustard–lime
  vinaigrette
Glass of red wine

DAY 14

BREAKFAST
Ezekiel French toast with
    maple syrup
Glass of pineapple juice
Coffee

SNACK
½ pink grapefruit
Rose hips tea

LUNCH
Grilled tuna salad sandwich
    on soy bread
Sliced apple
Water with lemon

SNACK
Tamari pumpkin seeds
Iced ginger tea

DINNER
Tofu and black bean stew
Steamed rice
Glazed turnips
Romaine salad with Caesar
    dressing
Herb tea

Everyday Menus for Type B

A Wonderfully Varied Diet

DAY 1	

BREAKFAST
Millet cereal with raisins,
  milk, and maple syrup
½ grapefruit
Ginger tea
 	
SNACK
Glass of kefir
Cherries
 	
LUNCH
Mashed sardines and
  lettuce on Ezekiel bread
Carrot sticks
Mineral water with lemon
	SNACK
	Blueberry spelt muffin
	Banana
	Coffee
	
	DINNER
	Stuffed peppers with spelt
	  berries and goat cheese
	Bean salad with red onion
	  and vinaigrette
	Steamed cauliflower with
	  lemon
	Glass of red wine

DAY 2

BREAKFAST
Fresh figs with goat cheese
2 slices of Ezekiel toast
    with raspberry preserves
Orange sections
Green tea

SNACK
Banana–pineapple yogurt
    drink

LUNCH
Gingered squash soup
Wasa bread with slice of
    cheese

SNACK
Cranberry spelt muffin
2 plums
Rose hips tea

DINNER
Liver with onions
Mashed potatoes with
    butter
Grilled eggplant
Mineral water

DAY 3

BREAKFAST
Single-egg omelet with feta
    cheese and chopped
    parsley
1 slice of Essene toast with
    apple butter
Papaya juice
Green tea

SNACK
Apricot–yogurt drink

LUNCH
Faro pilaf with goat cheese
Cucumber with oil and
    vinegar
Ginseng tea

SNACK
Rice cakes with almond
    butter
Grapes
Ginger tea

DINNER
Braised rabbit with orzo
Braised fennel with garlic
Tossed salad with olive oil
    and balsamic vinegar
Herb tea

DAY 4

BREAKFAST
Oatmeal with raisins, milk,
    and maple syrup
Pineapple juice
Coffee

SNACK
Glass of soy milk
Banana

LUNCH
Cherry–yogurt soup
2 plums
Ginger tea

SNACK
Pear spelt muffin
Green tea

DINNER
Sautéed monkfish
Brown rice pilaf
Sautéed peppers and
    shiitake mushrooms
Glass of white wine

DAY 5

BREAKFAST
Ricotta with sautéed
    bananas
Papaya juice
Coffee

SNACK
Slice of pineapple bread
Mixed berry salad
Green tea

LUNCH
Tuna salad and lettuce on
    Ezekiel bread
Carrot–cucumber juice

SNACK
Walnut cookies
Orange sections
Peppermint tea

DINNER
Venison stew
Braised greens with garlic
Pan-fried sweet potatoes
Glass of red wine

DAY 6

BREAKFAST
1 slice of almond-rice bread
  with plum
  preserves
Poached egg
½ grapefruit
Coffee

SNACK
Papaya–banana yogurt
  drink

LUNCH
Mixed roots soup
Grilled goat cheese
  sandwich

SNACK
Lemon squares
Green tea

DINNER
Broiled halibut with
  lemongrass
Basmati rice
Steamed beets with
  vinaigrette
Tropical salad
Mineral water

DAY 7

BREAKFAST
Oat flour–spelt pancakes
  topped with sautéed
  pears
Grape juice
Coffee

SNACK
Pineapple–yogurt smoothie

LUNCH
Poached fruit over ricotta
Mineral water with lemon

SNACK
Grapes
Green tea

DINNER
Broiled lamb chops with
  mint chutney
Brown rice
Carrots and parsnips with
  garlic, ginger, and
  cilantro
Sage tea

DAY 8

BREAKFAST
Yogurt with mixed plums
1 slice of Ezekiel bread
    with almond butter
Peppermint tea

SNACK
Mango–lime–soy smoothie

LUNCH
Tuna salad on spelt bread
Cole slaw
Carrot–celery juice

SNACK
Mixed fruit salad
Green tea

DINNER
Stuffed shells with pesto
Steamed broccoli with
    lemon
Tossed salad
Glass of wine

DAY 9

BREAKFAST
Single-egg omelet with
    Gruyère
1 slice of Ezekiel bread
    with butter
Pineapple juice
Coffee

SNACK
Yogurt with bananas and
    raisins

LUNCH
Cream of lima bean soup
Tossed salad
Mineral water with lemon

SNACK
Shortbread
Grapes
Green tea

DINNER
Sautéed squid with potatoes
Steamed beet leaves with
    lemon vinaigrette
Poached pears
Glass of white wine

DAY 10

BREAKFAST
Banana oat muffin
Papaya juice
Pineapple chunks
Coffee

SNACK
Cottage cheese and grapes
Peppermint tea

LUNCH
Spinach pasta with sautéed
  mushrooms and
  Parmesan
Tossed salad
Mineral water with lemon

SNACK
Wasa bread with goat
  cheese
Carrot–celery juice

DINNER
Curried lamb with
  vegetables
Basmati rice
Cucumber–yogurt soup
Cardamom tea

DAY 11

BREAKFAST
Single-egg omelet with feta
  and minced parsley
1 slice of rye bread with
  plum preserves
½ grapefruit
Green tea

SNACK
Banana–yogurt smoothie

LUNCH
Soft goat cheese and cherry
  preserves on almond-rice
  bread
Red grapes
Mineral water with lemon

SNACK
Rice pudding
2 plums
Ginger tea

DINNER
Roast turkey breast
Boiled red potatoes
Steamed beet leaves with
  raspberry vinaigrette
Glass of red wine

DAY 12

BREAKFAST
Cream of rice with dried
   cherries and soy-rice milk
Fresh pineapple
Coffee

SNACK
Glass of kefir
Fresh papaya

LUNCH
Almond butter and sliced
   bananas on Ezekiel bread
Grape juice

SNACK
Blueberry oat muffin
Bosc pear
Green tea

DINNER
Broiled lamb chops
Millet pilaf with shiitake
   mushrooms
Braised greens with garlic
Glass of red wine

DAY 13

BREAKFAST
Cottage cheese with fresh
   pineapple and papaya
1 slice of spelt bread with
   grape jelly
Green tea

SNACK
Glass of goat's milk
Banana

LUNCH
Quinoa pasta with sautéed
   mixed peppers and goat
   cheese
Mineral water

SNACK
2 walnut cookies
Green grapes
Coffee

DINNER
Broiled flounder
Steamed Brussels sprouts
   with butter, lemon, and
   parsley
Brown rice
Glass of white wine

DAY 14

BREAKFAST

Oat-spelt pancakes with
sautéed bananas

Orange and grapefruit
sections

Green tea

SNACK

Glass of soy milk

Dried figs and dates

LUNCH

Fish soup

1 slice of spelt baguette

Carrot–raisin salad

SNACK

Rice crackers with goat
cheese

Raspberry leaf tea

DINNER

Ricotta-stuffed shells with
pesto

Braised eggplant, peppers,
shiitake mushrooms, and
garlic

Mesclun salad with oil and
vinegar

Green tea

Everyday Menus for Type AB

The Best of Both Worlds

DAY 1

BREAKFAST
Wild rice pudding
Grapes
Coffee

SNACK
Papaya–kiwi soy shake

LUNCH
Peanut butter, raisins, and
   honey on Ezekiel bread
Cranberry juice

SNACK
Pineapple spelt muffin
Green tea

DINNER
Fried monkfish over pasta
   with parsley
Steamed broccoli with
   lemon
Sliced tomatoes, red onion,
   and lemon vinaigrette

DAY 2

BREAKFAST
Single-egg omelet with
   mozzarella and leftover
   steamed broccoli
Carrot juice
Green tea

SNACK
Apricot lassi

LUNCH
Onion soup with French
   bread and Gruyère
Tossed salad

SNACK
Lemon bread
Cherries
Coffee

DINNER
Grilled curried leg of lamb
Basmati rice
Braised greens
Cucumber salad
Green tea

DAY 3

BREAKFAST
Spelt pancakes with sautéed
   apples
Papaya juice
½ grapefruit
Coffee

SNACK
Pinapple–kiwi yogurt shake

LUNCH
Lentil soup
Tossed salad
Mineral water with lemon

SNACK
Wasa bread with goat
   cheese
Cherries
Green tea

DINNER
Salmon with garlic, ginger,
   and cilantro
Brown rice
Braised celery
Glass of white wine

DAY 4

BREAKFAST
Cottage cheese with fresh
    pineapple and kiwi
1 slice of soy bread with
    cherry preserves
Coffee

SNACK
Blueberry oat muffin
Ginger tea

LUNCH
Turkey soup
Rye bread with sliced goat
    cheese

SNACK
Kefir
Mixed plums

DINNER
Grilled rainbow trout
Mashed sweet potatoes
Grilled eggplant and
    zucchini
Glass of white wine
Grapes

DAY 5

BREAKFAST
Oatmeal with dried
    cranberries, maple syrup,
    and goat milk
Pineapple juice
Coffee

SNACK
Glass of soy milk
Grapes

LUNCH
Tuna salad with
    mayonnaise and alfalfa
    sprouts on rye bread
Carrot and celery sticks
Mineral water with lemon

SNACK
Blueberry spelt muffin
Apple
Green tea

DINNER
Liver with mushrooms
    and onions
Roasted new potatoes with
    herbs
Braised dandelion greens
    with garlic
Glass of wine

DAY 6

BREAKFAST
Single-egg omelet with feta,
tomato, and basil
1 slice of almond-rice bread
with apricot preserves
½ grapefruit
Coffee

SNACK
Yogurt with sliced kiwi
Green tea

LUNCH
Pinto bean chili
Brown rice
Mixed salad

SNACK
1 slice of pineapple bread
Cherries
Ginger tea

DINNER
Poached red snapper
Spinach pasta with
cauliflower and garlic
Sliced tomatoes, cucumbers,
and red onion with
lemon vinaigrette

DAY 7

BREAKFAST
Millet cereal with raisins
and soy milk
½ grapefruit
Coffee

SNACK
Handful of peanuts,
walnuts, and chocolate
chips
Pear

LUNCH
Bean salad with red onion,
goat cheese, and lemon
vinaigrette
Mineral water

SNACK
Baklava
Coffee

DINNER
Rabbit stew with carrots,
potatoes, celery, and
parsnips
Braised spinach with garlic
French bread
Tropical fruit salad

DAY 8

BREAKFAST
Yogurt with honey, walnut,
    and raisins
Grapefruit sections
Green tea

SNACK
Cottage cheese with
    pineapple
Rose hips tea

LUNCH
Sardines with lemon
    squeeze on rye bread
Carrot–celery juice

SNACK
Peanut butter cookies
Peach and apricots

DINNER
Turkey breast with
    pineapple chutney
Wild rice salad with
    walnuts
Boiled, mashed plantains
Glass of white wine

DAY 9

BREAKFAST
2 poached eggs
Fresh figs with goat cheese
1 slice of sprouted-wheat
    toast with grapefruit
    marmalade
Green tea

SNACK
Glass of soy-rice milk
Apple

LUNCH
Stewed fruit on ricotta
Papaya juice

SNACK
Spelt-bread pudding
Coffee

DINNER
Tuna steak with cherry
    tomatoes
Brown basmati rice
Braised turnips
Wilted greens salad with
    goat cheese
Mineral water

DAY 10

BREAKFAST
Citrus salad
Pineapple juice
Ginger tea

SNACK
Date–prune shake

LUNCH
Spelt berry salad with
    cucumber, parsley, and
    feta cheese
Carrot–celery juice

SNACK
Peanut butter on rice
    crackers
Grapes
Coffee

DINNER
Grilled marinated tempeh
Eggplant garlic stew
Steamed quinoa
Halved red and yellow
    cherry tomatoes with
    lemon vinaigrette

DAY 11

BREAKFAST
Spelt-bread pudding
Grapes
Coffee

SNACK
Glass of goat's milk
Cherries and pineapple

LUNCH
Miso soup with tofu
Brown rice
Cucumber salad

SNACK
Peanut butter candy
Green tea

DINNER
Broiled lamb chops
Mashed sweet potatoes
Braised cauliflower with
    garlic

DAY 12

BREAKFAST
Citrus salad
Grapefruit juice
Coffee

SNACK
Yogurt with fresh kiwis
Mineral water

LUNCH
Pinto bean salad with garlic
  dressing
Celery–carrot juice
Rye crackers with sheep
  cheese

SNACK
Pumpkin bread with
  walnuts
Coffee

DINNER
Grouper with peanut crust
Basmati rice
Braised dandelion greens
  with garlic
Glass of white wine
Plum cake

DAY 13

BREAKFAST
Scrambled egg
2 slices of turkey bacon
2 slices of oat toast with
  grapefruit marmalade
Green tea

SNACK
Glass of soy milk
Green grapes

LUNCH
Tuna salad on rye bread
  with alfalfa sprouts
Carrot–celery juice

SNACK
Fruit salad with peanut
  dressing
Ginsing tea

DINNER
Lasagna with Portobello
  mushrooms and pesto
Tossed salad with lemon
  vinaigrette
Spelt baguette
Glass of red wine

DAY 14

BREAKFAST
Oat-spelt pancakes with
   maple syrup
½ grapefruit
Coffee

SNACK
Yogurt with walnuts,
   raisins, and honey drizzle
Ginger tea

LUNCH
Lentil salad with sheep
   cheese
Mineral water

SNACK
Cherry muffin
Green tea

DINNER
Rabbit stew
Braised greens with garlic
Pear cake
Glass of red wine

Blood Types at a Glance

TYPE O: *The Hunter*

strong ▪ *self-reliant* ▪ *leader*

STRENGTHS	WEAKNESSES	MEDICAL RISKS	DIET PROFILE	WEIGHT-LOSS KEY	SUPPLEMENTS	EXERCISE REGIMEN
Hardy digestive tract	Intolerant to new dietary, environ- ment conditions	Blood- clotting disorders	High protein: Meat eaters	Avoid: wheat corn kidney beans	vitamin B vitamin K calcium iodine licorice	Intense physical exercise, such as: *aerobics
Strong immune system	Immune system can be *over*active and attack itself	Inflam- matory diseases— arthritis	meat fish vegetables fruit	navy beans lentils cabbage Brussels sprouts	kelp	*martial arts *contact sports
Natural defenses against infections		Low thyroid production	Limited: grains, beans, legumes	cauliflower mustard greens		*running
System designed for efficient metabolism and preser- vation of nutrients		Ulcers Allergies		Aids: kelp seafood salt liver red meat kale spinach broccoli		

TYPE A: *The Cultivator*

settled ■ *cooperative* ■ *orderly*

STRENGTHS	WEAKNESSES	MEDICAL RISKS	DIET PROFILE	WEIGHT-LOSS KEY	SUPPLEMENTS	EXERCISE REGIMEN
Adapts well to dietary and envi-ronmental changes	Sensitive digestive tract	Heart disease	Vegetarian	Avoid:	vitamin B_{12}	Calming, centering exercises, such as:
		Cancer	vegetables	meat		
			tofu	dairy	folic acid	
	Vulnerable		seafood	kidney beans		
	immune	Anemia	grains	lima beans	vitamin C	*Yoga
Immune	system,		beans	wheat		
system pre-serves and	open to microbial	Liver and gallbladder	legumes		vitamin E	*Tai chi
metabolizes	invasion	disorders	fruit	Aids:		
nutrients				vegetable oil	hawthorn	
more easily				soy foods		
		Type I Diabetes		vegetables	echinacea	
				pineapple		
					quercitin	
					milk thistle	

TYPE B: *The Nomad*

balanced ▪ *flexible* ▪ *creative*

STRENGTHS	WEAKNESSES	MEDICAL RISKS	DIET PROFILE	WEIGHT-LOSS KEY	SUPPLEMENTS	EXERCISE REGIMEN
Strong immune system	No natural weak-nesses, but imbalance causes tendency toward auto-immune breakdowns and rare viruses	Type I diabetes	Balanced omnivore	Avoid: corn lentil peanuts sesame seeds buckwheat wheat	magnesium licorice ginkgo lecithin	Moderate physical, with mental balance— such as:
Versatile adaptation to dietary and envi-ronmental changes		Chronic fatigue syndrome	meat (no chicken) dairy grains beans legumes vegetables fruit			*hiking *cycling *tennis *swimming
Balanced nervous system		Auto-immune disorders— Lou Gehrig's disease, lupus, multiple sclerosis		Aids: greens eggs venison liver licorice tea		

TYPE AB: *The Enigma*

rare ■ *charismatic* ■ *mysterious*

STRENGTHS	WEAKNESSES	MEDICAL RISKS	DIET PROFILE	WEIGHT-LOSS KEY	SUPPLEMENTS	EXERCISE REGIMEN
Designed for modern conditions	Sensitive digestive tract	Heart disease	Mixed diet in modera-tion	Avoid: red meat kidney beans	vitamin C	Calming, centering exercises, such as:
		Cancer		lima beans	hawthorn	
Highly tolerant immune system	Tendency for over-tolerant immune system, allowing microbial invasion	Anemia	meat seafood dairy tofu beans legumes grains vegetables fruit	seeds corn buckwheat	echinacea	*Yoga
					valerian	*Tai chi
Combines benefits of Type A and Type B				Aids: tofu seafood dairy greens kelp pineapple	quercitin	Combined with moderate physical, such as:
	Reacts negatively to A-like and B-like conditions				milk thistle	*hiking *cycling *tennis

Answers to Your Questions

It has been my experience that most people respond with great enthusiasm and curiosity when they learn about the blood type connection. Yet it is far easier to embrace a provocative idea than it is to immerse oneself in the gritty details.

The Blood Type Plan is revolutionary, and as such requires many fundamental adjustments. Some people find it easier than others, depending on how much they're already living according to the needs of their blood type. Most of the questions people ask me have similar themes. I've included the most common ones here. They may help you get a clearer sense of what this diet will mean for you.

Where does my blood type come from?

Blood is universal, yet it is also unique. Like the color of your eyes or hair, your blood type is determined by two sets of genes—the inheritance you receive from your mother and father. It is from those genes commingling that your blood type is selected, at the moment of your conception.

Like genes, some blood types are dominant over others. In the cellular creation of a new human being, Type A and Type B are dominant over Type O. If at conception the embryo is given an A gene from the mother and an O gene from the father, the infant will be Type A, although it will continue to carry the father's O gene unexpressed in its DNA. When the infant grows up and passes these genes to its offspring, half of the genes will be for Type A blood and half will be for Type O blood.

Because A and B genes are equally strong, you are Type AB if you received an A gene from one parent and a B gene from the other.

Finally, because the O gene is recessive to all the others, you are Type O only if you receive an O gene from each parent.

It is possible for two Type A parents to conceive a child who is Type O. This happens when the parents each have one A gene and one O gene and both pass the O gene on to the offspring. In the same way two brown-eyed parents can conceive a blue-eyed offspring if each carries the sleeping recessive gene for blue eyes.

Blood type genetics can sometimes be used to help determine the paternity of a child. There is one catch, however. Blood type can only prove that a man is *not* the father of a child. It cannot be used to prove that a man *is* the child's father (although newer DNA technology can do that). Consider this example, a paternity case: An infant is Type A, the mother is Type O, and the man alleged to be the father is Type B. As both A and B genes are dominant to O, the child's father could not be Type B. Think about it. The child's A gene could not have come from the father, who, because he was Type B, would have either two B genes or a B gene and an O gene. Nor could the A gene come from the mother, because people with Type O blood always carry two O genes. The A gene had to come from someone else. These were the exact circumstances surrounding the famous paternity suit against Charlie Chaplin in 1944. Unfortunately, Chaplin was subjected to a tumultuous trial, because the use of blood type to determine paternity was not yet acceptable in a California court of law. Even though blood type had clearly shown that Chaplin was not the father of the child, the jury still decided in favor of the mother, and he was forced to pay child support.

Do I have to make all of the changes at once for my Blood Type Diet to work?

No. On the contrary, I suggest you start slowly, gradually eliminating the foods that are not good for you, and increasing those that are highly beneficial. Many diet programs urge you to plunge in headfirst and radically change your lifestyle immediately. I think it's more realistic and ultimately more effective if you engage in a learning process. Don't just take my word for it. You have to learn it in your body.

Before you begin your Blood Type Diet, you may know very little about which foods are good or bad for you. You're used to making your choices according to your taste buds, family traditions, and fad diet books. Chances are you are eating some foods that are good for you, but the Blood Type Diet provides you with a powerful tool for making informed choices every time.

Once you know what your optimal eating plan is, you have the freedom to veer from your diet on occasion. Rigidity is the enemy of joy; I certainly am not a proponent of it. The Blood Type Diet is designed to make you feel great, not miserable and deprived. Obviously, there are going to be times when common sense tells you to relax the rules a bit—like when you're eating at a relative's house.

I'm Blood Type A and my husband is Blood Type O. How do we cook and eat together? I don't want to prepare two separate meals.

My wife, Martha, and I have exactly the same situation. Martha is Type O and I am Type A. We find that we can usually share about two-thirds of a meal. The main difference is in the protein source. For example, if we make a stir-fry, Martha might separately prepare some chicken, while I'll add cooked tofu. We have also found that many Type O and Type A foods are beneficial for both of us, so we emphasize those foods. For example, we might have a meal that includes salmon, rice, and broccoli. It has become relatively easy for us because we are quite familiar with the specifics of each other's Blood Type Diet. It will help you to spend some time getting familiar with your spouse's food lists. You can even make a separate list of foods that you can share. You might be surprised at how many there are.

People worry a lot about what they fear will be impossible limitations on the Blood Type Diet. But think about it. There are more than two hundred foods listed for each diet—many of them compatible across the board. Considering that the average person eats only about twenty-five foods, the Blood Type Diets actually offer more, not fewer, options.

My family is Italian, and you know the kinds of foods we like to eat. Being Type A, I don't see how I can still enjoy my favorite Italian foods—especially, no tomato sauce!

We tend to associate ethnic foods with one or two of the most commonly available—like spaghetti with meat balls and tomato sauce. But the Italian diet, like most others, includes a wide variety of different foods. Many southern Italian dishes, usually prepared with olive oil instead of heavy sauces, are wonderful choices for both Type A and Type AB. Instead of a plate of pasta drenched in red sauce, try the more delicate flavors of olive oil and garlic, a complex pesto, or a light white wine sauce. Fresh fruits or flavorful but light Italian ices are preferable to rich pastries.

My seventy-year-old husband has a history of heart problems, and has had bypass surgery. He still has a hard time staying away from the wrong foods. He's Type B and I think the Type B Diet would be perfect for him. But he's very resistant to diets. Is there a good way to introduce the diet without a lot of fuss?

It isn't easy to radically change your diet at age seventy—which is probably why your husband has had so much trouble eating healthily, even after surgery. Rather than nagging, which is usually counterproductive, begin to gradually incorporate the beneficial Type B foods into his diet, while slowly eliminating those that aren't good for Type Bs. It's likely that your husband will develop preferences for the good foods as his digestive tract adjusts to their positive qualities.

Why do you list different portion recommendations according to ancestry?

The portion listings according to ancestry are merely refinements to the diet that you may find helpful. In the same way that men, women, and children have different portion standards, so too do people according to their body size and weight, geography, and cultural food preferences. These suggestions will help you until you are comfortable enough with the diet to naturally eat the appropriate portions.

The portion recommendations also take into account specific problems that people of different ancestries tend to have with food. African-Americans, for example, are often lactose intolerant, and most Asians are unaccustomed to eating dairy foods, so they may have to introduce these foods slowly to avoid negative reactions.

I'm allergic to peanuts, but you say they're a highly beneficial food for my blood type. Are you saying I should eat them? I'm Type A.

No. Type As have plenty of great protein sources without peanuts. These reactions are generated by the immune system, which creates antibodies that resist the food. Chances are, a person with Type A blood would not be allergic to peanuts, which contain friendly, A-like properties. You may, however, be intolerant to peanuts. That means you have digestive distress when you eat them. This could be caused by any number of factors, including an overall poor diet. Maybe you once ate peanuts, along with other problem foods, and blamed the peanuts.

Again, you don't need to include peanuts in your diet, but you may find that you tolerate them quite well once you've adjusted to the Type A Diet.

I'm Type B and my meat choices are very strange to me. It looks as though all I can eat are lamb, mutton, venison, and rabbit— which I NEVER eat. Why no chicken?

The elimination of chicken is the toughest adjustment for most people I've treated who are Type B. Not only is chicken a protein staple of many ethnic groups, but most of us have been conditioned to think that chicken is healthier than beef and other meats. Once again, however, there is no single rule that works for everyone. Chicken contains a lectin in its muscle meat that is very detrimental to Type Bs. On the brighter side, you can eat turkey and a wide variety of seafood.

What does "neutral" mean? Are these foods good for me?

The three categories are designed to focus on the foods that are most and least beneficial to you, according to your blood type reaction to certain lectins. The highly beneficial foods act as a medicine; the foods to avoid act as a poison. The neutral foods simply act as foods. While the neutral foods may not have the special health benefits of some other foods, they're certainly good for you in the sense that they contain many nutrients that your body needs.

Must I eat all of the foods marked "highly beneficial"?

It would be impossible to eat everything on your diet! Think of your Blood Type Diet as a painter's palette from which you may choose colors in different shades and combinations. However, do try to reach the weekly amount of the various food groups if possible. Frequency is probably more important than the individual portion sizes, so if you are Type O and have a very small build, try to have animal protein five to seven times weekly, but cut back on the portions, perhaps using two to three ounces instead of four to five ounces. This ensures that the most valuable nutrients will continue to be delivered into the bloodstream at a constant rate.

Is food combining helpful on the Blood Type Diet?

Some diet plans recommend food combining, which involves eating certain food groups in combination for better digestion. Many of these books are full of bunk and hokum, with a lot of unnecessary rules and regulations. Perhaps the only real food-combining rule is to avoid eating animal proteins, such as meats, with large amounts of starches, such as breads and potatoes. This is important because animal products are digested in the stomach in a high-acid environment, while starches are digested in the intestines in a high-alkaline environment. When these foods are combined, the body alternately nibbles at the protein, then the starch, then back to the protein, then back to the starch; not a very efficient method. By keeping these food groups separated, the stomach can concentrate its full functions on the job at hand. Substitute low-starch, high-fiber vegetable side dishes, such as greens. Protein–starch avoidance doesn't apply to tofu and other vegetable proteins, which are essentially predigested.

What should I do if a food to avoid is the fourth or fifth ingredient in a recipe?

That depends on the severity of your condition, or the degree of your compliance. If you have food allergies, or colitis, you may want to practice complete avoidance. Many high-compliance patients avoid these foods altogether, although I think this might be too extreme. Unless they suffer from a specific allergic condition, it won't hurt most people to occasionally eat a food that is not on their diet.

Will I lose weight on the Blood Type Diet?

When you read your Blood Type Plan, you will find specific recommendations for weight loss. They differ from blood type to blood type. That's because the lectins in various foods have a different effect. For example, for Type O, meat is efficiently digested and metabolized, while for Type A it slows the digestive and metabolic processes.

Your Blood Type Diet is tailor-made to eliminate any imbalances that lead to weight gain. If you follow your Blood Type Diet, your metabolism will adjust to its normal level and you'll burn calories more efficiently; your digestive system will process nutrients properly and reduce water retention. You'll lose weight immediately.

In my practice, I've found that most of my patients who have weight problems also have a history of chronic dieting. One would think that constant dieting would lead to weight loss, but that's not true if the structure of the diet and the foods it includes go against everything that makes sense for your specific body.

In our culture, we tend to promote "one size fits all" weight-loss programs, and then we wonder why they don't work. The answer is obvious! Different blood types respond to food in different ways. In conjunction with the recommended exercise program, you should see results very quickly.

Do calories matter on the Blood Type Diet?

As with most general diet issues, concerns about calories are automatically taken care of by following your specific Blood Type Diet. Most new patients who follow the guidelines concerning diet and exercise lose some weight. Some people even complain that they are losing too much weight. There is an adjustment period on this diet, and over time you'll be able to find the food amounts that suit your needs. However, the charts in each food category give you a place to start.

It's important to be aware of portion sizes. No matter what you eat, if you eat too much of it you'll gain weight. This probably seems so obvious that it doesn't even bear mentioning. But overeating has become one of America's most difficult and dangerous health problems. Millions of Americans are bloated and dyspeptic because of the amounts of food they eat. When you eat excessively, the walls of your stomach stretch like an inflated balloon. Although stomach muscles are elastic and were created to contract and expand, when they are grossly enlarged, the cells of the abdominal walls undergo a tremendous strain. If you are eating until you feel full, and you normally feel sluggish after a meal, try to reduce your portion sizes. Learn to listen to what your body is telling you.

I have heart problems and I've been told to totally avoid any fat and cholesterol. I'm Type O. How can I eat meat?

First, realize that it is grains, not meats, that are the cardiovascular culprits for Type O. This is especially interesting because almost everybody who has or is attempting to prevent heart disease is advised to go on a diet based largely on complex carbohydrates!

For Type Os, a high intake of certain carbohydrates, usually wheat breads, increases the insulin levels. In response, your body stores more fat in the tissues, and fat levels are elevated in the blood.

Also bear in mind that your blood cholesterol level is only moderately controlled by the dietary intake of foods that are high in cholesterol content. Approximately 85 to 90 percent is actually controlled by the manufacture and metabolism of cholesterol in your liver.

I'm Type O and don't want to eat much fat in my diet. What do you suggest?

A high-protein diet does not automatically mean one that is high in fat, especially if you avoid heavily marbleized meats. Although more expensive, try to find free-range meats that have been raised without the excessive use of antibiotics and other chemicals. Our ancestors consumed rather lean game or domestic animals that grazed on alfalfa and other grasses; today's high-fat meats are produced by using high amounts of corn feed.

If you can't afford or can't find free-range meats, choose the leanest cuts available and remove all excess fat before cooking. Type Os also have many other good protein choices that are naturally lower in fat—such as chicken and seafood. The fat in the oil-rich fish is composed of omega-3 fatty acids, which seem to promote lower cholesterol and healthier hearts.

How can I be sure to buy the most natural and the freshest foods?

Within the last few years, many consumers have banded together to create food co-ops, groups of people who buy in bulk. Very often this bulk purchasing power results in great savings and high-quality produce. Most food co-ops require a small membership fee and a few hours of work at the co-op per month. Savings, especially on items such as grains, spices, beans, vegetables, and oils, can be substantial.

Health-food stores can be a valuable place to buy fresh foods, but don't fall into the trap of thinking that because you are in a health-food store you can relax your guard. Many health-food stores, especially the smaller ones, do not have the rapid turnover of a busy greengrocer or supermarket, and their foods might not be so fresh.

Are organic foods more healthy than nonorganic foods?

A good rule of thumb is to use organic vegetables if they are not exorbitantly priced. They do taste better and are more healthy. However, if you are on a fixed income and cannot find competitively priced organic produce, high-quality, properly cleaned, fresh nonorganic produce will do just fine.

More and more supermarkets seem to be stocking organic produce, mostly from California, a state with specific laws concerning the use of the term organic. Interestingly, in one supermarket in my neighborhood, organic vegetables and fruits are displayed next to the nonorganic versions, and are priced identically! I suspect that market pressures will continue to push more and more vegetable and fruit growers toward the organic way, if for no other reason than the cost of commercial fertilizers, made from petrochemicals, will eventually make them more expensive to produce than naturally grown products.

Will eating canned food hurt my diet?

Commercially canned foods, subject to high heat and pressure, lose most of their vitamin content, especially the antioxidants, such as vitamin C. They do retain the vitamins that are not heat sensitive, such as vitamin A. Canned foods typically are lower in fiber than their fresh counterparts and higher in salt, usually added to offset the loss of flavors in production. Soggy, with little of the "life" we find in fresh foods and vegetables, and few natural enzymes (which are destroyed by the canning process), canned foods should be used sparingly, if at all. You pay much more per weight for canned food, and don't get back much in return.

Other than fresh, frozen foods are your best second bet. Freezing does not change the nutritional content of the food very much (its preparation before freezing may), although the taste and texture are often blunted.

Why is stir-frying so beneficial?

The quick frying of Asian-style cooking is healthier than deep frying. Less oil is used, and the oil itself, typically sesame oil, is more resistant to high temperatures than safflower or canola oils. The idea behind stir-frying is to quickly braise the food on its outside, which has the added effect of sealing in flavors.

Most types of meals can be prepared in this manner using a wok. The deep, cone-shaped design of the wok concentrates the heat at a small area at its base, which allows food to be cooked there and then moved to the cooler edges of the pan. Wok cooking usually mixes vegetables and seafoods or meats. Cook the meats and vegetables that require longer heating first, then move them to the outside of the pan, adding the vegetables that require less cooking to the center.

Steaming vegetables is also a quick and effective method of cooking, and helps to keep the nutrients in the food. Use a simple steamer basket, purchased at any hardware or department store, fitted inside a large pot filled with water to the level of the basket bottom. Add vegetables, cover, and heat. Don't cook until soggy! Crisp means better taste, better texture, and better nutrition.

Should I take a multivitamin every day on the Blood Type Diet?

If you are in good health and are following your Blood Type Diet, you shouldn't really need a supplement, although there are exceptions. Pregnant women should supplement their diet with iron, calcium, and folic acid. Most women also need extra calcium—especially if their diet doesn't include many dairy foods.

Those engaged in heavy physical activity, people in stressful occupations, the elderly, those who are ill, heavy smokers—all should be on a supplementation program. More specific details are available in your individual Blood Type Plan.

How important are herbs and herbal teas?

That depends on your blood type. Type Os respond well to soothing herbs, Type As to the more stimulating ones, and Type Bs do quite nicely without most of them. Type ABs should follow the herbal protocols laid down for Type As, with the added proviso that Type ABs shun those herbs that both Type As and Type Bs are asked to avoid.

Why are vegetable oils so limited on the Blood Type Diet? I thought all vegetable oils were good for you.

What you've probably heard is advertisers hawking the news that vegetable oils have "No Cholesterol!" Well, that's not news to anyone with even a modicum of knowledge about nutrition. Plants and vegetables do not manufacture cholesterol, which is found only in products derived from animals. Your cholesterol-free oil may have little else to recommend it.

Here are the facts. Always avoid tropical oils, such as coconut oil, as they are high in saturated fat, which can be harmful to the cardiovascular system. Most oils sold today, including safflower and canola (rapeseed), are polyunsaturated, which makes them an improvement over lard and tropical oils. However, there is some concern that overconsumption of polyunsaturated fats may be linked to certain types of cancer, especially if they're subjected to the high temperatures of cooking. In general, I prefer to use olive oil as much as possible in cooking. I believe that olive oil has proven to be the most tolerated and beneficial of fats. As a monounsaturated oil it seems to have positive effects on the heart and arteries. There are many different blends of olive oil available. The finest quality is the extra-virgin grade. It is slightly greenish in color and almost odorless—although when gently heated, the perfume of the olives is sensational. Olive oil is usually cold-pressed rather than extracted using heat or chemicals. The less processed an oil is, the better its quality.

Tofu seems like a very unappealing food. Must I eat it if I'm Type A?

Many Type A and Type AB people raise their eyebrows and grimace with disgust when I recommend that they make tofu a staple of their diets. Well, tofu is not a glamour food. I admit it. When I was an impoverished Type A college student, I ate tofu with vegetables and brown rice almost every day for years. It was cheap, but I actually liked it.

I think the real problem with tofu is the way it is usually displayed in the markets. Tofu—in soft or hard cakes—sits with its other tofu friends in a large plastic tub, immersed in cold water. When people manage to overcome their initial aversion and actually purchase one or two tofu cakes (calling them cakes has a rather bitter irony), many people take it home, pop it on a plate, and break off a hunk to give it a try. This is a bad way to experience tofu! It might be comparable to tossing a whole raw egg into your mouth and chewing . . . not a very pleasant experience.

If you are going to use tofu, it is best cooked and combined with vegetables and strong flavors that you enjoy, such as garlic, ginger, and soy sauce.

Tofu is a nutritionally complete meal that is filling and extremely inexpensive. Type As take note: The path to your good health is paved with bean curd!

I've never heard of many of the grains you mention. Where do I find out more?

If you're looking for alternative grains, health food stores are a bonanza. In recent years, many ancient grains, largely forgotten, have been rediscovered and are now being produced. Examples of these are amaranth, a grain from Mexico, and spelt, a variation of wheat that seems to be free of the problems found with whole wheat. Try them! They're not bad. Spelt flour makes a hearty, chewy bread that is quite flavorful, while several interesting breakfast cereals are now being made with amaranth. Another alternative is to use sprouted-wheat breads, sometimes referred to as Ezekiel or Essene bread, as the gluten lectins found principally in the seed coat are destroyed by the sprouting process. These breads spoil rapidly and are usually found in the refrigerator cases of health-food stores. They are a live food, with many beneficial enzymes still intact. Beware of commercially produced sprouted-wheat breads, as they usually have a minority of sprouted wheat and a majority of whole wheat in their formulas. Sprouted bread is somewhat sweet tasting, as the sprouting process also releases sugars, and it is moist and chewy. This bread makes wonderful toast.

I'm Type A and I've been a runner for many years. Running seems to be a great way to reduce stress. I'm confused about your advice that I shouldn't exercise heavily.

There is a great deal of evidence that your blood type informs your unique reaction to stress, and that Type As tend to do better with less intense exercise. My father has observed this thousands of times in his thirty-five years studying the connection. However, there is much we don't yet know, so I would hesitate to say absolutely that you shouldn't run.

I would ask you to reevaluate your health and energy levels. I often have patients who say things like, "I've always been a runner," or "I've always eaten chicken," as if that were all the proof they needed that an activity or a food was beneficial. Often, these very people are suffering from an assortment of physical problems and stresses that they've never thought to associate with specific activities or foods. You may be a Type A with a twist—one who thrives on intense physical activity. Or you may discover that you're running on empty.

Terms You Should Know

ABO BLOOD GROUP SYSTEM: THE MOST IMPORTANT OF THE blood-typing systems, the ABO blood group is the determinant for transfusion reactions and organ transplantation. Unlike the other blood-typing systems, the ABO blood types have far-ranging significance other than transfusion or transplantation, including the determination of many of the digestive and immunological characteristics of the body. The ABO blood group is comprised of four blood types: O, A, B, and AB. Type O has no true antigen, but carries antibodies to both A and B blood. Type A and Type B carry the antigen named for their blood type and make antibodies to each other. Type AB does not manufacture any antibodies to other blood types because it has both A and B antigens.

Anthropologists use the ABO blood types extensively as a guide to the development of early peoples. Many diseases, especially digestive disorders, cancer, and infection, express preferences, choosing between the ABO blood types. These expressions are not generally understood or appreciated by either physicians or the general population.

Agglutinate: Derived from the Latin word "to glue." The process by which cells are made to adhere to one another, usually through the actions of an agglutinin, such as an antibody or a lectin. Certain viruses and bacteria also are capable of agglutinating blood cells. Many agglutinins, particularly the food lectins, are blood type specific. Certain foods clump only the cells of one blood type, but do not react with the cells of another type.

Anthropology: The study of the human race in relation to distribution, origin, and classification. Anthropologists study physical characteristics, the relationship of races, environmental and social relations, and culture. The ABO blood types are extensively used by anthropologists in the study of early human populations.

Antibody: A class of chemicals, called the immunoglobulins, made by the cells of the immune system to specifically tag or identify foreign material within the body of the host. Antibodies combine with specific markers—antigens—found on viruses, bacteria, or other toxins, and agglutinate them. The immune system is capable of manufacturing millions of different antibodies against a wide variety of potential invaders. Individuals of Type O, Type A, or Type B blood carry antibodies to other blood types. Type AB, the universal recipient, manufactures no antibodies to other types.

Antigen: Any chemical that generates an antibody by the immune system in response to it. The chemical markers that determine blood type are considered blood type antigens because other blood types may carry antibodies to them. Antigens are commonly found on the surface of germs, and are used by the immune system to detect foreign material. Specialized antigens are often made by cancer cells, these being called tumor antigens. Many germs and cancer antigens are clever impersonators that can mimic the blood type of the host in an effort to escape detection.

Antioxidant: Vitamins that are believed to strengthen the immune system and prevent cancer by fighting off toxic compounds (called free radicals) that attack cells. Vitamins C, E, and beta-carotene are believed to be the most powerful antioxidants.

Cro-Magnon: The first truly modern human. Originating around 70,000 to 40,000 B.C., Cro-Magnon migrated extensively from Africa into Europe and Asia. A master hunter, Cro-Magnon led a largely hunter-gatherer existence. Most of the digestive characteristics of people with Type O blood are derived from Cro-Magnon.

Differentiation: The cellular process by which cells develop their specialized characteristics and functions. Differentiation is controlled by the genetic machinery of the cell. Cancer cells, which often have defective genes, usually de-evolve, and lose many of the characteristics of a normal cell, often reverting to earlier embryologic forms long repressed since early development.

Gene: A component of the cell that controls the transmission of hereditary characteristics by specifying the construction of a particular protein or enzyme. Genes are composed of long chains of deoxyribonucleic acid (DNA) contained in the chromosomes of the cell nucleus.

Indo-European: An early Caucasian people who migrated westward to Europe from their early homelands in Asia and the Middle East around 7000 to 3500 B.C. The Indo-Europeans were probably the progenitors for Type A blood in western Europe.

Ketosis: A state that is achieved with a high-protein, low-carbohydrate diet. The high-protein diets of our early Type O ancestors forced the burning of fat for energy and the production of ketones—a sign of rapid metabolic activity. The state of ketosis allowed early humans to maintain high energy, metabolic efficiency, and physical strength—all qualities needed for hunting game.

Lectin: Any compound, usually a protein, found in nature, that can interact with surface antigens found on the body's cells, causing them to agglutinate. Lectins are often found in common foods, and many of them are blood type specific. Because cancer cells often manufacture copious amounts of antigens on their surface, many lectins will agglutinate them in preference to normal cells.

Mucus: Secretions manufactured by specialized tissues, called mucous membranes, that are used to lubricate and protect the delicate internal linings of the body. Mucus contains antibodies to protect against germs. In secretors, large amounts of blood type antigens are secreted in mucus, which serves to filter out bacteria, fungi, and parasites with opposing blood type characteristics.

Naturopathic doctor (N.D.): A physician trained in natural healing methods. Naturopathic doctors receive four-year postgraduate training at an accredited college or university, and function as primary-care providers.

Neolithic: The period of early human development characterized by the development of agriculture and the use of pottery and polished tools. The radical change in human lifestyle, from the previous hunter-gatherer existence, probably was a major stimulus to the development of Blood Type A.

Panhemaglutinans: Lectins that agglutinate all blood types. An example is the tomato lectin.

Phytochemical: Any natural product with specific health applications. Most phytochemicals are traditional herbs and plants.

Polymorphism: Literally means "many shapes." A polymorphism is any physical manifestation between a species of living organisms that is variable through genetic influence. The blood types are a well-known polymorphism.

Triglycerides: The body's fat stores, also contained in the bloodstream. High tryglycerides—or high blood fats—are considered a risk for heart disease.

The Blood Sub-Groups

MORE THAN 90 PERCENT OF ALL FACTORS ASSOCIATED WITH BLOOD type are related to your major ABO type. There are, however, many minor blood subtypes, most of them playing insignificant roles. Of all the subtypes, only three will have any impact on your profile or affect your health and diet. I mention them only because they occasionally pop up as a useful refinement in your health plan. But let me stress: Knowing whether you are Type O, Type A, Type B, or Type AB is the only blood type information you really need.

The three subtypes that play minor roles are:

- Secretor/nonsecretor status
- RH Positive (RH+) and RH Negative (RH–)
- The MN blood group system

Secretors and Nonsecretors

Although everyone carries a blood type antigen on their blood cells, some people also have blood type antigens that float around freely in their body secretions. These people are called secretors, because they secrete their blood type antigens into their saliva, mucous, sperm, and other body fluids. In addition to their blood, it's possible to learn the blood type of a secretor from these other fluids. Secretors comprise about 80 percent of the population, nonsecretors, 20 percent.

Secretor status has important implications in law enforcement. A semen sample taken from a rape victim can be used to help convict the rapist if he is a secretor and his blood type matches the blood type identified in the semen. However, if he is in the small population of nonsecretors, his blood type cannot be identified from any fluids except the blood.

People who do not secrete their blood type antigens in other fluids besides blood are called nonsecretors. Being a secretor or a nonsecretor is independent of your ABO blood type; it is controlled by a different gene. Thus one person could be a Type A secretor, and another a Type A nonsecretor.

Because secretors have more places to put their blood type antigens, they have more blood type expression in their bodies than nonsecretors. Finding out whether or not you are a secretor is as easy as finding out your ABO blood type. The most common way to determine secretor status involves testing saliva for the presence of blood type activity. It is not a common test, although there are several laboratories (listed in the back of the book) that will perform it for a small fee. I suggest that until you find out your secretor status for certain, play the numerical odds and assume you are a secretor.

If you are tested for secretor status, something called the Lewis System will probably be used. It's a quick and dirty way to identify secretors and nonsecretors, and I mention it here only so you can recognize it if you see it on a blood type report.

In the Lewis System there are two possible antigens that can be produced, called Lewis "a" and Lewis "b" (not to be confused with the A and B of the ABO system) and their interplay determines your secretor status. LEWIS a+ b– equals non-secretor. LEWIS a– b+ equals secretor.

Positive or Negative

When we blood-type patients in my office, they almost immediately ask if they are negative or positive. Many people don't realize that this is an additional separate blood grouping called the Rhesus or Rh system, and it really has nothing to do with your ABO blood type— although it does have one important ramification for pregnant women.

The Rh system is named for the Rhesus monkey, a commonly used laboratory animal, in whose blood it was first discovered. For many years it remained a mystery to doctors why some women who had normal first pregnancies developed complications in their second and subsequent pregnancies, often resulting in miscarriage and even the death of the mother. In 1940, it was discovered (again by the amazing Dr. Landsteiner) that these women were carrying a different blood type than their babies, who took their blood type from the father. The babies were Rh+, meaning that they carried the Rh antigen on their blood cells. Their mothers were Rh–, which meant that this antigen was missing from their blood. Unlike the ABO system where the antibodies to other blood types develop from birth, Rh– people do not make an antibody to the Rh antigen unless they are first sensitized. This sensitization usually occurs when blood is exchanged between the mother and infant during birth, so the mother's immune system does not have enough time to react to the first baby. However, should a subsequent conception result in another Rh+ baby, the mother, now sensitized, will produce antibodies to the baby's blood type. Reactions to the Rh factor can only occur in Rh– women who conceive the children of Rh+ fathers. Rh+ women, 85 percent of the population, have nothing to worry about. Even though the Rh system doesn't figure prominently when it comes to diets or diseases, it is certainly a factor for childbearing women who are Rh–.

IF YOU HAVE	BUT DO NOT HAVE	YOU ARE
The Rh antigen	The anti-Rh antibody	Rh+
The anti-Rh antibody	The Rh antigen	Rh–

The MN Blood Group System

The MN Blood Group System is virtually unknown because it is not a major factor in transfusions or organ transplants, and is of little interest in the day-to-day practice of medicine. This is deceiving, however, because a variety of diseases are associated with them—if only in a minor way.

In this system, a person can type out as MM, NN or MN, depending upon whether their cells have only the M antigen (which would make them MM), the N antigen (NN), or both (MN). This system will pop up occasionally in our discussions, especially when we talk about cancer and heart disease. Around 28 percent of the population is typed as MM, 22 percent as NN, and 50 percent as MN.

IF YOU HAVE	BUT DO NOT HAVE	YOU ARE
The M antigen	The N antigen	Type MM
The N antigen	The M antigen	Type NN
The M and N antigens		Type MN

Your Blood Type Pedigree

These three subtype systems are often used in my office, and they are often a part of various lab panels in use by other doctors. Although you can find almost all of the information you will ever need by simply knowing your ABO type, these systems offer a further refinement that allows a much deeper understanding of your blood's characteristics.

This results in what I call the blood type pedigree, a string of letters that is a patient's profile. In many ways, it is as specific as a fingerprint. One look at the pedigree points me in the proper direction and guides me in devising a diet and disease prevention strategies. An example of one person's pedigree is:

BLOOD TYPE	SECRETOR STATUS	NEG/POS	MN
O	Lewis a+ b– (non-secretor)	Rh–	MM

Another is:

BLOOD TYPE	SECRETOR STATUS	NEG/POS	MN
A	Lewis a– b+ (secretor)	Rh+	MM

The Anthropology
of Blood Type

ANTHROPOLOGY IS THE STUDY OF HUMAN DIFFERENCES, CUL-
TURAL and biological. Most anthropologists divide the field into two
categories: cultural anthropology, which looks at the manifestations
of culture, such as language or ritual; and physical anthropology,
the study of the evolutionary biology of our species, *Homo sapiens*.
Physical anthropologists attempt to trace human historical development through hard scientific methods, such as the blood types. A
central task in physical anthropology has been to document the
sequence of how the human line evolved from early primate ancestors. The use of blood types to study early societies has been termed
paleoserology, the study of ancient blood.

Physical anthropology is also concerned with how humans adapted
to environmental pressures. Traditional physical anthropology relied
heavily on the measuring of skull shape, stature, and other physical
characteristics. Blood type became a powerful tool for this type of
analysis. In the 1950s, as emphasis shifted to genetic characteristics,
interest shifted to the blood types and other markers that have known
genetic bases. A. E. Mourant, a physician and anthropologist, has
published two key works, *Blood Groups and Disease* (1978), and
Blood Relations: Blood Groups and Anthropology (1985), which have
collected much of the available material on the subject.

In addition to Mourant, I've used a variety of other source material for this appendix, including earlier anthropology sources such as
William Boyd's *Genetics and the Races of Man* (1950), and a series
of studies that were published in various journals of forensic medicine from 1920 to 1945.

It is possible to map the occurrence of the various blood groups in ancient populations by blood typing grave exhumations. Small amounts of blood type materials can be reconstituted from the remains, and the blood type determined. By studying the blood types of human populations, anthropologists gain information about that population's local history, movement, intermarriage, and diversification.

Many national and ethnic groups have unique blood type distributions. In certain more isolated cultures, a clear majority of one blood type over another can still be seen. In other societies, the distribution may be more even. In the United States, for example, the equal rates of Type O and Type A blood reflect masses of immigration. The United States also has a higher percentage of Type B than the western European countries, which probably reflects the influx of more eastern nationalities.

For the purpose of this analysis, we can divide humankind into two basic races—Ethiopian and Palearctic. The Palearctic can be further broken down to Mongolians and Caucasians, although most people lie somewhere in between. Each race is physically characterized by its environment and occupies distinct geographic areas. Ethiopians, probably the oldest race, are dark-skinned Africans, inhabiting the southern third of Arabia and sub-Saharan Africa. The Palearctic region comprises Africa north of the Sahara, then Europe, most of Asia (with the exception of southern Arabia), India, Southeast Asia, and southern China.

The roughest guesswork places the beginnings of human migration from Africa to Asia at about 1 million years ago. In Asia, most likely, modern *Homo sapiens* species split from a trunk of the ancestral Ethiopians into the Caucasians and Mongolians, but we know almost nothing about when or why it occurred.

Each of the basic races has its own homeland—a geographic area where it is preeminent. The Ethiopian homeland was Africa; the Caucasian, Europe and northern Asia; and the Mongolian, central and southern Asia.

As human groups migrated and interbred, intermediate populations evolved in the creases and crevices between these ancestral homelands. The area bound by the Sahara, the Middle East, and Somalia, for example, was home to a blending of the African and Caucasian races; the Indian subcontinent, a blend of the more northerly Caucasians and the more southerly Mongolians. These groups, which then split into innumerable, often temporary populations, were subject to the pressures of disease, food sources, and climate. They may have existed for thousands of years in the spaces between the homelands. Although the result of migration was to spread Type O blood far and wide around the world, it was from these spaces that the later blood types emerged.

There may be more physical differences between Africans and the other races, but the blood type differences between Caucasians and Mongolians are more clear cut—a good reason to reexamine racial stereotypes.

It would also be a mistake to think of the early Type O people as primitives. More intellectual development occurred in the Cro-Magnon age than in any time before or after. The Cro-Magnons created our early societies and rituals, more than the rudiments of communication, and the original wanderlust. Although we trace the genetic heritage of Type O blood back to early prehistory, it still remains a very workable chemistry, largely because of its simplicity and the fact that animal protein diets still account for a great portion of the world's current food intake.

The first attempt at using blood type to describe racial and nationality characteristics was undertaken by a husband-and-wife team of physicians, the Hirszfelds, in 1918. During the First World War both had served as doctors in the Allied armies that had concentrated in the area of Salonika, Greece.

Working with a multinational force, and with large amounts of refugees of different ethnic backgrounds, the Hirszfelds systematically blood-typed large numbers of people while also recording their race and nationality. Each group contained over five hundred or more subjects.

They found, for example, that the rate of Blood Type B ranged from a low of 7.2 percent of the population of English subjects, to a high of 41.2 percent in Indians, and that western Europeans in general had a lower incidence of Type B than Balkan Slavs, who had a lower incidence than Russians, Turks, and Jews; who again had a lower occurrence than Vietnamese and Indians. The distribution of Blood Type AB essentially followed the same pattern, with a low of 3 to 5 percent in western Europeans, and a high of 8.5 percent in Indians.

In subcontinental India, Type ABs makes up 8.5 percent of the population—remarkably high for a blood type that averages between 2 and 5 percent worldwide. This prevalence of Type AB is probably due to subcontinental India's location as an invasion route between the conquered lands to the west and the Mongolian homelands to the east.

Blood Type O and Type A were essentially the reverse of Type B and Type AB. The percentage of Type A remained fairly consistent (40 percent) among Europeans, Balkan Slavs, and Arabs, while being quite low in west Africans, Vietnamese, and Indians. Forty-six percent of the English population tested were Type O, which accounted for only 31.3 percent of the Indians tested.

Modern analysis (largely the result of records kept by blood banks), encompasses the blood types of more than 20 million individuals from around the world. Yet these large numbers can do no more than confirm the original observations of the Hirszfelds. No scientific journals saw fit to publish their material at that time. For a while, the Hirszfelds' study languished in an obscure anthropology journal; for more than thirty years this fascinating and important work was overlooked.

Apparently, there was little interest in using this knowledge of the blood types as an anthropological probe into the history of humanity.

Racial Classifications Based on Blood Type

In the 1920s several anthropologists first attempted racial classification based on blood groups. In 1929 Laurance Snyder published a book called *Blood Grouping in Relationship to Clinical and Legal Medicine*. In it, Snyder proposed a comprehensive classification system based on blood type. It is especially interesting because it focuses largely on the distribution of the ABO groups, the only tool to be had at the time.

The racial classifications—as Snyder saw them—were:

THE EUROPEAN TYPE: High frequency of Blood Type A, low frequency of Type B, perhaps the result of Type A blood originating in western Europe. This category included English, Scots, French, Belgians, Italians, and Germans.

INTERMEDIATE TYPE: A sort of blend between western (high Type A) and central (high Type B) European populations. Higher incidence of Blood Type O overall. This category included the Finns, Arabs, Russians, Spanish Jews, Armenians, and Lithuanians.

HUNAN TYPE: Oriental groups with a high incidence of Blood Type A, possibly the result of an infusion of Caucasian elements, including the Ukrainians, Poles, Hungarians, Japanese, Romanian Jews, Koreans, and southern Chinese.

INDOMANCHURIAN TYPE: Contain population groups with a high incidence of Blood Type B over Type A. This type includes the subcontinental Indians, Gypsies, Northern Chinese, and Manchus.

AFRICO-MALAYSIAN TYPE: Moderately higher incidence of Type A and Type B overall, with normal incidence of Type O. This category includes Javanese, Sumatrans, Africans, and Moroccans.

PACIFIC-AMERICAN TYPE: Including Filipinos, North and South American Indians, and Eskimos. Extremely high incidence of Type O and Rh+ blood types, very small incidence of Type A, and almost absent incidence of Type B.

AUSTRALASIAN TYPE: Principally the Australian Aborigines, this classification shows high incidence of Type A (almost equivalent to western Europe), almost no Type B, and a high incidence of Type O, although not so high as found with the Pacific-American type.

Because he could only rely on ABO blood types, Snyder's classifications made for some strange pairings, such as the Hunan type containing both Koreans and Romanian Jews. Later, researchers began using the Rh and MN blood types, in addition to the ABO in their classifications, trying to refine these categories. They were aware that racial classification based merely on ABO groups would, in many cases, give results that would not coincide with older ideas about race, so they also incorporated MN types and occasional other blood factors to distinguish populations not clearly differentiated by ABO.

One classification, based on these newer criteria, distinguished the following races:

Europeans (Nordics and Alpines of Europe/Near East)
Mediterranean
Mongolian (Central Asia and Eurasia)
African
Indonesian
American Indian
Oceanic (including Japanese)
Australian

Another racial classification, based largely on ABO and Rh factors:

CAUCASIAN GROUP: Highest incidence of Rh–, relatively high Type A, moderately high incidence of all other blood types.

NEGROID GROUP: Highest incidence of rare Rh types, moderate frequency of Rh–, high relative incidence of Blood Type A2, and the rare intermediates of Type A—Ax and A Bantu.

MONGOLIAN GROUP: Virtual absence of blood types Rh– and Type A2. Using MN data further classified the Mongolian group into the Asiatic group, Pacific Island and Australian group, American Indian and Eskimo group.

William Boyd, in his 1950 book *Genetics and the Races of Man*, proposed a more accurate classification based on this earlier classification:

EARLY EUROPEAN GROUP: Possessing the highest incidence (over 30 percent) of the Rh–, and probably no Type B. A relatively high incidence of Blood Type O. The gene for subtype N possibly somewhat higher than in present-day Europeans. Represented today by their modern descendants, the Basques.

EUROPEAN (CAUCASOID) GROUP: Possessing the next-highest incidence of the Rh− gene and a relatively high incidence of Blood Type A2, with moderate frequencies of other blood group genes. Normal frequencies of the gene for subtype M.

AFRICAN (NEGROID) GROUP: Possessing a tremendously high incidence of a rare Rh+ blood type gene, Rh0, and a moderate frequency of Rh−; relatively high incidence of Type A2 and the rare intermediate types of A, and a rather high incidence of Blood Type B.

ASIATIC (MONGOLIAN) GROUP: Possessing high frequencies of Blood Type B, but little if any of the genes for Blood Type A2 and Rh−.

AMERICAN INDIAN GROUP: Possessing little or no Type A, and probably no Type B or Rh−. Very high rates of Blood Type O.

AUSTRALOID GROUP: Possessing high incidence of Blood Type Al, but not Type A2, or Rh−. High incidence of gene for N subtype.

Boyd's classification made more sense than the earlier classification systems, because it also fit the geographic distributions of the individual races more accurately.

Recent work by Dr. Luigi Cavalli-Sforza at Stanford University has tracked the genetic drift of the ancient human migrations, using even more sophisticated methods based on the new DNA technology. Many of his findings have confirmed the earlier observations of Mourant, the Hirszfelds, Snyder, and Boyd concerning the distribution of blood types worldwide.

Where to Learn More

RATHER THAN FILL THIS BOOK WITH ENDLESS FOOTNOTES, I'VE collected the most important influences on it and listed them here where they might be most easily referred to. They are grouped into several categories and listed alphabetically by author.

Blood types, general information

American Association of Blood Banks. *Technical Manual*, 10th ed. 1990.

D'Adamo, P. "Gut ecosystems III: The ABO and other polymorphic systems." *Townsend Ltr. for Doctors*, Aug. 1990.

Marcus, D. M. "The ABO and Lewis blood-group system." *New England J. Med.*, 280 (1969): 994–1005.

Diet and lifestyle

Atkins, R., and Herwood, R. W. *Dr. Atkins's Diet Revolution*. New York: Bantam, 1972.

D'Adamo, J. *The D'Adamo Diet*. Montreal: McGraw-Hill Ryerson, 1989.

———. *One Man's Food*. New York: Marek, 1980. (out of print).

Kushi, M., and Jack, A. *The Cancer Prevention Diet*. New York: St. Martin's, 1983.

Nomi, T., and Besher, A. *You Are Your Blood Type*. New York: Pocket, 1983.

Pritikin, N., and McGrady, P. *The Pritikin Program for Diet and Exercise*. New York: Grosset & Dunlap, 1979.

Schmid, R. *Traditional Foods Are Your Best Medicine*. New York: Ballantine, 1987.

Blood types and anthropology

Boyd, W. C. *Genetics and the Races of Man: An Introduction to Modern Physical Anthropology.* Boston: Little, Brown, 1950.

Brues, A. M. "Tests of blood group selection." *Amer. J. Forensic Medicine,* 1929: 287–289.

Childe, V. G. *Man Makes Himself.* London: Watts, 1936.

Coon, C. S. *The Races of Europe.* New York: Macmillan, 1939.

Gates, R. R. *Human Ancestry.* Cambridge, MA: Harvard University Press, 1948.

Hirszfeld, L., and Hirszfeld, H. *Lancet,* 2 (1919): 675.

Livingstone, F. R. "Natural selection disease and ongoing human evolution as illustrated by the ABO groups." Source unknown (copy in author's possession).

McNeil, W. H. *Plagues and Peoples.* New York: Doubleday/Anchor, 1975.

Mourant, A. E. *Blood Relations: Blood Groups and Anthropology.* Oxford, England: Oxford University Press, 1983.

Mourant, A. E., Kopec, A. C., and Domaniewska-Sobczak, K. *Blood Groups and Disease,* 4th ed. Oxford, England: Oxford University Press, 1984.

Muschel, L. "Blood groups, disease and selection." *Bacteriological Rev.,* 30, 2 (1966): 427–441.

Race, R. R., and Sanger, R. *Blood Groups in Man.* Oxford, England: Blackwell Scientific, 1975.

Sheppard, P. M. "Blood groups and natural selection." *Brit. Med. Bull.,* 15 (1959): 132–139.

Soulsby, E. H. L. "Antigen-antibody reactions in helminth infections." *Adv. Immunol.,* 2 (1962): 265–308.

Wyman, L. C., and Boyd, W. C. "Blood group determinations of pre-historic American Indians." *Amer. Anthropol.,* 39 (1937): 583–592.

———. "Human blood groups and anthropology." *Amer. Anthropol.,* 37 (1935): 181.

Blood types and lectins

D'Adamo, P. "Gut ecosystems II: Lectins and other mitogens." *Townsend Ltr. for Doctors,* 1991.

Freed, D. L. F. "Dietary lectins and disease." *Food Allergy and Intolerance*, 1987: 375–400.

———. "Lectins." *British Med. J.*, 290 (1985): 585–586.

Helm, R., and Froese, A. "Binding of receptors for IgE by various lectins." *Int. Arch. Allergy Appl. Immunology*, 65 (1981): 81–84.

The Lectins: Properties, Functions and Applications in Biology and Medicine. New York: Harcourt Brace Jovanovich/Academic Press, 1986.

———. "Lectins in the U.S. diet: Isolation and characterization of a lectin from the tomato (*Lycopersicon esculentum*)." *J. Biol. Chem.*, 255 (1980): 2056–2061.

Nachbar, M. S., et al. "Lectins in the U.S. diet: A survey of lectins in commonly consumed foods and a review of the literature." *Amer. J. Clin. Nut.*, 33 (1980): 233845.

Norn, S., et al. "Intrinsic asthma and bacterial histamine release via lectin effect." *Agents and Action*, 12, 2/3 (1983).

Sharon, N., and Halina, L. "The biochemistry of plant lectins (phytohemaglutinins A)." *Ann. Rev. Biochem.*, 42 (1973): 541–574.

———. "Lectins: Cell agglutinating and sugar-specific proteins." *Science*, 177 (1972): 949–959.

Shechter, Y. "Bound lectins that mimic insulin produce persistent insulin-like effects." *Endocrinology*, 113 (1983): 1921–1926.

Triadou, N., and Audron, E. "Interaction of the brush border hydrolases of the human small intestine with lectins." *Digestion*, 27 (1983): 1–7.

Uhlendruck, G., et al. "Love to lectins: Personal history and priority hysterics." *Lectins and Glycoconjugates in Oncology.* New York: Springer-Verlag, date.

Uimer, A. J., et al. "Stimulation of colony formation and growth factor production of human lymphocytes by wheat germ lectin." *Immunology*, 47 (1982): 551–556.

Wagner, H., et al. "Immunostimulant action of polysaccharides (heteroglycans) from higher plants." *Arzneimittelforschung* 34 (1984): 659–661 (German abstract in English).

Waxdal, M. J. "Isolation, characterization and biological activities of five mitogens from pokeweed." *Biochemistry*, 13 (1974): 3671–3675.

Zafrini, D., et al. "Inhibitory activity of cranberry juice on adherence of type 1 and type P fimbriated *E. coli* to eucaryotic cells." *Antimicrobial Agents and Chemotherapy*, 33 (1989): 92–98.

Disease associations with blood type

Addi, G. J. "Blood groups in acute rheumatism." *Scottish Med. J.*, 4 (1959): 547.

Aird, I., et al. "Blood groups in relation to peptic ulceration and carcinoma of the breast, colon, bronchus and rectum." *Brit. Med. J.*, 1954: 315–342.

Allan, T. M., and Dawson, A. A. "ABO blood groups and ischemic heart disease in men." *Brit. Heart J.*, 30 (1968): 377–382.

Billington, B. P. "Note on the distribution of ABO blood groups in bronchiectasis and portal cirrhosis." *Australian Ann. Med.*, 5 (1956): 20–22.

"Blood groups and susceptibility to disease: A review." *Brit. J. Prev. Soc. Med.*, 11 (1957): 107–125.

"Blood groups and the intestine" (editorial). *Lancet*, 7475 (Dec. 3, 1966).

Buchanan, J. A., and Higley, E. T. "The relationship of blood groups to disease." *Brit. J. Exper. Pathol.*, 2 (1921): 247–253.

Buckwalter, et al. "Ethnologic aspects of the ABO blood groups: Disease associations." *JAMA*, 1957: 327.

———. "ABO blood groups and disease." *JAMA*, 1956: 1210–4.

Camps, E. E., and Dodd, B. E. "Frequencies of secretors and non-secretors of ABH group substances among 1000 alcoholic patients." *Brit. Med. J.*, 4 (1969): 457–459.

———. "Increase in the incidence of non-secretors of ABH blood group substances among alcoholic patients." *Brit. Med. J.* 1 (1967): 30–31.

D'Adamo, P. "Blood types and diseases, a review." Clinical rounds presentation, Bastyr University, 1982.

———. "Combination naturopathic treatment of primary biliary cirrhosis." *J. Naturopathic Med.*, 4, 1 (1993): 24–25.

D'Adamo, P., Zampieron, E. "Does ABO bias in natural immunity imply an innate difference in T-cell response?" *J. Naturopathic Med.*, 2 (1991): 11–17.

Fraser Roberts, J. A. "Some associations between blood types and disease." *Brit. Med. Bull.*, 15 (1959): 129–133.

Harris, R., et al. "Vaccine virus and human blood group A substance." *Acta Genetica*, 13 (1963): 44–57.

Havlik, R., et al. "Blood groups and coronary heart disease" (letter). *Lancet*, Aug. 2, 1969: 269–270.

Hein, O. H., et al. "Alcohol consumption, Lewis phenotypes, and the risk of ischemic heart disease." *Lancet*, Feb. 13, 1993: 392–396.

"An insight is gained on how ulcers develop." *The New York Times*, Dec. 17, 1993.

Koskins, L. C., et al. "Degradation of blood group antigens in human colon ecosystems." *J. Clin. Invest*, 57 (1976): 63–73.

Langman, M. J. S., et al. "ABO and Lewis blood groups and serum cholesterol." *Lancet*, Sept. 20, 1969: 607–609.

Lim, W., et al. "Association of secretor status and rheumatic fever in 106 families." *Amer. J. Epidemiology*, 82 (1965): 103–111.

Martin, N. G., et al. "Do the MN and JK systems influence environmental variability in serum lipid levels?" *Clinical Genetics*, 24 (1983): 1–14.

McConnell, R. B., et al. "Blood groups in diabetes mellitis." *Brit. Med. J.*, 1 (1956): 772–776.

McDuffie and Hart. "The behavior in the Coombs test of anti-A and anti-B produced by immunization with various blood group specific substances and by heterospecific pregnancy." *J. Immunology*, 77 (1956): 61–71.

Myrianthopolous, N. C., et al. "Relation of blood groups and secretor factor to amyotrophic lateral sclerosis." *Amer. J. Human Genetics*, 19 (1967): 607–616.

"O! My aching stomach!" Witby *Republican*, Dec. 12, 1993.

Ratner, et al. "ABO group uropathogens and urinary tract infection." *Amer. J. Med. Sci.*, 292 (1986): 84–92.

Roath, S., et al. "Transient acquired blood group B antigen associated with diverticular bowel disease." *Acta Haematologica*, 77 (1987): 188–190.

Springer, G. F. "Relation of blood group active plant substances to human blood groups." *Acta Haem.*, 20 (1958): 147–155.

Springer, G. F. and Horton, R. E. "Erythrocyte sensitization by blood group specific bacterial antigens." *J. Gen. Physio.*, 47 (1964): 1229–1249.

Struthers, D. "ABO groups of infants and children dying in the west of Scotland (1949–51)." *Brit. J. Soc. Prev. Med.*, 5 (1951): 223–228.

Young, V. M., Gillem, H. G., and Akeroyd, J. H. "Sensitization of infant red cells by bacterial polysaccharides of *E. coli* during enteritis." *J. Ped.*, 60 (1962): 172–176.

Blood types and cancer

Aird, E., et al. "Blood groups in relationship to peptic ulceration, and carcinoma of the colon, rectum, breast and bronchus." *Brit. Med. J.*, 2 (1954): 315–321.

——. "Relationship between ABO group and cancer of the stomach." *Brit. Med. J.*, 1 (1954): 799–801.

——. "ABO blood groups and cancer of the esophagus, cancer of the pancreas and pituitary adenoma." *Brit. Med. J.*, 1 (1960): 1163–1166.

Bazeed, M. A., et al. "Effect of lectins on KK-47 bladder cancer cell line." *Urology*, 32, 2 (1988): 133–135.

Boland, C. R. "Searching for the face of cancer." *J. Clin. Gastroenterology*, 10, 6 (1988): 599–604.

Brooks, S. A. "Predictive value of lectin binding on breast cancer recurrence and survival." *Lancet*, May 9, 1987: 1054–1056.

Brooks, S. A. and Leathem, A. J. C. "Prediction of lymph node involvement in breast cancer by detection of altered glycosylation in the primary tumor." *Lancet*, 8759, 338 (1991): 71–74.

Cameron, C., et al. "Acquisition of a B-like antigen by red blood cells." *Brit. Med. J.*, July 11, 1959: 29–34.

D'Adamo, P. "Possible alteration of ABO blood group observed in non-Hodgkin's lymphoma." *J. Naturopath. Med.*, 1 (1990): 39–43.

Dahiya, R., et al. "ABH blood group antigen expression, synthesis and degradation in human colonic adenocarcinoma cell lines." *Cancer Res.*, 49, 16 (1989): 4550–4556.

——. "ABH blood group antigen synthesis in human colonic adenocarcinoma cell lines" (meeting abstract). *Proc. Ann. Mtg. Amer. Assoc. Cancer Res.*, 30 (1989): A1405.

Davis, D. L., et al. "Medical hypothesis: Xenoestrogens as preventable causes of breast cancer." *Environ. Health Persp.*, 101, 5, (1993): 372–777.

Feinmesser, R., et al. "Lectin binding characteristics of laryngeal cancer." *Otolaryngeal Head Neck Surgery*, 100, 3 (1989): 207–209.

Fenlon, S., et al. "*Helix pomatia* and *Ulex europeus* lectin binding in human breast carcinoma." *J. Pathology*, 152 (1987): 169–176.

Kvist, E., et al. "Relationship between blood groups and tumors of the upper urinary tract." *Scand. J. Urol. Nephrol.*, 22, 4 (1988): 289–291.

Langkilde, N. C., et al. "Binding of wheat and peanut lectins to human transitional cell carcinoma." *Cancer*, 64, 4 (1989): 849–853.

Lemon, H. "Clinical and experimental aspects of anti-mammary carcinogenic activity of estriol." *Front. Hormone Res.*, 5 (1978): 155–73.

———. "Pathophysiological considerations in the treatment of menopausal patients with estrogens: The role of estriol in the prevention of mammary carcinoma." *Acta Endocrin. Supp.*, 233 (1980): 17–27.

Marth, C., and Daxenbichiler, G. "Peanut agglutinin inhibits proliferation of cultured breast cancer cells." *Oncology*, 45 (1988): 47–50.

Morecki, S., et al. "Removal of breast cancer cells by soybean agglutinin in experimental model for purging human marrow." *Canc. Res.*, 48 (1988): 4573–4577.

Motzer, R. J., et al. "Blood group related antigens in human germ cell tumors." *Cancer Res.*, 48, 18 (1988): 5342–5347.

Murata, K., et al. "Expression of blood group related antigens ABH, Lewis a, Lewis b, Lewis x, Lewis y, Ca19-9 and CSLEX1 in early cancer, intestinal metaplasia and uninvolved mucosa of the stomach." *Amer. J. Clin. Path.*, 98 (1992): 67–75.

Osborne, R. H., and DeGeorge, F. V. "ABO blood groups and neoplastic disease of the ovary." *Amer. J. Human Genetics*, 15 (1963): 380–388.

Renton, P. H., et al. "Red cells of all four ABO groups in a case of leukemia." *Brit. Med. J.*, Feb. 2, 1962: 294–297.

Roberts, T. E., et al. "Blood groups and lung cancer" (letter). *Brit. J. Cancer*, 58, 2 (1988): 278.

Romodanov, S. A., et al. "Efficacy of chemo and immunochemistry in neuro-oncological patients with different ABO system blood group." *ZH-Vopr-Neirkhiir Im Nn Burdenko*, 53/1, 17–20 (1989).

Stachura, J., et al. "Blood group antigens in the distribution of pancreatic cancer." *Folia Histochem. Cytobiol.*, 27, 1 (1989): 49–55.

Springer, G., et al. "Blood group MN antigens and precursors in normal and malignant human breast glandular tissue." *J. Nat. Cancer Instit.*, 54, 2 (1975): 335–339.

———. "T/Tn antigen vaccine is effective and safe in preventing recurrence of advanced breast cancer." *Cancer Detection and Prevention* (1993).

Tryggvadottir, L., et al. "Familial and sporadic breast cancer cases in Iceland: A comparison related to ABO blood groups and risk of bilateral breast cancer." *Inter. J. Cancer*, 42, 4 (1988): 499–501.

Tzingounis, V. A., et al. "Estriol in the management of menopause." *JAMA*, 239, 16 (1978): 1638.

Wolf, G. T., et al. "A9 and ABH antigen expression predicts outcome in head and neck cancer." *Proc. Ann. Mtg. Amer. Assoc. Cancer Res.*, 30 (1989): A902.

Get Help Here

Dr. Peter D'Adamo and his staff continue to accept new patients on a limited basis. To find out more about scheduling an appointment, please contact:

The D'Adamo Clinic
2009 Summer Street
Stamford, CT 06905
203 348 4800

Note: Please do not submit questions regarding Dr. D'Adamo's work or questions seeking personal advice on health matters to Dr. D'Adamo at the clinic. Dr. D'Adamo maintains an Internet website (http://www.dadamo.com) which has an interactive message board and archives of past posts and questions to the boards. This is currently the only vehicle available for additional information on Dr. D'Adamo's ongoing research on blood type and individuality.

www.dadamo.com

The World Wide Web has proven to be a valuable venue for exploring and applying the tenets of the Blood Type Diet and Lifestyle. Since January 1997 hundreds of thousands have visited the site to participate in the ABO chat groups, to peruse the scientific archives, to share experiences and recipes, and to learn more about the science of blood type.

One of the most important features on the Web page is the Blood Type Outcome Registry, which has facilitated the collection of data on the measurable effects of the Blood Type Diet on a wide range of medical conditions.

I invite you to share your outcome at the website. It is actually quite simple. When you visit *www.dadamo.com*, scroll down the main page until you locate "Share Your Outcome." Click on "Share Your Outcome" and you will be taken to the Blood Type Outcome Registry.

I appreciate your taking the time to provide feedback about experiences you have had with the program. Your feedback can be critical in showing indicators and trends which can then be further studied. All information shared on the website Blood Type Outcome Registry will be held in complete confidence.

Self Testing

Home Blood Typing Kits

North American Pharmacal, Inc is the official distributor of Home Blood Type Testing Kits. Each kit costs $7.95 and is a single-use disposable educational device capable of determining one individual's ABO and rhesus blood type. Results are obtained within about 4-5 minutes. If you have several friends or family members who need to learn their blood type, you will need to order a separate home blood-typing kit for each individual.

All U.S. orders are shipped via UPS ground (shipping and handling cost is $5.25 per order irrespective of the number of kits ordered). Expedited shipping methods (UPS 2nd day or next day) are available but cost more. Please contact the customer service department to inquire about rates for expedited shipping to your area.

If you are ordering a kit to be shipped outside of the U.S., shipping rates can vary dramatically and can be quite expensive. Please contact our customer service department prior to placing your order for an estimate of shipping charges for non-U.S. orders.

To order a single Home Blood Typing Kit please enclose $7.95 + 5.25 for shipping and handling and send to:

North American Pharmacal, Inc.
5 Brook Street
Norwalk, CT 06851
Tel: 203-866-7664
Fax: 203-838-4066
Toll free: 877-ABO TYPE (877-226-8973)
www.4yourtype.com

North American Pharmacal, Inc. offers a range of other self-tests to monitor aspects of health, such as secretor status, stress hormone levels, female hormone levels, mineral balance, and antioxidant status. For prices and ordering information please contact North American Pharmacal, Inc.

Health Products and Supplements

North American Pharmacal, Inc., is the official distributor of Blood Type Specialty Products. The product line includes supplements, books, tapes, teas, meal replacement bars, cosmetics, and support material that makes eating and living right for your type easier.

Included in this product line are New Chapter® D'Adamo 4 Your Type Products™. These whole-food vitamins, herbs, and other food supplements have been specifically crafted to address the unique requirements of each blood type.

Also included are Sip Right 4 Your Type™ teas, Deflect™ lectin-blocking formulas, and a range of additional blood type specific and blood type friendly health products which have been formulated in partnership with The Republic of Tea and New Chapter. Product information and price lists are available from North American Pharmacal, Inc.

Naturopathic Physicians

Dr. Peter D'Adamo's father, James D'Adamo, ND, who pioneered the early clinical work on blood type continues to practice. He may be reached at:

Dr. James D'Adamo, ND
44-46 Bridge Street
Portsmouth, NH 03801

An Easy At-Home
Blood Test

NORTH AMERICAN PHARMACAL, INC., IS THE OFFICIAL DISTRIBUTOR of the Home Blood Type Kits and Blood Type Specialty Products. The product line includes supplements, books, audiotapes, a bi-monthly newsletter, meal replacement bars, protein powders and support materials that make "eating right for your type" easier to incorporate into your life. One of the most popular items North American Pharmacal distributes is the At-Home Blood Type Kit, which allows you to find out your blood type in five minutes. Each single-use kit is $7.95 plus shipping and handling.

Product information and price lists are available from:

North American Pharmacal, Inc.
5 Brook Street
Norwalk, CT 06851
Tel: 203-866-7664
Fax: 203-838-4066
Toll free: 1-877-ABO-TYPE (877-226-8973)

Or, if you prefer, you can contact the company through the Internet at www.4yourtype.com.

DR. PETER J. D'ADAMO is an eminent naturopathic physician and researcher with a wide international following. His first book, *Eat Right 4 (for) Your Type*, has consistently been on best-seller lists since its publication in 1996 and has been translated into more than 40 languages. For his work on blood type and nutrition, Dr. D'Adamo was selected 1990 Physician of the Year by the American Association of Naturopathic Physicians. In 1999, respected industry analysts named *Eat Right 4 Your Type* one of the ten most influential health books ever and Dr. D'Adamo the most intriguing health author of the year. The founder and editor emeritus of *The Journal of Naturopathic Medicine*, he maintains a small private practice in Stamford, Connecticut.

Index

Barbeque sauce, with tempeh
kabobs, 264–65
Barley:
and mushroom soup with
spinach, 316–17
and spelt pancakes, 331
Barley malt sweetners, and Type B,
126
Basic turkey stock, 309–10
Basic vegetable stock, 310
Basil:
pesto, 369
swordfish with cherry tomatoes,
red onion, and, 253
Basmati:
rice pudding, 358
and spelt berry rice pilaf, 289
and wild rice pilaf, 287
Beans, 279–82
adzuki beans, and pumpkin
soup, 313–14
black beans:
Cuban black bean soup, 319
dip, 384
soup, Cuban, 319
and tofu chili, 266
black-eyed peas with leeks, 281
green beans:
beef stew with carrots and,
312–13
with chevre and walnuts,
340
stewed, with tomatoes and
garlic, 298–99
legumes, 279–80
lentil salad, 281–82
lima beans, with goat cheese and
scallions, 280, 289
navy bean soup, 313–14
pinto beans, pureed with garlic,
282
and Type A, 84–85
and Type AB, 146–47
and Type B, 118
and Type O, 52–53

white beans, and wilted greens
soup, 315
See also Legumes
Beef:
brisket, 238
meat loaf, 247
pot roast, 246–47
sirloin, with cellophane noodles
and green vegetables,
275–76
stew, with green beans and
carrots, 312–13
Beer, and Type O, 64
Berries:
and Type A, 91
and Type AB, 152
and Type O, 59
Besher, Alexander, 38
Beverages:
and Type A, 96–97
and Type AB, 158
and Type B, 129–30
and Type O, 64–65
Biscotti, cranberry, 354–55
Black bean chili, and tofu,
266
Black beans:
Cuban Black Bean Soup,
319
dip, 384
soup, Cuban, 319
and tofu chili, 266
Blackberries, and Type O, 59
Black cherry juice:
and Type A, 93
and Type AB, 154
and Type O, 60
Black-eyed peas:
with leeks, 281
and Type B, 118
Black pepper, and Type O, 61
Blackstrap molasses, and Type A,
93, 100
Bladder wrack, and Type O, 61,
68–69

Green tea:
   and Type A, 95, 96
   and Type AB, 157, 158
   and Type O, 64–65
Green Vegetable Pasta, 271–72
Green vegetables, and Type B, 111
Grilled curried leg of lamb, 241–42
Grilled goat cheddar on Ezekiel or
   spelt bread, 343
Grilled lamb sausages, fettuccine
   and vegetables with, 273–74
Grilled loin lamb chops, with
   tamari-mustard marinade, 244
Grilled Portobello mushrooms, 306
Grilled sirloin, with cellophane
   noodles and green vegetables,
   275–76
Grilled sweet-potato salad, 338–39
Grilled wild-rice tempeh, 267–68
Ground rice, and Type AB, 148
Grouper, sauteed, 252
Guava, and Type AB, 153

H

Ham, 230
   and Type A, 78
Hand-kneaded breads, 323–24
   French, 323
   raisin-pumpernickel, 324
Harmful lectins, 21–24
   detecting, 22–24
Hatha yoga, and Type A, 104
Hawthorn:
   and Type A, 95, 101
   and Type AB, 157, 160–61
Health-food stores, checking "sell
   by" date in, 228
Heartburn, 234
Hearty fish soup, 314–15
Heavily fatted meats, avoiding,
   225–26
Herbal teas:
   and Type A, 95–96
   and Type AB, 157

   and Type B, 128–29
   and Type O, 63–64
Herbs/phytochemicals, and Type
   AB, 160–62
Herring, pickled. 230
Highly Beneficial, use of term, 236
Highly Beneficial category of
   foods, 29
Highly Beneficial foods list,
   224–25
High-protein diets, 30
Home blood-testing kit, 259–61
Honey, 229
   and Type B, 126
   and Type O, 61
Honeydew melons, and Type A,
   91
Honey and lemon dressing, 370
Hot dogs, 230
   and Type A, 78
Huangki:
   and Type A, 101
   and Type AB, 161
Humankind, story of, 4–5
Hunter, *See* Type O
Hypothyroidism, 45

I

Immune, origin of term, 14
Immune-enhancing herbs:
   and Type A, 101
   and Type AB, 161
Indian lamb stew with spinach,
   311
Indican Scale, 23–24
Indonesian Broiled Swordfish, 254
Infections, 4–5
Informative material, 259
Injera, 285
Iodine, 45
   and Type O, 67–68
Iodized salt, and weight loss, 46
Iron, and Type A, 99–100
Iron citrate, and Type A, 100

Neutral list, 229
Niacin, 32
Nightshade vegetables, and
    Type O, 57
Nitrates, 231
Nitrites, 24
    and Type A, 78
Nomad, *See* Type B
Nomi, Toshitaka, 38
North American Pharmacal, Inc.,
    259, 261
Nut butters:
    and Type AB, 146
    and Type O, 52
Nuts:
    and Type A, 83
    and Type B, 117
    and Type O, 51–52
    See also Almonds; Walnuts
Nuts and seeds, and Type AB,
    145–46

O

Oatmeal, and Type AB, 148, 150
Oils and fats:
    and Type A, 82
    and Type AB, 145
    and Type B, 116
    and Type O, 51
Old-Fashioned Yankee Pot Roast,
    246–47
Olive oil:
    and lemon dressing, 370
    and Type A, 82
    and Type AB, 145
    and Type O, 51, 63
Olive-oil mayonnaise, 364–65
Olives:
    fermented, and Type O, 57
    and Type B, 122
Omelet:
    alternative fillings for, 345–46
    single-egg, 345

Onions:
    carmelized, frittata with pasta
        and, 346–47
    glazed turnips and, 294–95
    swordfish with cherry tomatoes
        and basil, 253
    and Type A, 89
    Vidalia, dressing, 371
Oranges:
    and Type A, 91
    and Type AB, 153
    and Type O, 59
Organic foods, 227
    finding, 228
    fruits, 229
    purchasing, 228–29
    vegetables, 229
Organic meats, 44

P

Pancakes, 330–33
    amaranth, 332
    barley and spelt, 331
    brown rice and spelt, 333
    millet, spelt, and soy, 331–32
    sweet potato, 296
Pancreatic enzymes, and Type O, 69
Panhemaglutinan:
    and Type A, 89
    and Type AB, 151
Panhemaglutinans:
    and Type AB, 139
    and Type O, 57
Papaya, and Type A, 91
Parasites, 4–5
Parboiling, 231–32
Parmesan, and pasta, 270
Parsley:
    cauliflower with garlic and, 297
    and tofu dressing, 368
    and Type O, 61
Parsnips, and carrots, with garlic,
    ginger and cilantro, 295–96